ACP | MKSAP® 17
Medical Knowledge Self-Assessment Program®

Nephrology

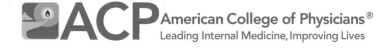
American College of Physicians®
Leading Internal Medicine, Improving Lives

Welcome to the Nephrology Section of MKSAP 17!

In these pages, you will find updated information on the clinical evaluation of kidney function, fluids and electrolytes, acid-base disorders, hypertension, chronic tubulointerstitial diseases, glomerular diseases, kidney manifestations of gammopathies, genetic disorders and kidney disease, acute kidney injury, kidney stones, the kidney in pregnancy, and chronic kidney disease. All of these topics are uniquely focused on the needs of generalists and subspecialists *outside* of nephrology.

The publication of the 17th edition of Medical Knowledge Self-Assessment Program (MKSAP) represents nearly a half-century of serving as the gold-standard resource for internal medicine education. It also marks its evolution into an innovative learning system to better meet the changing educational needs and learning styles of all internists.

The core content of MKSAP has been developed as in previous editions–newly generated, essential information in 11 topic areas of internal medicine created by dozens of leading generalists and subspecialists and guided by certification and recertification requirements, emerging knowledge in the field, and user feedback. MKSAP 17 also contains 1200 all-new, psychometrically validated, and peer-reviewed multiple-choice questions (MCQs) for self-assessment and study, including 108 in Nephrology. MKSAP 17 continues to include *High Value Care* (HVC) recommendations, based on the concept of balancing clinical benefit with costs and harms, with links to MCQs that illustrate these principles. In addition, HVC Key Points are highlighted in the text. Also highlighted, with blue text, are *Hospitalist*-focused content and MCQs that directly address the learning needs of internists who work in the hospital setting.

MKSAP 17 Digital provides access to additional tools allowing you to customize your learning experience, including regular text updates with practice-changing, new information and 200 new self-assessment questions; a board-style pretest to help direct your learning; and enhanced custom-quiz options. And, with MKSAP Complete, learners can access 1200 electronic flashcards for quick review of important concepts or review the updated and enhanced version of Virtual Dx, an image-based self-assessment tool.

As before, MKSAP 17 is optimized for use on your mobile devices, with iOS- and Android-based apps allowing you to sync your work between your apps and online account and submit for CME credits and MOC points online.

Please visit us at the MKSAP Resource Site (mksap.acponline.org) to find out how we can help you study, earn CME credit and MOC points, and stay up to date.

Whether you prefer to use the traditional print version or take advantage of the features available through the digital version, we hope you enjoy MKSAP 17 and that it meets and exceeds your personal learning needs.

On behalf of the many internists who have offered their time and expertise to create the content for MKSAP 17 and the editorial staff who work to bring this material to you in the best possible way, we are honored that you have chosen to use MKSAP 17 and appreciate any feedback about the program you may have. Please feel free to send us any comments to mksap_editors@acponline.org.

Sincerely,

Philip A. Masters, MD, FACP
Editor-in-Chief
Senior Physician Educator
Director, Clinical Content Development
Medical Education Division
American College of Physicians

Nephrology

Committee

Hasan Bazari, MD, FACP, Section Editor[2]
Program Director Emeritus, Internal Medicine Residency
Massachusetts General Hospital
Boston, Massachusetts

Virginia U. Collier, MD, MACP, Associate Editor[2]
Hugh R. Sharp, Jr. Chair of Medicine
Christiana Care Health System
Newark, Delaware
Professor of Medicine
Sidney Kimmel Medical College at Thomas Jefferson
    University
Philadelphia, Pennsylvania

Kerry Cho, MD, FACP[1]
Fellowship Program Director
Associate Professor of Clinical Medicine
Division of Nephrology
University of California San Francisco
San Francisco, California

Jai Radhakrishnan, MD, MS[2]
Professor of Medicine
Columbia University Medical Center
Clinical Director, Division of Nephrology
New York, New York

Michael Ross, MD[2]
Associate Professor
Division of Nephrology
Icahn School of Medicine at Mount Sinai
New York, New York
Chief, Renal Section
James J. Peters VA Medical Center
Bronx, New York

Ashita Tolwani, MD[2]
Professor of Medicine
Division of Nephrology
University of Alabama at Birmingham
Birmingham, Alabama

Alexander Wiseman, MD, FACP[2]
Professor of Medicine
Division of Renal Diseases and Hypertension
Medical Director
Kidney and Pancreas Transplant Programs
University of Colorado School of Medicine
Denver, Colorado

Consulting Authors

David Mount, MD[2]
Associate Division Chief
Director of Dialysis Services and Director of Clinical
    Services
Renal Division, Brigham and Women's Hospital
Staff Physician, Renal Division
VA Boston Healthcare System
Boston, Massachusetts

James E. Novak, MD, PhD, FACP[1]
Associate Director
Training Program and Medical Director
Home Dialysis
Division of Nephrology and Hypertension
Henry Ford Hospital
Detroit, Michigan

Editor-in-Chief

Philip A. Masters, MD, FACP[1]
Senior Physician Educator
Director, Clinical Content Development
American College of Physicians
Philadelphia, Pennsylvania

Director, Clinical Program Development

Cynthia D. Smith, MD, FACP[2]
American College of Physicians
Philadelphia, Pennsylvania

Nephrology Reviewers

Richard Fatica, MD[1]
Barri J. Fessler, MD, MSPH, FACP[1]
John D. Goldman, MD, FACP[2]
Kent A. Kirchner, MD, FACP[1]
Janis M. Orlowski, MD, MACP[1]
Adrian Sequeira, MD, FACP[2]
Asher Tulsky, MD, FACP[1]

Nephrology ACP Editorial Staff

Megan Zborowski[1], Senior Staff Editor
Margaret Wells[1], Director, Self-Assessment and Educational
    Programs
Becky Krumm[1], Managing Editor

ACP Principal Staff

Patrick C. Alguire, MD, FACP[2]
Senior Vice President, Medical Education

Sean McKinney[1]
Vice President, Medical Education

Margaret Wells[1]
Director, Self-Assessment and Educational Programs

Becky Krumm[1]
Managing Editor

Katie Idell[1]
Manager, Clinical Skills Program and Digital Products

Valerie A. Dangovetsky[1]
Administrator

Ellen McDonald, PhD[1]
Senior Staff Editor

Megan Zborowski[1]
Senior Staff Editor

Randy Hendrickson[1]
Production Administrator/Editor

Linnea Donnarumma[1]
Staff Editor

Susan Galeone[1]
Staff Editor

Jackie Twomey[1]
Staff Editor

Julia Nawrocki[1]
Staff Editor

Kimberly Kerns[1]
Administrative Coordinator

Rosemarie Houton[1]
Administrative Representative

---

1. Has no relationships with any entity producing, marketing, reselling, or distributing health care goods or services consumed by, or used on, patients.

2. Has disclosed relationship(s) with any entity producing, marketing, reselling, or distributing health care goods or services consumed by, or used on, patients.

Disclosure of Relationships with any entity producing, marketing, reselling, or distributing health care goods or services consumed by, or used on, patients.

Patrick C. Alguire, MD, FACP
Consultantship
National Board of Medical Examiners
Royalties
UpToDate
Stock Options/Holdings

Amgen Inc., Bristol-Myers Squibb, GlaxoSmithKline, Stryker Corporation, Zimmer Orthopedics, Teva Pharmaceuticals, Medtronic, Covidien, Inc., Express Scripts

Hasan Bazari, MD, FACP
Stock Options/Holdings
Pfizer

Virginia U. Collier, MD, MACP
Stock Options/Holdings
Celgene, Pfizer, Merck, Schering Plough, Abbott, Abbevie, Johnson and Johnson, Medtronic, McKesson, Amgen, Wellpoint, Roche, Sanofi, Novartis, Covidian, Stryker, Amerisource Bergen

John D. Goldman, MD, FACP
Employment
Pinnacle Health

David Mount, MD
Other (Co-author for publication in CKD)
Takeda

Jai Radhakrishnan, MD, MS
Consultantship
Eli Lilly, Merck

Michael Ross, MD
Consultantship
Bristol-Myers Squibb

Adrian Sequeira, MD, FACP
Employment
LSU Health Shreveport School of Medicine

Cynthia D. Smith, MD, FACP
Stock Options/Holdings
Merck and Co.; spousal employment at Merck

Ashita Tolwani, MD
Consultantship
Baxter Gambro

Alexander Wiseman, MD, FACP
Consultantship
Tolera, Astellas, Bristol-Myers Squibb, Veloxis
Honoraria
Novartis

Acknowledgments

The American College of Physicians (ACP) gratefully acknowledges the special contributions to the development and production of the 17th edition of the Medical Knowledge Self-Assessment Program® (MKSAP® 17) made by the following people:

Graphic Design: Michael Ripca (Graphics Technical Administrator) and WFGD Studio (Graphic Designers).

Production/Systems: Dan Hoffmann (Director, Web Services & Systems Development), Neil Kohl (Senior Architect), Chris Patterson (Senior Architect), and Scott Hurd (Manager, Web Projects & CMS Services).

MKSAP 17 Digital: Under the direction of Steven Spadt, Vice President, Digital Products & Services, the digital version of MKSAP 17 was developed within the ACP's Digital Product Development Department, led by Brian Sweigard (Director). Other members of the team included Dan Barron (Senior Web Application Developer/Architect), Chris Forrest (Senior Software Developer/Design Lead), Kara Kronenwetter (Senior Web Developer), Brad Lord (Senior Web Application Developer), John McKnight (Senior Web Developer), and Nate Pershall (Senior Web Developer).

The College also wishes to acknowledge that many other persons, too numerous to mention, have contributed to the production of this program. Without their dedicated efforts, this program would not have been possible.

MKSAP Resource Site (mksap.acponline.org)

The MKSAP Resource Site (mksap.acponline.org) is a continually updated site that provides links to MKSAP 17 online answer sheets for print subscribers; the latest details on Continuing Medical Education (CME) and Maintenance of Certification (MOC) in the United States, Canada, and Australia; errata; and other new information.

ABIM Maintenance of Certification

Check the MKSAP Resource Site (mksap.acponline.org) for the latest information on how MKSAP tests can be used to apply to the American Board of Internal Medicine for Maintenance of Certification (MOC) points.

Royal College Maintenance of Certification

In Canada, MKSAP 17 is an Accredited Self-Assessment Program (Section 3) as defined by the Maintenance of Certification (MOC) Program of The Royal College of Physicians and Surgeons of Canada and approved by the Canadian Society of Internal Medicine on December 9, 2014. Approval extends from July 31, 2015 until July 31, 2018 for the Part A sections. Approval extends from December 31, 2015 to December 31, 2018 for the Part B sections.

Fellows of the Royal College may earn three credits per hour for participating in MKSAP 17 under Section 3. MKSAP 17 also meets multiple CanMEDS Roles, including that of Medical Expert, Communicator, Collaborator, Manager, Health Advocate, Scholar, and Professional. For information on how to apply MKSAP 17 Continuing Medical Education (CME) credits to the Royal College MOC Program, visit the MKSAP Resource Site at mksap.acponline.org.

The Royal Australasian College of Physicians CPD Program

In Australia, MKSAP 17 is a Category 3 program that may be used by Fellows of The Royal Australasian College of Physicians (RACP) to meet mandatory Continuing Professional Development (CPD) points. Two CPD credits are awarded for each of the 200 *AMA PRA Category 1 Credits*™ available in MKSAP 17. More information about using MKSAP 17 for this purpose is available at the MKSAP Resource Site at mksap.acponline.org and at www.racp.edu.au. CPD credits earned through MKSAP 17 should be reported at the MyCPD site at www.racp.edu.au/mycpd.

Continuing Medical Education

The American College of Physicians (ACP) is accredited by the Accreditation Council for Continuing Medical Education (ACCME) to provide continuing medical education for physicians.

The ACP designates this enduring material, MKSAP 17, for a maximum of 200 *AMA PRA Category 1 Credits*™. Physicians should claim only the credit commensurate with the extent of their participation in the activity.

Up to 19 *AMA PRA Category 1 Credits*™ are available from December 31, 2015, to December 31, 2018, for the MKSAP 17 Nephrology section.

Learning Objectives

The learning objectives of MKSAP 17 are to:
- Close gaps between actual care in your practice and preferred standards of care, based on best evidence
- Diagnose disease states that are less common and sometimes overlooked or confusing
- Improve management of comorbid conditions that can complicate patient care
- Determine when to refer patients for surgery or care by subspecialists
- Pass the ABIM Certification Examination
- Pass the ABIM Maintenance of Certification Examination

Target Audience

- General internists and primary care physicians
- Subspecialists who need to remain up-to-date in internal medicine and in areas outside of their own subspecialty area
- Residents preparing for the certification examination in internal medicine
- Physicians preparing for maintenance of certification in internal medicine (recertification)

Earn "Instantaneous" CME Credits Online

Print subscribers can enter their answers online to earn instantaneous Continuing Medical Education (CME) credits. You can submit your answers using online answer sheets that are provided at mksap.acponline.org, where a record of your MKSAP 17 credits will be available. To earn CME credits, you need to answer all of the questions in a test and earn a score of at least 50% correct (number of correct answers divided by the total number of questions). Take any of the following approaches:

1. Use the printed answer sheet at the back of this book to record your answers. Go to mksap.acponline.org, access the appropriate online answer sheet, transcribe your answers, and submit your test for instantaneous CME credits. There is no additional fee for this service.

2. Go to mksap.acponline.org, access the appropriate online answer sheet, directly enter your answers, and submit your test for instantaneous CME credits. There is no additional fee for this service.

3. Pay a $15 processing fee per answer sheet and submit the printed answer sheet at the back of this book by mail or fax, as instructed on the answer sheet. Make sure you calculate your score and fax the answer sheet to 215-351-2799 or mail the answer sheet to Member and Customer Service, American College of Physicians, 190 N. Independence Mall West, Philadelphia, PA 19106-1572, using the courtesy envelope provided in your MKSAP 17 slipcase. You will need your 10-digit order number and 8-digit ACP ID number, which are printed on your packing slip. Please allow 4 to 6 weeks for your score report to be emailed back to you. Be sure to include your email address for a response.

If you do not have a 10-digit order number and 8-digit ACP ID number or if you need help creating a user name and password to access the MKSAP 17 online answer sheets, go to mksap.acponline.org or email custserv@acponline.org.

Disclosure Policy

It is the policy of the American College of Physicians (ACP) to ensure balance, independence, objectivity, and scientific rigor in all of its educational activities. To this end, and consistent with the policies of the ACP and the Accreditation Council for Continuing Medical Education (ACCME), contributors to all ACP continuing medical education activities are required to disclose all relevant financial relationships with any entity producing, marketing, reselling, or distributing health care goods or services consumed by, or used on, patients. Contributors are required to use generic names in the discussion of

therapeutic options and are required to identify any unapproved, off-label, or investigative use of commercial products or devices. Where a trade name is used, all available trade names for the same product type are also included. If trade-name products manufactured by companies with whom contributors have relationships are discussed, contributors are asked to provide evidence-based citations in support of the discussion. The information is reviewed by the committee responsible for producing this text. If necessary, adjustments to topics or contributors' roles in content development are made to balance the discussion. Further, all readers of this text are asked to evaluate the content for evidence of commercial bias and send any relevant comments to mksap_editors@acponline.org so that future decisions about content and contributors can be made in light of this information.

Resolution of Conflicts

To resolve all conflicts of interest and influences of vested interests, the American College of Physicians (ACP) precluded members of the content-creation committee from deciding on any content issues that involved generic or trade-name products associated with proprietary entities with which these committee members had relationships. In addition, content was based on best evidence and updated clinical care guidelines, when such evidence and guidelines were available. Contributors' disclosure information can be found with the list of contributors' names and those of ACP principal staff listed in the beginning of this book.

Hospital-Based Medicine

For the convenience of subscribers who provide care in hospital settings, content that is specific to the hospital setting has been highlighted in blue. Hospital icons (H) highlight where the hospital-based content begins, continues over more than one page, and ends.

High Value Care Key Points

Key Points in the text that relate to High Value Care concepts (that is, concepts that discuss balancing clinical benefit with costs and harms) are designated by the HVC icon (**HVC**).

Educational Disclaimer

The editors and publisher of MKSAP 17 recognize that the development of new material offers many opportunities for error. Despite our best efforts, some errors may persist in print. Drug dosage schedules are, we believe, accurate and in accordance with current standards. Readers are advised, however, to ensure that the recommended dosages in

MKSAP 17 concur with the information provided in the product information material. This is especially important in cases of new, infrequently used, or highly toxic drugs. Application of the information in MKSAP 17 remains the professional responsibility of the practitioner.

The primary purpose of MKSAP 17 is educational. Information presented, as well as publications, technologies, products, and/or services discussed, is intended to inform subscribers about the knowledge, techniques, and experiences of the contributors. A diversity of professional opinion exists, and the views of the contributors are their own and not those of the American College of Physicians (ACP). Inclusion of any material in the program does not constitute endorsement or recommendation by the ACP. The ACP does not warrant the safety, reliability, accuracy, completeness, or usefulness of and disclaims any and all liability for damages and claims that may result from the use of information, publications, technologies, products, and/or services discussed in this program.

Publisher's Information

Unauthorized Use of This Book Is Against the Law

MKSAP 17 ISBN: 978-1-938245-18-3
(Nephrology) ISBN: 978-1-938245-28-2

Printed in the United States of America.

For order information in the United States or Canada call 800-523-1546, extension 2600. All other countries call 215-351-2600, (M-F, 9 AM – 5 PM ET). Fax inquiries to 215-351-2799 or email to custserv@acponline.org.

Errata

Errata for MKSAP 17 will be available through the MKSAP Resource Site at mksap.acponline.org as new information becomes known to the editors.

Table of Contents

Glomerular Diseases

Kidney Manifestations of Gammopathies

Genetic Disorders and Kidney Disease

Acute Kidney Injury

Kidney Stones

The Kidney in Pregnancy

Chronic Kidney Disease

Nephrology High Value Care Recommendations

The American College of Physicians, in collaboration with multiple other organizations, is engaged in a worldwide initiative to promote the practice of High Value Care (HVC). The goals of the HVC initiative are to improve health care outcomes by providing care of proven benefit and reducing costs by avoiding unnecessary and even harmful interventions. The initiative comprises several programs that integrate the important concept of health care value (balancing clinical benefit with costs and harms) for a given intervention into a broad range of educational materials to address the needs of trainees, practicing physicians, and patients.

HVC content has been integrated into MKSAP 17 in several important ways. MKSAP 17 now includes HVC-identified key points in the text, HVC-focused multiple choice questions, and, for subscribers to MKSAP Digital, an HVC custom quiz. From the text and questions, we have generated the following list of HVC recommendations that meet the definition below of high value care and bring us closer to our goal of improving patient outcomes while conserving finite resources.

High Value Care Recommendation: A recommendation to choose diagnostic and management strategies for patients in specific clinical situations that balance clinical benefit with cost and harms with the goal of improving patient outcomes.

Below are the High Value Care Recommendations for the Nephrology section of MKSAP 17.

- The presence of both leukocyte esterase and nitrites on urine dipstick is highly suggestive of a urinary tract infection (UTI), and uncomplicated patients with these findings may be treated empirically with antibiotics; the absence of both has a high negative predictive value for a UTI, and most patients will not need antibiotics.
- Urinalysis should not be used to screen for bladder cancer in asymptomatic patients.
- Ultrasonography is typically the first imaging test in the evaluation of the kidneys and upper urinary tract because of its safety, cost effectiveness, and general utility.
- The initial treatment of asymptomatic patients with the syndrome of inappropriate antidiuretic hormone secretion includes management of the underlying cause if possible and fluid restriction without limiting sodium intake (see Item 63).
- Echocardiography is not routinely indicated in the assessment of hypertension except in patients with known heart disease, the presence of left bundle branch block on electrocardiogram, or suspected white coat hypertension.
- Identification of prescription and nonprescription medications that may be contributing to blood pressure elevation is necessary in patients with elevated blood pressure not yet defined as hypertension (see Item 79).
- Prehypertension is managed with lifestyle modifications and annual follow-up visits to monitor blood pressure (see Item 1).
- In patients with white coat hypertension, close observation for the emergence of sustained hypertension or end-organ damage is recommended; drug therapy is not usually required (see Item 42).
- Lifestyle modifications are indicated for all patients with hypertension, which can produce reductions in blood pressure that are equivalent to antihypertensive agents (see Item 11).
- A combination of two hypertensive agents at moderate dose is often more successful at achieving blood pressure goals than one agent at maximal dose, which can help minimize the side effects more commonly noted at higher doses.
- For patients with chronic kidney disease, the eighth report from the Joint National Committee recommends a blood pressure target goal of <140/90 mm Hg using a medication regimen that includes an ACE inhibitor or angiotensin receptor blocker (see Item 13 and Item 68).
- The eighth report of the Joint National Committee recommends a treatment goal of <150/90 mm Hg for patients with hypertension who are ≥60 years (see Item 38).
- The risk of complications, morbidity, and mortality related to lower blood pressure in frail individuals may supersede the potential benefit of lower blood pressure goals (see Item 64).
- Adequate blood pressure control and use of an ACE inhibitor or angiotensin receptor blocker has been shown to slow the progression of diabetic nephropathy (see Item 45).
- Medical management is the primary therapeutic intervention in most patients with renal artery stenosis.
- Ultrasonography is increasingly being used as an initial diagnostic study for nephrolithiasis due to availability, lack of radiation exposure, and low cost; it is also the preferred modality during pregnancy.
- Ultrasonography is an appropriate imaging modality for patients with chronic kidney disease to avoid adverse events such as contrast-induced nephropathy or nephrogenic systemic fibrosis (see Item 2).

- For patients with kidney stones ≤10 mm in diameter, conservative management, including analgesia, hydration, and expulsive therapy, may be attempted.
- Very elderly patients who have end-stage kidney disease with a high burden of comorbid conditions and poor functional status may live as long or longer with non-dialytic therapy that is focused on alleviating symptoms and maximizing quality of life (see Item 18).
- The incidence of dialysis initiation is increasing most rapidly among patients over the age of 75 years; decisions regarding initiation of renal replacement therapy in an older patient with impending end-stage kidney disease must take into account comorbid medical conditions, functional status, expected outcomes, and patient preferences regarding goals of care.
- Management of infection-related glomerulonephritis typically only consists of treatment of the underlying infection (see Item 12).
- Trimethoprim is known to interfere with creatinine secretion without affecting the glomerular filtration rate and can cause increases in serum creatinine of up to 0.5 mg/dL (44.2 µmol/L); this rise therefore does not reflect a drop in actual kidney function and does not require an extensive work-up (see Item 34).
- Patients with isolated hematuria with a family history of hematuria may require serial measurements of kidney function and urine protein because kidney failure may occur later in life (see Item 14).
- Proton pump inhibitors are a potentially treatable cause of chronic tubulointerstitial disease and should be discontinued to see if kidney function improves (see Item 50).
- For patients with autosomal dominant polycystic kidney disease, screening for intracranial cerebral aneurysms using MR angiography is only recommended for those with a family history of aneurysm or subarachnoid hemorrhage, those with a previous rupture, or those with high-risk occupations in which a rupture would affect the lives of others and should not be done routinely (see Item 62).
- Observation with serial blood pressure measurements, urine studies, and serum creatinine levels is appropriate for patients with IgA nephropathy with low-risk features for progression (see Item 85).
- In obese patients with likely secondary focal segmental glomerulosclerosis, weight loss is sometimes associated with a drop in proteinuria, as is the use of ACE inhibitors or angiotensin receptor blockers, and is the preferred initial therapy (see Item 87).
- An extensive evaluation for cancer is not indicated in patients with membranous glomerulopathy beyond age-appropriate cancer screening except for those with symptoms suggestive of a cancer diagnosis or significant risk factors for specific malignancies (see Item 106).

Nephrology

Clinical Evaluation of Kidney Function

Assessment of Kidney Function

Glomerular filtration rate (GFR) is the net sum of the filtration rates of thousands of nephrons, providing a quantitative measure of the flow rate of filtered fluid through the kidney per minute. Normal GFR is influenced by gender and body size, with a steady decline with aging. Assessment of GFR in patients with kidney disease provides an index of the severity of kidney functional impairment. There is not an exact correlation between the loss of functioning nephrons and GFR due to compensatory hypertrophy and increased flow in residual nephrons. Consequently, patients may have significant structural kidney disease with a normal GFR and/or progression of structural kidney disease without a significant change in measured GFR.

Biochemical Markers of Kidney Function

Serum creatinine is generated from the metabolism of creatine in muscle and from dietary meat. It is freely filtered by the glomerulus without metabolism or reabsorption by renal tubules. Although some creatinine is secreted by organic cation transport mechanisms in the proximal tubule, it is useful as an endogenous marker of GFR.

Measurement of serum creatinine concentration has been used for almost a century as an indicator of kidney function. Although it is the most commonly used marker of GFR, it is an imperfect measure. The relationship between GFR and serum creatinine is not linear, but inversely proportional (**Figure 1**). In patients who become functionally anephric, the serum creatinine typically increases 1.0 to 1.5 mg/dL (88.4-133 µmol/L) per day.

Reduction of muscle mass, as seen in amputees and those with malnutrition or muscle wasting, can result in a lower serum creatinine concentration without a change in GFR. Because of decreased muscle mass, serum creatinine overestimates kidney function in elderly persons, especially women. Young persons, men, and black persons often have higher muscle mass and higher serum creatinine concentration at a given GFR compared with older persons. Patients with advanced liver disease produce lower amounts of creatine (the precursor of creatinine) and have muscle wasting, resulting in a correspondingly lower serum creatinine at a given GFR. Certain medications (such as cimetidine and trimethoprim) inhibit organic cation transporters and block tubular secretion of creatinine, resulting in a higher serum creatinine without a change in GFR. Conversely, in patients who have chronic kidney disease (CKD) with intact tubular function, creatinine secretion increases, thus leading to a progressive overestimation of GFR.

Creatinine clearance is a measure of the volume of plasma that is cleared of creatinine by the kidney per unit of time and can be directly measured from a 24-hour urine collection to approximate the GFR (**Table 1**). The "adequacy" or "completeness" of the collection is estimated by the total excreted creatinine per 24 hours. For a 20- to 50-year-old man, creatinine excretion should be 18.5-25.0 mg/kg body weight and 16.5-22.4 mg/kg body weight for a woman of the same age. Because of the secretion of creatinine in the proximal tubule, the direct measurement of creatinine clearance tends to overestimate GFR. Nonetheless, the 24-hour urine collection with an adequate collection judged by the creatinine excreted is used to estimate GFR as well as excretion of other electrolytes and metabolic products such as calcium, phosphate, and urate.

Blood urea nitrogen (BUN) is derived from the metabolism of proteins. BUN concentration is a poor marker of kidney function because it is not produced at a constant rate and is reabsorbed along the tubules; furthermore, alterations in renal blood flow markedly influence tubular reabsorption and excretion. Urea clearances significantly underestimate GFR but may be useful in estimating GFR <15 mL/min/1.73 m^2.

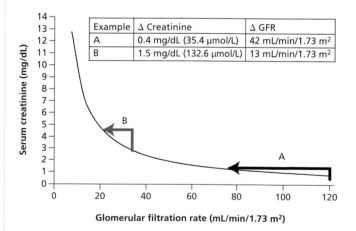

Example	Δ Creatinine	Δ GFR
A	0.4 mg/dL (35.4 µmol/L)	42 mL/min/1.73 m^2
B	1.5 mg/dL (132.6 µmol/L)	13 mL/min/1.73 m^2

FIGURE 1. The relationship between serum creatinine and glomerular filtration rate (GFR). Example A illustrates that a small increase in the serum creatinine level in the reference range (in this case, 0.8 to 1.2 mg/dL [70.7-106 µmol/L]) reflects a relatively large change in GFR (120 to 78 mL/min/1.73 m^2). Example B illustrates that a relatively greater increase in the serum creatinine level (in the high range of 3.0 to 4.5 mg/dL [265-398 µmol/L]) reflects a proportionately smaller change in GFR (35 to 22 mL/min/1.73 m^2).

TABLE 1. Methods for Estimating Kidney Function

Method	Considerations	Application
Creatinine Clearance		
U_{Cr} (mg/dL) × 24-hour urine volume (mL/24 h)/S_{Cr} (mg/dL) × 1440 (min/24 h)	Overestimates GFR 10%-20% Incomplete or excessive 24-hour urine collections limit accuracy	Useful in pregnancy, extremes of age and weight, amputees, and patients with cirrhosis
Serum Cystatin C		
	Levels are affected by thyroid status, diabetic status, inflammation, and glucocorticoid use	More accurate in elderly population and patients with cirrhosis
Modification of Diet in Renal Disease (MDRD) Study Equation[a]		
$GFR = 175 \times (S_{Cr})^{-1.154} \times (age)^{-0.203} \times 0.742$ (if female) or × 1.212 (if black)	Most accurate when eGFR is 15-60 mL/min/1.73 m² Underestimates GFR when GFR >60 mL/min/1.73 m² Less accurate in populations with normal or near normal eGFR, extremes of age and weight, amputees, in pregnancy, and in patients with cirrhosis	Chronic kidney disease when eGFR is 15-60 mL/min/1.73 m²
Chronic Kidney Disease Epidemiology (CKD-EPI) Collaboration Equation[a]		
$GFR = 141 \times \min(S_{Cr}/\kappa, 1)^{\alpha} \times \max(S_{Cr}/\kappa, 1)^{-1.209} \times 0.993^{age} \times 1.018$ (if female) × 1.159 (if black)[b]	Superior to CGE and MDRD equations in patients with eGFR >60 mL/min/1.73 m²	More accurate than MDRD equation in elderly population
Cockcroft-Gault Equation (CGE)		
$CrCl = \dfrac{(140 - age) \times (weight\ in\ kg) \times (0.85\ if\ female)}{(72 \times S_{Cr})}$	Most accurate when eGFR is 15-60 mL/min/1.73 m² Underestimates GFR in obesity Overestimates GFR when BMI <25 Takes into account lean body weight, age, and gender	Improved accuracy when age is <65 years
Radionuclide Kidney Clearance Scanning		
Iothalamate GFR scan Diethylenetriamine pentaacetic acid (DTPA) GFR scan	Most precise method; expensive	Kidney donor evaluation if eGFR is borderline for donation; research; prediction of eGFR following nephrectomy

CrCl = creatinine clearance; eGFR = estimated glomerular filtration rate; GFR = glomerular filtration rate; S_{Cr} = serum creatinine (mg/dL); U_{Cr} = urine creatinine (mg/dL).

[a]Mathematical equations recommended by the National Kidney Foundation Kidney Disease Outcomes Quality Initiative for estimation of GFR.

[b]κ is 0.7 for women and 0.9 for men; α is -0.329 for women and -0.411 for men; min = the minimum of S_{Cr}/κ or 1; max = the maximum of S_{Cr}/κ or 1.

Serum cystatin C is an alternative marker of GFR less influenced than serum creatinine by age, gender, muscle mass, and body weight. Cystatin C is produced by all nucleated cells, completely filtered by glomeruli, and then metabolized by renal tubules; serum levels thus provide an index of GFR, without the need to measure urine excretion. Serum cystatin C is more sensitive in identifying milder decrements in kidney function than serum creatinine.

Estimation of Glomerular Filtration Rate

Isotopic markers that are filtered and not secreted (for example, iothalamate) provide very accurate estimates of GFR but are expensive and not available in routine clinical practice. However, the correlation of these forms of measurement with serum creatinine, age, race, and gender has led to the development of equations that provide a more accurate estimation of GFR than creatinine clearance (see Table 1).

Three estimation equations are commonly used: the Cockcroft-Gault equation (CGE), the Modification of Diet in Renal Disease (MDRD) study equation, and the Chronic Kidney Disease Epidemiology (CKD-EPI) Collaboration equation. Each equation was developed in different study populations and uses different variables to provide an estimation of the GFR. Because of this, these equations tend to be more accurate when used in specific clinical circumstances. For example, the MDRD study equation has been validated in multiple populations with CKD but frequently underestimates GFR when it is >60 mL/min/1.73 m². The CKD-EPI equation performs better at higher (normal) values of GFR. Despite its long history and widespread use, the CGE equation is slightly less accurate than these newer equations for estimating GFR. Accurate estimation of GFR is important for appropriate adjustment of drug dosing in the elderly population and in patients with kidney disease. Historically, drug-dosing guidelines have been developed based on the estimated creatinine clearance derived from the CGE equation. For the purposes of drug dosing, the CGE equation correlates adequately with GFR as estimated by the MDRD study equation.

Most clinical laboratories employ the MDRD study equation to estimate GFR, with higher levels of GFR reported as ">60 mL/min/1.73 m²." Physicians may therefore ignore other signs or symptoms of CKD (such as proteinuria) after erroneously assuming that a level reported as normal means an absence of structural kidney disease. Conversely, the appropriateness of labeling a patient who has a stable GFR around 55 mL/min/1.73 m² (apart from guiding appropriate drug dosing) as having stage 3 CKD, with no other signs of kidney disease, remains unclear.

> **KEY POINT**
>
> - The Modification of Diet in Renal Disease study equation has been validated in multiple populations with chronic kidney disease but frequently underestimates the glomerular filtration rate (GFR) when it is >60 mL/min/1.73 m², whereas the Chronic Kidney Disease Epidemiology Collaboration equation performs better at higher (normal) values of GFR; the Cockcroft-Gault equation is slightly less accurate than these newer equations for estimating GFR but is the basis for drug dosing guidelines.

Interpretation of the Urinalysis

Dipstick analysis and microscopic examination of the urine are indicated in the clinical evaluation of kidney function for both acute and chronic kidney disease (**Table 2**). The sample is best collected without contamination, which requires a "clean catch" midstream collection or a bladder catheterization, and should be examined within 1 hour to minimize the breakdown of formed elements.

Urine Dipstick or Automated Urinalysis
Specific Gravity

Specific gravity is the ratio of the weight of urine to an equal quantity of the weight of water. Normal specific gravity of urine is approximately 1.010, and the typical range of 1.005 to 1.030 varies depending on hydration status and the capacity of the kidneys to maximally dilute and concentrate the urine. Specific gravity is used to estimate the urine osmolality, with a specific gravity of 1.010 approximating a urine osmolality of 300 mOsm/kg H_2O, indicating isosmolar urine; higher or lower values reflect concentrated and dilute urine, respectively.

pH

A typical high-protein American diet results in the need to excrete a high acid load, primarily via the kidneys. The urine in this case is relatively more acidic, ranging from 5.0 to 6.0. An alkaline pH of ≥7.0 can occur in strict vegetarians, postprandially, in type 1 (distal) renal tubular acidosis, or with infections caused by urease-splitting organisms such as *Proteus* and *Pseudomonas* species.

Albumin

Albumin is the predominant protein detected on urine dipstick, which detects albumin excretion graded as trace (5-30 mg/dL), 1+ (30 mg/dL), 2+ (100 mg/dL), 3+ (300 mg/dL), and 4+ (>1000 mg/dL). Highly alkaline urine specimens can produce false-positive results on dipstick testing for protein. The sulfosalicylic acid (SSA) test can be used to detect the presence of not only albumin but also other proteins that are not detected with the urine dipstick, such as urine light chains or immunoglobulins. The possibility of cast nephropathy should be raised in patients with acute kidney injury (AKI) when the urine dipstick reads negative or trace for protein, but the urine shows increased positivity for protein by the SSA test. This should be confirmed by immunoelectrophoresis, which can detect urine light chains or Bence-Jones proteins.

Glucose

Glycosuria typically occurs when the plasma glucose concentration is >180 to 200 mg/dL (10.0-11.1 mmol/L). Generalized proximal tubular dysfunction (termed *Fanconi syndrome*) may result in glycosuria in the absence of hyperglycemia or in pregnancy with a change in threshold for glucose.

Ketones

Ketones in the urine are associated with diabetic ketoacidosis, salicylate toxicity, isopropyl alcohol poisoning, and states of starvation such as alcoholic ketoacidosis. Because the urine dipstick detects acetoacetate but not β-hydroxybutyrate, patients who are ketotic with β-hydroxybutyrate as the only ketone body do not display a positive urine dipstick for

TABLE 2.	Findings on Urinalysis	
	Reference Range	**Comments**
Dipstick		
Specific gravity	1.005-1.030	Low with dilute urine; high with concentrated urine or hypertonic product excretion such as with glycosuria and contrast dye
pH	5.0-6.5	Elevated with low acid ingestion, alkaline tide postprandial, inability to excrete acid load (renal tubular acidosis), urease-splitting organisms
Blood	None	False positives with myoglobin or intravascular hemolysis
Albumin	None to trace	Most dipsticks detect primarily albumin but not other proteins; trace positive can be normal in a concentrated specimen; specialized dipsticks designed to detect small amounts of albumin for detection of moderately increased albuminuria (microalbuminuria) are available
Glucose	None	Positive when plasma glucose level exceeds 180 mg/dL (10.0 mmol/L) with lower threshold in pregnancy or Fanconi syndrome
Ketones	None	Positive for acetoacetic acid, not acetone or β-hydroxybutyrate
Nitrites	None	Detects nitrite converted from dietary nitrate by bacteria; normally, no nitrites are present in urine
Leukocyte esterase	None	Detects the presence of leukocytes in the urine; positive test requires at least 3 leukocytes/hpf
Microscopy		
Erythrocytes	0-3/hpf	Urine microscopy should be performed to evaluate erythrocyte morphology
Leukocytes	0-3/hpf	The presence of any leukocytes may be abnormal depending on clinical circumstances
Casts	None or hyaline	Hyaline casts are indicative of poor kidney perfusion but can be benign or reversible; other casts are indicative of intrinsic injury
Crystals	None	Most common include calcium oxalate, calcium phosphate, uric acid, and struvite; occur when urine is supersaturated with a specific substance

ketones; this scenario may occur in patients with alcoholic ketoacidosis. Drugs such as captopril have sulfhydryl groups that can result in a false-positive urine dipstick for ketones.

Blood

The urine dipstick detects both free hemoglobin and intact erythrocytes via measurement of peroxidase activity. One to three erythrocytes/hpf are usually required for a positive result. Other substances with peroxidase activity can cause false-positive reactions, including myoglobin, bacteria expressing peroxidase activity, hypochlorite, rifampin, chloroquine, and certain forms of iodine. Ascorbic acid can cause a false-negative result. A positive urine dipstick for blood but without evidence of erythrocytes on microscopic urinalysis should raise suspicion for hemolysis or rhabdomyolysis; urine myoglobin levels can be measured to confirm rhabdomyolysis.

Leukocyte Esterase and Nitrites

Leukocyte esterase is an enzyme present in leukocytes. The urine dipstick is usually positive for leukocyte esterase when approximately 3 leukocytes/hpf are present. Nitrites result from the conversion of nitrates to nitrites, which occur in urinary tract infections (UTIs) caused by gram-negative organisms, including Escherichia coli, Klebsiella pneumoniae, and the Proteus and Pseudomonas species. False-negative results for nitrites can occur in the setting of a UTI caused by gram-

positive organisms such as Enterococcus species. The presence of both leukocyte esterase and nitrites on urine dipstick is highly suggestive of a UTI; the absence of both has a high negative predictive value for a UTI.

Bilirubin

Conjugated bilirubin is not usually present in the urine of patients with normal serum bilirubin levels. The presence of conjugated bilirubin is suggestive of severe liver disease or obstructive jaundice. False-positive results occur with chlorpromazine, and false-negative results occur with ascorbic acid.

Urobilinogen

Urobilinogen is produced in the gut from the metabolism of bilirubin and is then reabsorbed and excreted in the urine. A positive urine dipstick for urobilinogen usually results from hemolytic anemia or hepatic necrosis but not from obstructive causes.

KEY POINTS

- Albumin is the predominant protein detected on urine dipstick.
- The presence of both leukocyte esterase and nitrites on urine dipstick is highly suggestive of a urinary tract infection (UTI); the absence of both has a high negative predictive value for a UTI.

HVC

Urine Microscopy

Microscopic assessment of urine sediment is indicated for patients with abnormalities on urine dipstick or automated urinalysis, AKI, suspicion for glomerulonephritis, or newly diagnosed CKD. Cells, casts, and crystals are possible findings in patients with kidney disease.

Erythrocytes

Erythrocytes in the urine can originate at any location along the genitourinary tract, from the glomerulus to the urethra. Assessment of erythrocyte morphology is a key component in the evaluation of hematuria (see Clinical Evaluation of Hematuria). Isomorphic erythrocytes are of the same size and shape and usually arise from a urologic process causing bleeding into the genitourinary tract such as a tumor, stone, or infection. Dysmorphic erythrocytes have varying sizes and shapes. Acanthocytes, a specific form of dysmorphic erythrocytes, are characterized by vesicle-shaped protrusions (**Figure 2**) and suggest a glomerular source of bleeding. Acanthocytes and erythrocyte casts are highly specific for glomerulonephritis and should prompt evaluation.

Leukocytes

Pyuria refers to excess leukocytes in the urine and is defined as ≥4 leukocytes/hpf. The most common cause of pyuria is a UTI. Sterile pyuria refers to the presence of leukocytes in the urine in the setting of a negative bacterial culture. *Mycobacterium tuberculosis* is an important infectious cause of sterile pyuria. Acute interstitial nephritis is associated with sterile pyuria and low-grade proteinuria; it is often caused by antibiotics, NSAIDs, or proton pump inhibitors. Kidney stones and kidney transplant rejection can also cause sterile pyuria.

Eosinophils

Urine eosinophils are visualized via Wright or Hansel stains. The presence of eosinophils in the urine can be indicative of an allergic reaction, atheroembolic disease, rapidly progressive glomerulonephritis, small-vessel vasculitis, UTI, prostatic disease, or parasitic infections. Poor sensitivity and specificity limit the utility of assays for urine eosinophils in the diagnosis of interstitial nephritis.

Epithelial Cells

Renal tubular epithelial cells have large, central nuclei and are 1.5 to 3 times larger than leukocytes; these can be seen, along with pigmented casts, in the setting of acute tubular necrosis (ATN). Transitional epithelial cells originate anywhere from the renal pelvis to the proximal urethra and are slightly larger than renal tubular epithelial cells. Squamous epithelial cells are large and irregular in shape with small central nuclei and are derived from the distal urethra or external genitalia; their presence denotes urine contaminated by genital secretions.

Casts

Urine casts consist of a matrix comprised of Tamm-Horsfall mucoprotein (also known as uromodulin), which may contain cells, cellular debris, or lipoprotein droplets. Casts are formed within the tubular lumen and are therefore cylindrical. Documentation of particular types of casts is instrumental in the diagnostic evaluation of AKI. ATN may lead to deposition of pigmented epithelial tubular debris in the proteinaceous matrix of the cast, with the formation of pigmented granular (muddy brown) casts (**Figure 3**). An abundance of these casts and renal tubular epithelial cells correlates with the severity of AKI. Erythrocyte casts are highly specific, but not particularly sensitive, for glomerulonephritis. Tubulointerstitial inflammation of the kidney, including pyelonephritis, can lead to the formation of leukocyte casts.

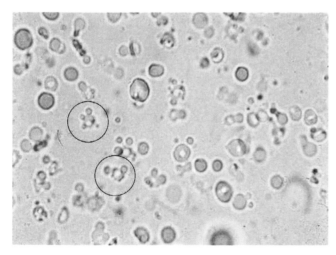

FIGURE 2. Urine microscopy demonstrating acanthocytes, indicated in the red circles. Acanthocytes, one form of dysmorphic erythrocytes, are characterized by vesicle-shaped protrusions.

Courtesy of J. Charles Jennette, MD.

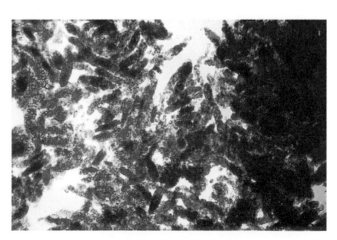

FIGURE 3. Tubular injury (for example, acute tubular necrosis) may lead to deposition of pigmented epithelial tubular debris in the proteinaceous matrix of the cast, with the formation of pigmented granular (muddy brown) casts.

Crystals

Table 3 highlights the crystals commonly observed in the urine, along with morphology and associated conditions. Certain medications, including sulfadiazine, intravenous acyclovir, methotrexate, and indinavir, can result in crystals in the urine.

TABLE 3. Urine Crystals		
Type	**Morphology/ Shape**	**Associated Conditions**
Calcium oxalate	Envelope; dumbbell; needle	Hypercalciuria; hyperoxaluria; calcium oxalate stones; ethylene glycol poisoning
Calcium phosphate	Prism; needle; star-like clumps	Distal renal tubular acidosis; urine pH >6.5; tumor lysis syndrome; acute phosphate nephropathy
Uric acid	Rhomboid; needle; rosette	Diabetes mellitus; obesity; gout; hyperuricemia; tumor lysis syndrome; urine pH <6.0
Magnesium ammonium phosphate (struvite)	Coffin-lid	Chronic urinary tract infection with urease-producing organisms
Cystine	Hexagonal	Cystinuria

Measurement of Albumin and Protein Excretion

Proteinuria is most commonly comprised of albumin, but other proteins, including kidney-derived low-molecular-weight proteins, monoclonal immunoglobulins and light chains, myoglobin, and hemoglobin, may be present. Low-molecular-weight proteinuria is more common in tubulointerstitial disease or in generalized proximal tubular dysfunction (termed *Fanconi syndrome*), whereas a predominance of albuminuria favors a glomerular process.

Protein detected by urine dipstick should always be quantified. Quantification of proteinuria has traditionally been performed with a 24-hour urine collection, which measures all proteins present in the urine. Due to challenges in feasibility, accuracy, and patient adherence, measurement of proteinuria is now typically performed by determining the ratio of protein or albumin to creatinine on random urine samples. These ratios are easily obtained and correlate well with timed collections. See **Table 4** for the definitions of proteinuria and albuminuria.

The urine protein-creatinine ratio measures all proteins present in the urine, and a value of ≤150 mg/g is considered

TABLE 4. Definitions of Proteinuria and Albuminuria			
Total Urine Protein			
Urine Collection Method	**Normal**	**Clinical Proteinuria**	
24-Hour Excretion	<150 mg/24 h	≥150 mg/24 h	
Spot Urine Protein-Creatinine Ratio[a]	≤150 mg/g ≈ ≤150 mg/24 h	>150 mg/g ≈ >150 mg/24 h	
Urine Albumin			
Urine Collection Method	**Normal**	**Moderately Increased Albuminuria (Microalbuminuria)**	**Severely Increased Albuminuria (Macroalbuminuria)**
24-Hour Excretion	<30 mg/24 h	30-300 mg/24 h	>300 mg/24 h
Conventional Spot Urine Dipstick[b]	Negative	Negative	Positive
Albumin-Specific Spot Urine Dipstick[c]	<3.0 mg/dL Negative	≥3.0 mg/dL Positive	Positive
Spot Urine Albumin-Creatinine Ratio[a]	<30 mg/g ≈ <30 mg/24 h	30-300 mg/g ≈ 30-300 mg/24 h	>300 mg/g ≈ >300 mg/24 h

[a]Because of the difficulty of obtaining a 24-hour urine collection, urine protein-creatinine ratio or urine albumin-creatinine ratio on random (spot) urine samples are used to estimate 24-hour excretion. Measurement of either urine protein or albumin concentration in a sample is divided by the creatinine concentration of the same sample to derive a unitless value. These ratios correlate well with the 24-hour excretion of protein or albumin. Although these calculations are technically dimensionless, they may be expressed by different laboratories with their units of calculation, such as mg/g (mg protein or albumin/g creatinine) or with units to reflect the proportional 24-hour excretion amount (mg or g protein or albumin/g creatinine).

[b]Conventional urine dipsticks are more sensitive for detection of albumin than non-albumin proteins; the detection limit is approximately 30 mg/dL, although they are not highly accurate for determining the degree of albuminuria if present.

[c]Urine dipsticks designed specifically to detect small amounts of albuminuria. Similar to conventional urine dipsticks, these dipsticks detect albumin above a concentration threshold but are sensitive to the presence of albumin at lower levels and can be used to indicate the presence of moderately increased albuminuria (microalbuminuria).

normal. Levels of proteinuria may be diagnostically helpful. Urine protein-creatinine ratios >150 mg/g but <200 mg/g may indicate either tubulointerstitial disease or glomerular disease, whereas nephrotic-range proteinuria, defined as a urine protein-creatinine ratio >3500 mg/g, usually indicates a glomerular process. In patients with evidence of proteinuria, at least two samples on different days should be collected to confirm the diagnosis. It is important to characterize the proteinuria (such as in suspected cast nephropathy) with urine electrophoresis with immunofixation of monoclonal immunoglobulins when indicated.

The urine albumin-creatinine ratio measures only albumin in the urine and is helpful in evaluating for diabetic kidney disease. Because albuminuria is one of the earliest indicators of diabetic kidney disease, the American Diabetes Association (ADA) recommends annual assessment of urine albumin excretion by measuring the urine albumin-creatinine ratio in patients with type 1 diabetes mellitus of 5 years' duration and in all patients with type 2 diabetes starting at the time of diagnosis. Normal albumin excretion by this method is considered <30 mg/g. Although screening for albuminuria is commonly performed in patients with diabetes, the American College of Physicians (ACP) found the current evidence insufficient to evaluate the benefits and harms of screening for CKD in asymptomatic adults with CKD risk factors, including diabetes, hypertension, and cardiovascular disease.

The terminology for describing abnormal albumin excretion has changed. A urine albumin-creatinine ratio of 30 to 300 mg/g, previously termed *microalbuminuria*, is now referred to as *moderately increased albuminuria*, and levels >300 mg/g, previously known as *macroalbuminuria* or *overt proteinuria*, are now termed *severely increased albuminuria*. The diagnosis of moderately increased albuminuria in patients with diabetes is made when two or three random samples obtained over 6 months show a urine albumin-creatinine ratio of 30 to 300 mg/g; the use of ACE inhibitors or angiotensin receptor blockers in these patients has been shown to delay progression of CKD, underscoring the importance of early detection. Once a diagnosis of moderately increased albuminuria has been established and treatment initiated, the ACP recommends against further screening for albuminuria because it will not significantly influence management decisions.

In other patients at increased risk for kidney disease, the urine protein-creatinine ratio is appropriate to evaluate for suspected proteinuria. Transient proteinuria is common and is associated with febrile illnesses or rigorous exercise; it requires no further evaluation. Orthostatic proteinuria occurs when proteinuria increases when the patient is in an upright position and decreases when the patient is recumbent; this benign condition, more common in adolescents, can be assessed with a split urine collection. This test should be obtained in patients younger than 30 years of age who appear to have persistent proteinuria.

Clinical Evaluation of Hematuria

Hematuria is defined as >3 erythrocytes/hpf and may be either macroscopic (grossly visible) or microscopic (detectable only on urine testing). Hematuria has many potential causes and a wide range of clinical significance. False hematuria or hematuria mimics may be caused by contamination from menstrual bleeding or from substances that produce red-colored urine not due to erythrocytes or hemoglobinuria, including medications (rifampin, phenytoin), food (rhubarb, beets), acute porphyrias, and myoglobinuria. Hemoglobinuria results from the release of free hemoglobin intravascularly in conditions such as hemolysis from perivalvular leak and delayed transfusion reaction. Benign causes of hematuria include infections such as UTIs, nephrolithiasis, trauma, and exercise. Potentially life-threatening and often clinically urgent causes of hematuria include rapidly progressive glomerulonephritis and urinary tract malignancy. Glomerular causes of hematuria also include more benign or indolent diseases such as thin glomerular basement membrane disease, IgA nephropathy, and other forms of chronic glomerulonephritis.

Glomerular hematuria typically features brown- or tea-colored urine with dysmorphic erythrocytes (or acanthocytes) and/or erythrocyte casts on urine sediment examination. Urologic hematuria may include passage of blood clots or pure blood and nondysmorphic erythrocytes. Examination of the urine is not definitive in determining glomerular versus urologic sources of hematuria, especially in patients at risk for genitourinary tract malignancies. Patients with a bleeding diathesis or on anticoagulation merit a complete evaluation; hematuria should not be attributed to the coagulopathy or anticoagulation until other causes have been excluded.

Evaluation of the patient with hematuria begins with a careful history, especially for more benign causes (**Figure 4**). False hematuria should be excluded. Historical and/or laboratory clues may point to a glomerular etiology and the need for nephrology consultation. In patients with suspected glomerular hematuria, extrarenal manifestations of a systemic disease such as vasculitis should be sought.

The American Urological Association (AUA) guidelines for the evaluation of asymptomatic microhematuria recommend CT urography as the imaging modality of choice (**Table 5**, on page 9). The AUA guidelines also recommend cystoscopy for all patients over 35 years of age or those with risk factors for urologic malignancy. The AUA guidelines do not recommend urine cytology for routine evaluation of asymptomatic microhematuria. The U.S. Preventive Services Task Force recommends against using

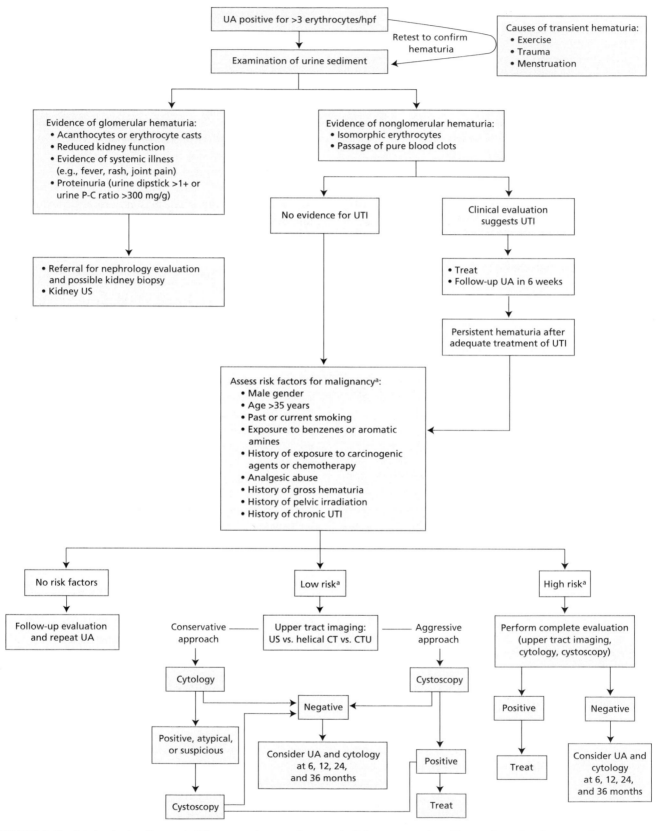

FIGURE 4. The clinical evaluation of hematuria. CTU = computed tomography urography; P-C = protein-creatinine; UA = urinalysis; US = ultrasonography; UTI = urinary tract infection.

[a]Modified from Urology. Grossfeld GD, Litwin MS, Wolf JS, et al. Evaluation of asymptomatic microscopic hematuria in adults: the American Urological Association best practice policy–part II: patient evaluation, cytology, voided markers, imaging, cystoscopy, nephrology evaluation, and follow-up. 2001 Apr;57(4):604-10. [PMID: 11306357] Copyright 2001, modified with permission from Elsevier.

TABLE 5.	Imaging Used in the Evaluation of Hematuria	
Study	**Advantages**	**Disadvantages**
CT urography (CTU)	High sensitivity (100%) and specificity (97%); image modality of choice	High radiation dose; Risk of CIN; contraindicated in pregnancy
MR urography	Useful in eGFR range of 30-60 mL/min/1.73 m² or when CTU is contraindicated	Contraindicated when eGFR <30 mL/min/1.73 m² (risk of gadolinium-induced nephrogenic systemic fibrosis); less sensitive than CTU for smaller cancers and stones
Ultrasonography	No contrast or radiation exposure; useful in pregnancy, lower cost	Limited sensitivity, especially for lesions <2 cm and ureteral lesions

CIN = contrast-induced nephropathy; eGFR = estimated glomerular filtration rate.

urinalysis for bladder cancer screening in asymptomatic patients, even those with risk factors.

KEY POINTS

- Potentially life-threatening and often clinically urgent causes of hematuria include rapidly progressive glomerulonephritis and urinary tract malignancy.

- Evaluation of asymptomatic microhematuria should include CT urography except in patients with chronic kidney disease, pregnant patients, or patients allergic to contrast; cystoscopy should be performed in patients over 35 years of age or those with risk factors for urologic malignancy.

- **HVC** Urinalysis should not be used to screen for bladder cancer in asymptomatic patients.

Imaging Studies

The four main modalities of kidney imaging (ultrasonography, CT, MRI, and radionuclide studies) provide information about structure and function of the urinary tract. Ultrasonography (US) is safe, noninvasive, relatively inexpensive, and easy to obtain. Often the first imaging test in the evaluation of kidney disease, US can assess kidney size and cortical thickness, detect renal cysts and tumors, and diagnose obstruction and hydronephrosis. US is useful for assessment of the bladder, postvoid residual, and the prostate in bladder outlet obstruction but is less helpful in evaluating diseases affecting the mid and distal ureter. Increased echogenicity of the kidney is nonspecific but implies parenchymal disease. Experienced centers have used Doppler US for detection of clinically relevant renal artery stenosis.

US is being increasingly used as an initial diagnostic study for uncomplicated nephrolithiasis. Although less sensitive than CT, particularly for detecting small stones and ureteral stones, it does not expose patients to radiation, is often more readily available, and is usually more cost-effective when compared with CT; it is also the indicated modality during pregnancy. A positive ultrasound may be adequate for initial diagnosis, with CT imaging for those with a nondiagnostic ultrasound or a more complicated clinical presentation.

Noncontrast abdominal helical CT has traditionally been the most commonly used imaging technique for suspected nephrolithiasis because it detects most stones, provides anatomic information, and visualizes the entire urinary tract; it may also suggest stone composition and potentially provide alternative diagnoses if nephrolithiasis is not detected. Contrast abdominal CT characterizes renal tumors and cysts, whereas CT urography is the preferred test for patients with unexplained urologic/nonglomerular hematuria. Intravascular iodinated contrast for CT and angiography may be complicated by contrast-induced nephropathy, especially in patients with CKD. The decision to use contrast depends on the clinical scenario, the patient's risk factors for contrast-induced nephropathy, and the availability and utility of alternative imaging modalities.

Kidney MRI can also identify renal masses, cysts, and renal vein thrombosis. MR angiography with gadolinium contrast can detect renal artery stenosis in the evaluation of possible renovascular hypertension, replacing standard angiography as the preferred modality. However, gadolinium can cause nephrogenic systemic fibrosis (NSF), a systemic fibrosing disorder that occurs predominantly in patients with CKD (typically stage 4 or 5), and gadolinium contrast must be avoided in patients with an estimated GFR <30 mL/min/1.73 m². See MKSAP 17 Dermatology for more information on NSF.

Often used for clinical research studies, radionuclide kidney imaging is the gold standard for measuring GFR and renal plasma flow and can be used in the evaluation of a kidney transplant donor candidate with borderline kidney function. In clinical practice, radionuclide scans are most useful for determining relative function of the kidneys, such as a hydronephrotic, atrophic, or cancerous kidney prior to nephrectomy.

KEY POINTS

- Ultrasonography is typically the first imaging test in the evaluation of the kidneys and upper urinary tract because of its safety, cost effectiveness, and general utility. **HVC**

- Contrast abdominal CT characterizes renal tumors and cysts, whereas CT urography is the preferred test for patients with unexplained urologic/nonglomerular hematuria.

H Kidney Biopsy

Kidney biopsy provides pathologic diagnostic information that can be useful for treatment, disease surveillance, and, potentially, prognosis. Kidney biopsy should be considered in patients with glomerular hematuria, severely increased albuminuria, acute or chronic kidney disease of unclear etiology, and kidney transplant dysfunction or monitoring. Some kidney diseases such as acute interstitial nephritis or atheroembolic disease may be occult and difficult to diagnose without biopsy. Direct visualization by ultrasound or CT is the standard for percutaneous kidney biopsy. Nonpercutaneous approaches for kidney biopsy include open, laparoscopic, or transjugular.

Contraindications to kidney biopsy include bleeding diatheses, severe anemia (especially with patient refusal of blood transfusions), UTI, hydronephrosis, uncontrolled hypertension, anatomic abnormalities, renal tumor, atrophic kidneys, and an uncooperative patient. Solitary native kidney and pregnancy are not absolute contraindications, but careful consideration of the risks and benefits is necessary. Significant complications include pain, macroscopic hematuria, hemorrhage (potentially requiring transfusions, angiography with embolization, and surgery such as nephrectomy), loss of kidney function, and death. H

KEY POINT

- Kidney biopsy should be considered in patients with glomerular hematuria, severely increased albuminuria, acute or chronic kidney disease of unclear etiology, and kidney transplant dysfunction or monitoring.

Fluids and Electrolytes
Osmolality and Tonicity

Plasma osmolality is determined by the concentration of sodium and its accompanying anions, plasma glucose, and blood urea nitrogen (BUN). Total osmolality can be directly measured with an osmometer or may be calculated:

$$\text{Plasma Osmolality (mOsm/kg H}_2\text{O)} =$$
$$2 \times \text{Serum Sodium (mEq/L)} + \text{Plasma Glucose}$$
$$\text{(mg/dL)}/18 + \text{BUN (mg/dL)}/2.8$$

Although both methods indicate the overall osmolality of plasma, urea is freely diffusible across most cell membranes and does not exert a significant osmotic effect. Therefore, the *effective* osmolality (tonicity) is determined by subtracting the measured concentration of urea (divided by 2.8, if in mg/dL) from the measured osmolality. Under normal conditions, the effective osmolality is maintained in the range of 275 to 295 mOsm/kg H$_2$O.

Disorders of osmolality are usually caused by abnormalities in the relative ratio of sodium to body water. Two key effectors in maintaining normal plasma osmolality are thirst and the level of circulating antidiuretic hormone (ADH; also

known as arginine vasopressin), which promotes water reabsorption in the distal tubule and collecting duct of the kidney and has a peripheral vasoconstricting effect. Thirst and ADH release are stimulated by increases in plasma osmolality through central osmoreceptors in the hypothalamus. ADH release is also influenced by volume status; hypovolemia is associated with higher circulating ADH levels at each level of plasma osmolality.

Disorders of Serum Sodium H
Hyponatremia

Hyponatremia, defined as a serum sodium concentration <136 mEq/L (136 mmol/L), most often results from an increase in circulating ADH in response to a true or sensed reduction in effective arterial blood volume with resulting fluid retention. Hyponatremia may also be caused by elevated ADH levels associated with the syndrome of inappropriate antidiuretic hormone secretion. Hyponatremia occurring with normal or suppressed ADH levels may be seen in the setting of very low solute intake (such as the "tea and toast" syndrome and "beer potomania"), in which inadequate amounts of solute are available to excrete an increased volume of ingested free water.

Evaluation

The initial evaluation of patients with hyponatremia includes measurement of plasma and urine osmolality and urine sodium as well as a careful assessment of the volume status.

Measurement of plasma osmolality is needed to exclude hyperosmolar hyponatremia and pseudohyponatremia (in which plasma osmolality is normal). Hyperosmolar hyponatremia results from elevated plasma glucose or from exogenously administered solutes such as mannitol or sucrose. Hyperglycemia causes the osmotic translocation of water from the intracellular to the extracellular fluid compartment, which results in a decrease in the serum sodium level by approximately 1.6 mEq/L (1.6 mmol/L) for every 100 mg/dL (5.6 mmol/L) increase in the plasma glucose above 100 mg/dL (5.6 mmol/L).

Pseudohyponatremia is the result of a laboratory error in the measurement of serum sodium. Clinical laboratories measure the amount of sodium present in a dilute serum sample. The serum sodium concentration is then calculated based on the assumption that plasma is 93% water. However, in patients with extreme hyperlipidemia and/or hyperproteinemia, this assumption may not be correct because lipids or protein make up a greater percentage of overall plasma volume. This may result in the reporting of a falsely low serum sodium concentration.

In patients with hypotonic hyponatremia, further evaluation is based on urine osmolality (**Figure 5**). Urine osmolality <100 mOsm/kg H$_2$O is consistent with appropriately suppressed ADH release as seen in primary polydipsia or inadequate solute intake. Urine osmolality >100 mOsm/kg H$_2$O indicates that ADH excess is playing a dominant role. Hypotonic

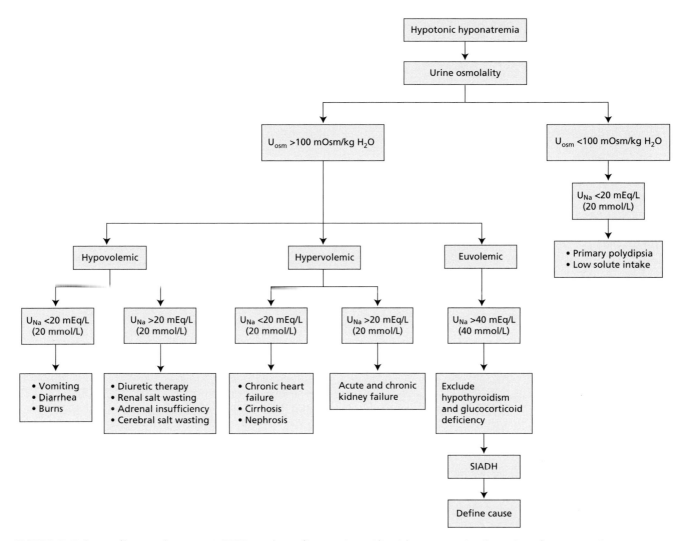

FIGURE 5. Evaluation of hypotonic hyponatremia. SIADH = syndrome of inappropriate antidiuretic hormone secretion; U_{Na} = urine sodium concentration; U_{osm} = urine osmolality.

CONT.

hyponatremia with a urine osmolality >100 mOsm/kg H_2O is classified into three groups based on the clinical volume status: hypovolemic, hypervolemic, and euvolemic.

Hypovolemic Hyponatremia
Hypovolemia causes stimulation of the sympathetic nervous system, activation of the renin-angiotensin-aldosterone (RAA) axis, and release of ADH. These adaptive responses allow volume maintenance at the expense of a low serum sodium with excessive water intake.

Extrarenal causes of hypovolemia are common and include loss of sodium from the gastrointestinal tract (vomiting or diarrhea) and insensible loss of sodium chloride (sweating, burns, respiratory tract); in these conditions, the urine sodium concentration is typically <20 mEq/L (20 mmol/L). Renal causes of hypovolemic hyponatremia result in excessive loss of salt and water in the urine with volume depletion; the urine sodium concentration is typically >20 mEq/L (20 mmol/L). Diuretic therapy is the most common cause. Less common are

adrenal insufficiency and salt-wasting nephropathies with impaired renal tubular function; typical causes include reflux nephropathy, interstitial nephropathies, post-obstructive uropathy, cystic kidney diseases, and the recovery phase of acute tubular necrosis. The syndrome of cerebral salt wasting is a rare cause due to inappropriate natriuresis from intracranial disease such as subarachnoid hemorrhage, traumatic brain injury, craniotomy, encephalitis, and meningitis.

Hypervolemic Hyponatremia
Patients with hypervolemic hyponatremia have increased total body sodium and water, with the latter dominating and leading to a reduced serum sodium concentration. The pathophysiology of hyponatremia in sodium-avid edematous disorders (heart failure, cirrhosis, and the nephrotic syndrome) is similar to that in hypovolemic hyponatremia, with the kidney sensing a decreased arterial blood volume despite excess total body sodium and water. The urine sodium concentration is typically <20 mEq/L (20 mmol/L) in the absence of diuretic therapy.

CONT.

However, in patients with hypervolemic hyponatremia due to acute or chronic kidney failure, there is an inability to effectively manage both sodium and water, leading to an excess of water relative to sodium. In acute or chronic kidney failure, the urine sodium concentration is typically >20 mEq/L (20 mmol/L).

Euvolemic Hyponatremia

Euvolemic hyponatremia results from abnormalities in maintaining sodium and water balance in the setting of normal total volume or to a reset osmostat. Because the effective arterial blood volume is normal, the urine sodium concentration is usually >20 mEq/L (20 mmol/L). The most common cause of euvolemic hyponatremia is the syndrome of inappropriate antidiuretic hormone secretion (SIADH) **(Table 6)**. It is important to exclude hypothyroidism and glucocorticoid insufficiency in patients with euvolemic hyponatremia and suspected SIADH because thyroid hormone and endogenous glucocorticoid are necessary for normal free water excretion by the kidney.

Reset osmostat refers to a downward setting of the level at which sensors of plasma osmolality trigger the release of antidiuretic hormone and is associated with quadriplegia, tuberculosis, advanced age, pregnancy, psychiatric disorders, and chronic malnutrition. This lowered setpoint leads to mild hypo-osmolar euvolemic hyponatremia.

Clinical Presentation

Patients with acute symptomatic hyponatremia (occurring in <48 hours) often present with symptoms and signs ranging from headache, nausea, and/or vomiting, to altered mental

TABLE 6. Causes of the Syndrome of Inappropriate Antidiuretic Hormone Secretion

Central nervous system disorders: Guillain-Barré syndrome; hemorrhage[a]; infections; inflammatory disorders; mass lesions[a]; multiple sclerosis

Drugs: 3,4-methylenedioxymethamphetamine (also known as ecstasy)[a]; antipsychotic medications; carbamazepine; chlorpropamide; clofibrate; cyclooxygenase-2 inhibitors[a]; cyclophosphamide; desmopressin[a]; ifosfamide; nicotine; NSAIDs[a]; opiates[a]; phenothiazines; selective serotonin reuptake inhibitors[a]; serotonin-norepinephrine reuptake inhibitors[a]; tricyclic antidepressants; vasopressin[a]; vincristine

Endurance exercise (marathon running)

Familial disorders

Infections: HIV infection; Rocky Mountain spotted fever

Postoperative setting: anesthesia[a]; nausea[a]; pain[a]

Pulmonary disorders: infections[a]; inflammatory disorders; positive pressure mechanical ventilation[a]; respiratory failure

Tumors: gastrointestinal tract tumors; genitourinary tract tumors; lymphomas; respiratory tract tumors[a]; sarcomas; small cell cancer[a]; thymomas

[a]Most common causes.

status, seizures, obtundation, central herniation, or death. Acute symptomatic hyponatremia can occur in several clinical settings and is a medical emergency because a sudden drop in serum sodium concentration can overwhelm the capacity of the brain to regulate cell volume, leading to massive cerebral edema.

Due to cerebral adaptation, patients with chronic hyponatremia (developing over >48 hours) are less likely to exhibit severe symptoms and may be completely asymptomatic.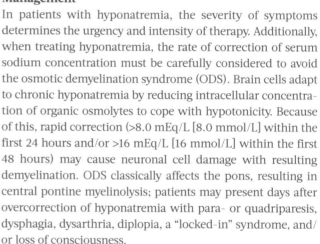

KEY POINTS

- Initial evaluation of hyponatremia includes measurement of plasma and urine osmolality and urine sodium as well as clinical assessment of volume status.

- Hypotonic hyponatremia evaluation begins with urine osmolality; urine osmolality <100 mOsm/kg H_2O suggests appropriately suppressed antidiuretic hormone (ADH), whereas urine osmolality >100 mOsm/kg H_2O suggests ADH excess.

Management

In patients with hyponatremia, the severity of symptoms determines the urgency and intensity of therapy. Additionally, when treating hyponatremia, the rate of correction of serum sodium concentration must be carefully considered to avoid the osmotic demyelination syndrome (ODS). Brain cells adapt to chronic hyponatremia by reducing intracellular concentration of organic osmolytes to cope with hypotonicity. Because of this, rapid correction (>8.0 mEq/L [8.0 mmol/L] within the first 24 hours and/or >16 mEq/L [16 mmol/L] within the first 48 hours) may cause neuronal cell damage with resulting demyelination. ODS classically affects the pons, resulting in central pontine myelinolysis; patients may present days after overcorrection of hyponatremia with para- or quadriparesis, dysphagia, dysarthria, diplopia, a "locked-in" syndrome, and/or loss of consciousness.

Acute Symptomatic Hyponatremia

Initial treatment of acute symptomatic hyponatremia includes hypertonic saline to acutely increase serum sodium concentration by 1.0 to 2.0 mEq/L (1.0-2.0 mmol/L) per hour to a total increase of 4.0 to 6.0 mEq/L (4.0-6.0 mmol/L) within the first 6 hours; this increase is typically sufficient to alleviate acute symptoms, avoiding overly rapid correction as previously discussed. The achieved serum sodium should be maintained at a constant level for the first 24 hours. Because the response to hypertonic saline can be highly unpredictable due to a rapid reduction in circulating ADH and the excretion of a dilute urine, frequent (every 1 to 2 hours) measurements of serum sodium concentration are necessary. Should the serum sodium concentration be inadvertently overcorrected, hyponatremia can be safely re-established by administration of the vasopressin agonist desmopressin and intravenous 5% dextrose in water, with monitoring of the serum sodium concentration.

Intravenous loop diuretics increase free water excretion by interfering with the renal countercurrent multiplication system and may facilitate acute treatment. Vasopressin antagonists do not have a role in the management of acute symptomatic hyponatremia.

Chronic Hyponatremia

In patients with hypovolemic hyponatremia, diagnosis and correction of the underlying cause of hypovolemia are indicated. In patients requiring specific treatment, volume repletion with oral salt supplementation or intravenous isotonic saline suppresses circulating ADH and induces a water diuresis.

Management of hypervolemic hyponatremia includes treatment of the underlying disorder, sodium and free water restriction (in practical terms, fluid restriction), and diuretic therapy. In patients with heart failure, vasopressin antagonists (such as tolvaptan and conivaptan) are effective in normalizing hyponatremia; however, use of these agents should be limited to patients with a serum sodium concentration <120 mEq/L (120 mmol/L) despite optimal therapy with diuresis and RAA system inhibition. Neither tolvaptan nor conivaptan is currently recommended for the treatment of hyponatremia associated with cirrhosis.

The initial treatment of euvolemic hyponatremia includes management of the underlying cause if possible. Fluid restriction without limiting sodium intake is a cornerstone of therapy. Patients who do not respond to fluid restriction can be treated with loop diuretics combined with oral salt supplementation.

Oral demeclocycline, which induces nephrogenic water loss, can be utilized to treat SIADH that fails fluid restriction or furosemide plus salt. However, demeclocycline can be associated with acute kidney injury from natriuresis and/or direct renal toxicity and is contraindicated in patients with cirrhosis. Vasopressin antagonists (oral tolvaptan and intravenous conivaptan) have been shown to be effective in normalizing serum sodium concentration in SIADH. Oral tolvaptan should be reserved for the management of serum sodium concentrations <120 mEq/L (120 mmol/L) and persistent SIADH that has failed fluid restriction and/or oral furosemide and salt tablets. Liver chemistry test abnormalities have been reported with chronic tolvaptan therapy; therefore, the use of this drug should be limited to less than 1 to 2 months, with close laboratory monitoring.

KEY POINTS

- Initial treatment of acute symptomatic hyponatremia includes hypertonic saline to acutely increase serum sodium concentration by 1.0 to 2.0 mEq/L (1.0-2.0 mmol/L) per hour to a total increase of 4.0 to 6.0 mEq/L (4.0-6.0 mmol/L) within the first 6 hours; the achieved serum sodium should be maintained for the first 24 hours. *(Continued)*

KEY POINTS (continued)

- Chronic asymptomatic hypervolemic hyponatremia management includes treatment of the underlying disorder, sodium and free water restriction, and diuretic therapy.

- First-line therapy of euvolemic hyponatremia includes treatment of the underlying cause and free water restriction, and second-line therapy includes loop diuretics combined with oral salt supplementation followed by oral demeclocycline; vasopressin antagonists should be reserved for patients with a serum sodium concentration <120 mEq/L (120 mmol/L) who are unresponsive to first- and second-line therapy.

HVC

Hypernatremia

Hypernatremia, defined as a serum sodium concentration >145 mEq/L (145 mmol/L), is often the result of a combined water and volume deficit, with losses of water in excess of sodium. Considerably less common than hyponatremia, hypernatremia is associated with mortality rates of approximately 40% to 60%. Elderly individuals with reduced thirst and/or diminished access to fluids are at the highest risk of developing hypernatremia. Patients with hypernatremia may rarely have a central defect in hypothalamic osmoreceptor function, with both decreased thirst and reduced ADH secretion.

More commonly, hypernatremia may develop following the loss of free water via renal or extrarenal routes. Insensible losses of water due to evaporation from the skin or respiratory tract may increase in the setting of fever, exercise, heat exposure, severe burns, or mechanical ventilation. Osmotic diarrhea and viral gastroenteritides typically generate hypo-osmotic stools, leading to significant free water loss and hypernatremia. Secretory diarrheas typically do not result in hypernatremia; rather, the isotonic stool loss causes hypovolemia with or without hypovolemic hyponatremia.

Common causes of renal water loss include osmotic diuresis secondary to hyperglycemia, post-obstructive diuresis, or drugs (contrast, mannitol). Water diuresis occurs in central or nephrogenic diabetes insipidus. Central diabetes insipidus results from inadequate secretion of ADH from the hypothalamus (see MKSAP 17 Endocrinology and Metabolism, Disorders of the Pituitary Gland). Nephrogenic diabetes insipidus results from resistance of the kidney to the action of ADH and has multiple causes. Gestational diabetes insipidus is a rare complication of pregnancy wherein increased activity of a placental protease with "vasopressinase" activity leads to reduced circulating ADH. See **Table 7** for more information.

Evaluation

In patients with hypernatremia, the history should focus on the presence or absence of thirst, polyuria, and/or an extrarenal source for water loss such as diarrhea. The physical examination should include a neurologic examination and assessment of volume status; accurate documentation of daily

TABLE 7.	Causes of Diabetes Insipidus

Central diabetes insipidus

   Autoimmune hypophysitis (idiopathic)[a]

   Malignancy (metastatic or primary)[a]

   Neurosurgery[a]

   Infiltration (sarcoidosis, histiocytosis X, lymphocytic hypophysitis, granulomatosis with polyangiitis [formerly known as Wegener granulomatosis], IgG4-related disease)[a]

   Trauma

   Following correction of supraventricular tachycardia

   Hypoxic encephalopathy

   Anorexia nervosa

   Sheehan syndrome

   Familial

Nephrogenic diabetes insipidus

   Lithium[a]

   Other medications (demeclocycline, cidofovir, foscarnet, didanosine, amphotericin B, ifosfamide, ofloxacin)[a]

   Electrolyte disorders (hypercalcemia, hypokalemia)[a]

   Urinary tract obstruction

   Sickle cell nephropathy

   Amyloidosis

   Sjögren syndrome

   Nephronophthisis

   Cystinosis

Gestational diabetes insipidus (placental "vasopressinase")

[a]Most common causes.

TABLE 8.	Correction of Hypernatremia

H₂O Deficit

Estimate total body water (TBW): 50%-60% body weight (kg) depending on body composition

Calculate free water deficit: $[(Na^+ - 140)/140] \times TBW$

Administer deficit over 48-72 h

Ongoing H₂O Losses

Calculate free water clearance (C_eH_2O):

$$V\left(1 - \frac{U_{Na} + U_K}{S_{Na}}\right)$$

Where V is urine volume, U_{Na} is urine sodium, U_K is urine potassium, and S_{Na} is serum sodium

Insensible Losses

~10 mL/kg/d: less if ventilated, more if febrile

Total

Add components to determine H₂O deficit and ongoing H₂O loss; correct the water deficit over 48-72 h and replace daily H₂O loss

Reproduced with permission from McGraw-Hill Education. Fauci A, Braunwald E, Kasper D, et al. Harrison's Manual of Medicine, 17th Edition. Electrolytes/Acid-Base Balance. 2009;8. New York, NY. Copyright 2009, McGraw-Hill Education.

CONT.

fluid intake and daily urine output is also required. Laboratory studies include measurement of plasma and urine osmolality as well as urine electrolytes. The appropriate renal response to hypernatremia and a plasma osmolality >295 mOsm/kg H₂O is the excretion of low volumes (<500 mL/24 h) of maximally concentrated urine (>800 mOsm/kg H₂O).

Most patients with hypernatremia and polyuria have a predominant water diuresis with hypotonic urine. However, those who have an osmotic diuresis as a cause of hypernatremia will demonstrate excessive excretion of sodium chloride, glucose, and/or urea, with a urine osmolality of >750 to 1000 mOsm/24 h (>15 mOsm/kg body water/24 h). In patients with hypotonic urine and suspected diabetes insipidus, differentiation between nephrogenic and central causes is made by the response of urine osmolality to desmopressin. For patients with hypernatremia due to renal loss of water, it is critical to quantify ongoing daily losses using the formula for electrolyte-free water clearance, in addition to calculation of the baseline water deficit (**Table 8**).

Management

The underlying condition leading to hypernatremia should be identified and addressed; patients diagnosed with desmopressin-sensitive nephrogenic diabetes insipidus should be started on chronic therapy. The approach to the management of hypernatremia is outlined in Table 8. The water deficit should be corrected over 48 to 72 hours to avoid neurologic compromise. Depending on the blood pressure or clinical volume status, initial treatment with hypotonic saline solutions (1/4 or 1/2 normal saline) may be appropriate; plasma glucose should be monitored in patients treated with large volumes of 5% dextrose in water. Calculation of urinary electrolyte-free water clearance is helpful to estimate daily, ongoing loss of free water in patients with nephrogenic or central diabetes insipidus.

KEY POINT

- Management of hypernatremia involves correction of the water deficit and replacement of daily water loss; the water deficit should be corrected slowly (over 48-72 hours) to avoid neurologic compromise.

Disorders of Serum Potassium

Hypokalemia

Hypokalemia is defined as a serum potassium concentration <3.5 mEq/L (3.5 mmol/L). Patients have minimal symptoms unless serum potassium levels are <3.0 mEq/L (3.0 mmol/L). Symptoms range from generalized weakness and malaise to paralysis, depending on the serum potassium level. Rhabdomyolysis can occur with serum potassium levels <2.5 mEq/L (2.5 mmol/L), and ascending paralysis with respiratory failure is seen with levels <2.0 mEq/L (2.0 mmol/L). Symptoms correlate with the

CONT.

rapidity of the decrease. In patients with heart conditions, mild to moderate hypokalemia increases the risk of cardiac arrhythmias.

Evaluation

Hypokalemia can occur from transcellular shift of potassium or from a decrease in total body potassium through decreased intake, renal loss, or extrarenal loss. The cause can be determined by a thorough history, physical examination, and measurement of serum and urine electrolytes (**Figure 6**). The history should focus on medications and history of vomiting or diarrhea. The blood pressure (including examination for orthostasis) and volume status should be assessed. Pseudohypokalemia, a laboratory artifact caused by uptake

of potassium by cells in the test tube from patients with leukemia, should be ruled out.

Abrupt development of hypokalemia suggests a transient shift of potassium from the extracellular compartment into cells. Medications commonly result in intracellular shifts, including sympathomimetic agents (epinephrine, decongestants, bronchodilators), phosphodiesterase inhibitors (theophylline, caffeine), and insulin. Systemic alkalosis (respiratory, metabolic) may also be associated with acute hypokalemia. Hypokalemic periodic paralysis is a rare familial or acquired disorder characterized by flaccid generalized weakness from a sudden intracellular potassium shift precipitated by strenuous exercise or a high-carbohydrate meal. The acquired form occurs with thyrotoxicosis and is found in

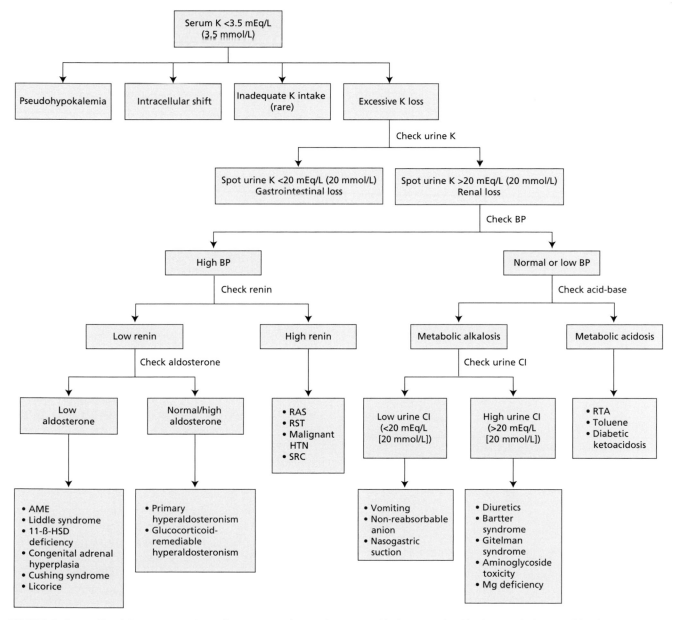

FIGURE 6. Causes of hypokalemia. AME= syndrome of apparent mineralocorticoid excess; BP = blood pressure; Cl = chloride; HSD = hydroxysteroid dehydrogenase; HTN = hypertension; K = potassium; Mg = magnesium; RAS = renal artery stenosis; RST = renin-secreting tumor; RTA = renal tubular acidosis; SRC = scleroderma renal crisis.

CONT.

men of Asian or Mexican descent. It is resolved with treatment of hyperthyroidism.

Hypokalemia from decreased total body potassium can be the result of extrarenal or renal losses. Because the kidneys can reduce urine potassium excretion to <20 mEq/24 h (20 mmol/24 h), hypokalemia from inadequate intake is uncommon. Urinary or gastrointestinal losses of potassium are most common. Assessment of urine potassium excretion is critical to establish renal potassium wasting. Urine potassium loss >20 mEq/24 h (20 mmol/24 h), a spot urine potassium >20 mEq/L (20 mmol/L), or a spot urine potassium-creatinine ratio >13 mEq/g (1.5 mEq/mmol) suggests excessive urinary losses. Conversely, urine potassium loss <20 mEq/24 h (20 mmol/24 h) suggests cellular shift, decreased intake, or extrarenal losses of potassium.

Urine potassium loss can be caused by enhanced sodium delivery and urine flow to the collecting duct and increased mineralocorticoid activity (**Table 9**). Blood pressure measurement can help define the cause; patients with increased mineralocorticoid activity have evidence of volume expansion with elevated blood pressure. The specific etiology can be further differentiated by plasma renin activity and aldosterone levels (see Figure 6). Patients with hypokalemia due to increased distal sodium delivery can have findings of volume depletion and low or normal blood pressure. The specific cause can be further determined by acid-base status and urine sodium and chloride levels (see Figure 6). Diuretics are the most common cause of increased distal sodium delivery.

TABLE 9. Causes of Renal Potassium Loss
Increased Urine Flow or Sodium Delivery to Distal Nephron
Diuretics: loop diuretics; thiazides; carbonic anhydrase inhibitors
Antibiotics: high-dose penicillin
Osmotic diuresis: diabetes mellitus; mannitol
Saline diuresis
Renal tubular acidosis
Gitelman syndrome
Bartter syndrome
Increased Mineralocorticoid Activity
Exogenous mineralocorticoid
Primary hyperaldosteronism: adrenal adenoma; bilateral adrenal hyperplasia; glucocorticoid-remediable aldosteronism
Congenital adrenal hyperplasia: 17-α-hydroxylase deficiency; 11-β-hydroxylase deficiency
Secondary hyperaldosteronism: renin-secreting tumor; renovascular disease
Liddle syndrome
11-β-hydroxysteroid dehydrogenase deficiency: congenital; acquired (licorice, carbenoxolone)
Cushing syndrome

Management

Patients with hypokalemia who have arrhythmias or symptomatic severe hypokalemia (serum potassium concentration <2.5 mEq/L [2.5 mmol/L]) should be promptly treated with intravenous potassium chloride at a rate no faster than 20 mEq/h (20 mmol/h) and a maximum concentration of 40 mEq/L (40 mmol/L). Patients with mild symptoms and serum potassium levels of 2.5 to 3.5 mEq/L (2.5-3.5 mmol/L) may only need oral potassium replacement. Potassium-sparing diuretics can be used in patients with normal kidney function who are prone to significant hypokalemia. Magnesium depletion should be corrected because it can cause and maintain renal potassium loss.

KEY POINTS

- Urine potassium loss >20 mEq/24 h (20 mmol/24 h) suggests excessive urinary losses; urine potassium loss <20 mEq/24 h (20 mmol/24 h) suggests cellular shift, decreased intake, or extrarenal losses.
- Hypokalemia due to increased mineralocorticoid activity can be associated with volume expansion and elevated blood pressure.
- Hypokalemia due to increased distal sodium delivery can be associated with volume depletion and low or normal blood pressure; diuretics are the most common cause.

Hyperkalemia

Hyperkalemia is defined as a serum potassium level >5.0 mEq/L (5.0 mmol/L). Any level >6.0 mEq/L (6.0 mmol/L) can be life-threatening. Generally, a slowly rising serum potassium level is better tolerated than an abrupt rise. Signs and symptoms are related to adverse effects of serum potassium on skeletal and cardiac muscle cell membranes, including muscle weakness and cardiac conduction and rhythm abnormalities.

Evaluation

Initial evaluation of hyperkalemia begins with the history, medication review, and physical examination. Laboratory studies should be targeted toward the diagnosis suggested by the history and physical examination. Because of the potential cardiac effects of hyperkalemia, immediate electrocardiography (ECG) is indicated. The earliest ECG changes of hyperkalemia are peaking of the T waves and shortening of the QT interval. As hyperkalemia progresses, there is prolongation of the PR interval, loss of P waves, and eventual widening of the QRS complexes with a "sine-wave" pattern that can precede asystole.

Hyperkalemia can result from increased potassium intake, decreased urine potassium excretion, or a shift of potassium from the intracellular to extracellular space (**Figure 7**). Excessive intake and extracellular shift are uncommon as the sole causes of hyperkalemia. Often, multiple etiologies are present simultaneously, such as increased potassium intake in the setting of chronic kidney disease (CKD). Disorders causing transcellular

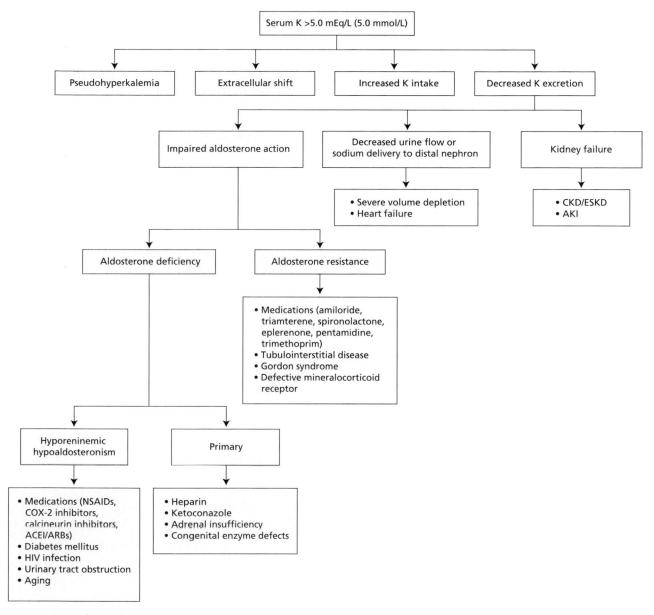

FIGURE 7. Causes of hyperkalemia. ACEI = angiotensin-converting enzyme inhibitor; AKI = acute kidney injury; ARB = angiotensin receptor blocker; CKD = chronic kidney disease; COX = cyclooxygenase; ESKD = end-stage kidney disease; K = potassium.

shifts include drug-induced (digoxin toxicity, succinylcholine, β-blockers, somatostatin) and non-drug–induced (metabolic acidosis, insulin deficiency, rhabdomyolysis, tumor lysis, hemolysis, hyperosmolarity, hyperkalemic periodic paralysis) causes. Pseudohyperkalemia occurs with a false rise in potassium values from cellular release of potassium during venipuncture due to hemolysis or prolonged tourniquet use. It also occurs with significant leukocytosis or thrombocytosis. Pseudohyperkalemia can be ruled out by checking serum and plasma potassium levels simultaneously, with the plasma level being normal.

Major underlying causes of persistent hyperkalemia are disorders in which urine potassium excretion is impaired. The most common cause is CKD with a glomerular filtration rate <20 mL/min/1.73 m² or acute kidney injury. Other causes include decreased distal sodium delivery and impaired aldosterone action; aldosterone is the primary hormone that facilitates urine potassium excretion (see Figure 7). Medications commonly associated with hyperkalemia from impaired aldosterone activity include potassium-sparing diuretics, trimethoprim, NSAIDs, and ACE inhibitors.

A spot urine test for potassium, creatinine, and osmolality should be obtained to calculate the transtubular potassium gradient (TTKG) and assess for impaired aldosterone action. The TTKG is an assessment of renal potassium handling and is calculated as follows:

$$\text{TTKG} = (\text{Urine Potassium} \div \text{Plasma Osmolality}) / (\text{Serum Potassium} \div \text{Urine Osmolality})$$

A TTKG <3 suggests decreased aldosterone effect on the collecting tubules with inadequate potassium excretion. A TTKG >8 suggests appropriate excretion by the kidneys. The TTKG is only valid if the urine osmolality exceeds plasma osmolality and if urine sodium is >20 mEq/L (20 mmol/L).

Management

Severe hyperkalemia with ECG changes requires immediate stabilization of the myocardial cell membrane, rapid shifting of potassium intracellularly, and total body potassium elimination. All sources of potassium should be removed. Intravenous calcium is used for membrane stabilization. Improvement in ECG changes occurs within minutes of calcium infusion with duration of action of 30 to 60 minutes. Repeated doses can be given while other measures are initiated. Calcium infusion is contraindicated in digoxin toxicity because it can worsen the myocardial effects. Shifting of potassium from extracellular to intracellular is done either with insulin or with high-dose inhaled β-adrenergic agonists. Insulin is given as 10 units intravenously with 50 mL of 50% dextrose; this acts in 10 to 20 minutes, and duration is 4 to 6 hours. In patients who are hyperglycemic, insulin alone may be sufficient. The onset of action of β-adrenergic agonists is 3 to 5 minutes and lasts for 1 to 4 hours. The effect of insulin and β-adrenergic agonists is additive. Sodium bicarbonate may be used to promote intracellular shift of potassium in the setting of metabolic acidosis.

Removal of total body potassium is achieved by drug therapy or dialysis. Potassium excretion can be increased with the use of loop diuretics in combination with saline infusion to ensure delivery of sodium to the distal nephron with normal kidney function. Sodium polystyrene sulfonate (SPS) binds potassium in the colon in exchange for sodium and can be given orally or as a retention enema, the latter form being faster. One of the potential adverse effects of sorbitol-containing SPS preparations is bowel necrosis. Hemodialysis is indicated for life-threatening hyperkalemia in severe CKD or unresponsiveness to standard therapy.

Long-term treatment of hyperkalemia should be directed at correcting the underlying cause in addition to initiating a low-potassium diet and discontinuing hyperkalemia-causing medications. Loop diuretics or fludrocortisone may be needed for patients who have hyporeninemic hypoaldosteronism with hyperkalemia. Chronic diuretic therapy can be used in patients with CKD and mild hyperkalemia. H

KEY POINT

- Severe hyperkalemia with electrocardiogram changes requires immediate stabilization of the myocardial cell membrane with intravenous calcium; rapid shifting of potassium intracellularly with insulin or β-adrenergic agonists; total body potassium elimination with loop diuretics, sodium polystyrene sulfonate, or dialysis; and removal of all sources of potassium.

Disorders of Serum Phosphate

Hypophosphatemia

Hypophosphatemia, defined as a serum phosphate concentration <3.0 mg/dL (0.97 mmol/L), is seen in patients with chronic alcohol use, malnutrition, or critical illness. Symptoms rarely occur unless the serum phosphate concentration is <2.0 mg/dL (0.65 mmol/L); severe symptoms occur with a serum phosphate concentration <1.0 mg/dL (0.32 mmol/L). Symptoms include weakness, myalgia, rhabdomyolysis, arrhythmias, heart failure, respiratory failure, seizures, coma, and hemolysis.

Evaluation

Hypophosphatemia occurs because of inadequate intake, intracellular shift, decreased intestinal absorption, or increased urine loss (**Table 10**). Spurious hypophosphatemia can be caused by interference of paraproteins with the phosphate assay. The Fanconi syndrome is characterized by a type 2 (proximal) renal tubular acidosis with urine loss of bicarbonate as well as phosphaturia, glucosuria, and aminoaciduria.

TABLE 10. Causes of Hypophosphatemia
Inadequate Intake
Intracellular Shift
Refeeding
Treatment of diabetic ketoacidosis
Respiratory alkalosis
Drugs: insulin; glucagon; epinephrine; β_2-agonists; glucocorticoids; xanthine derivatives
Rapid cell proliferation/uptake: hungry bone syndrome; acute leukemia
Decreased Intestinal Absorption
Phosphate-binding antacids (aluminum; sucralfate)
Vitamin D deficiency
Chronic diarrhea
Steatorrhea
Increased Urine Loss
Hyperparathyroidism
Vitamin D disorders: vitamin D deficiency; hypophosphatemic rickets
Oncogenic osteomalacia
Volume expansion
Fanconi syndrome: heavy metal intoxication; Wilson disease; hereditary fructose intolerance; multiple myeloma; tenofovir; ifosfamide
Diuretics: acetazolamide; metolazone
Osmotic diuresis
Metabolic acidosis
Kidney transplantation

CONT.

Hypophosphatemia also occurs in patients receiving continuous renal replacement therapy.

If the cause of hypophosphatemia is not evident from the history, a 24-hour urine phosphate collection or calculation of the fractional excretion of filtered phosphate (FEPO4) from a random urine sample can help differentiate renal from extrarenal causes. The FEPO4 can be calculated as follows:

$$FEPO4 = (Urine\ PO4 \times Serum\ Creatinine \times 100)/(Serum\ PO4 \times Urine\ Creatinine)$$

Urine phosphate excretion >100 mg/d or an FEPO4 >5% indicates renal phosphate wasting.

Management

Treatment of hypophosphatemia depends on the cause, severity, and duration. Mild or moderate hypophosphatemia can be managed with oral replacement therapy. Patients with severe hypophosphatemia and clinical findings should be treated with intravenous phosphate, with serum phosphate and calcium levels monitored every 6 hours.

KEY POINTS

- Hypophosphatemia symptoms rarely occur unless the serum phosphate concentration is <2.0 mg/dL (0.65 mmol/L) and include weakness, myalgia, rhabdomyolysis, arrhythmias, heart failure, respiratory failure, seizures, coma, and hemolysis.

- Mild or moderate hypophosphatemia can be managed with oral replacement therapy; severe symptomatic hypophosphatemia should be treated with intravenous phosphate, with serum phosphate and calcium levels monitored every 6 hours.

Hyperphosphatemia

Hyperphosphatemia is defined as a serum phosphate concentration >4.5 mg/dL (1.45 mmol/L). Most patients are asymptomatic.

Evaluation

Hyperphosphatemia is caused by excessive intake, acute extracellular shift of phosphate, or decreased urine excretion (**Table 11**). Spurious hyperphosphatemia can be caused by substances that interfere with the phosphate assay, including hyperglobulinemia, hyperbilirubinemia, hyperlipidemia, and in vitro hemolysis. The cause often can be determined from the clinical history and is most commonly due to CKD or acute kidney injury.

Management

Management of hyperphosphatemia includes treating the underlying cause. Phosphate excretion can be enhanced by forced saline diuresis if kidney function is intact. Patients with symptomatic hypocalcemia and decreased kidney function may need hemodialysis. Treatment of chronic hyperphosphatemia includes dietary phosphate restriction and phosphate binders.

TABLE 11.	Causes of Hyperphosphatemia
Excessive Intake	
Excessive use of phosphate-containing bowel preparations	
Vitamin D intoxication	
Milk-alkali syndrome	
Extracellular Shift	
Rhabdomyolysis	
Tumor lysis syndrome	
Acute hemolysis	
Acute acidosis	
Decreased Excretion	
Acute or chronic kidney failure	
Hypoparathyroidism	
Acromegaly	
Severe hypomagnesemia	
Familial tumoral calcinosis	
Bisphosphonates	

KEY POINT

- The most common causes of hyperphosphatemia are chronic kidney disease and acute kidney injury.

Acid-Base Disorders

Introduction

The systemic pH is controlled through renal and respiratory mechanisms, which preserve a stable internal milieu. Disturbances in acid-base balance lead to predictable responses that limit the magnitude of change of the blood pH. The cause is usually evident by reviewing results from arterial or venous blood gas studies (pH, P_{CO_2}) and venous electrolyte measurements (serum bicarbonate and anion gap).

Primary acid-base disorders are classified by their underlying mechanism (*metabolic* or *respiratory*) and their effect on acid-base balance (*acidosis* or *alkalosis*). In primary metabolic acidosis without additional acid-base disorders, the serum bicarbonate is below the normal range. In primary metabolic alkalosis, the serum bicarbonate is above normal. In primary respiratory acidosis, the arterial P_{CO_2} is above the normal range. In primary respiratory alkalosis, the P_{CO_2} is below normal.

Analysis of acid-base disorders involves identification of the likely primary acid-base disorder, followed by assessment of the compensatory response (**Table 12**). A mixed acid-base disorder is present when measured values fall outside the range of the predicted secondary response; multiple acid-base disturbances may coexist.

TABLE 12.	Compensation in Acid-Base Disorders
Condition	**Expected Compensation**
Metabolic acidosis	Acute: $P_{CO_2} = (1.5)[HCO_3] + 8$
	Chronic: $P_{CO_2} = [HCO_3] + 15$
	Failure of the P_{CO_2} to decrease to the expected value = complicating respiratory acidosis; excessive decrease of the P_{CO_2} = complicating respiratory alkalosis
	Quick check: P_{CO_2} = value should approximate last two digits of pH
Metabolic alkalosis	For each ↑ 1.0 mEq/L (1.0 mmol/L) in $[HCO_3]$, P_{CO_2} ↑ 0.7 mm Hg (0.09 kPa)
Respiratory acidosis	Acute: 1.0 mEq/L (1.0 mmol/L) ↑ $[HCO_3]$ for each 10 mm Hg (1.3 kPa) ↑ in P_{CO_2}
	Chronic: 3.5 mEq/L (3.5 mmol/L) ↑ $[HCO_3]$ for each 10 mm Hg (1.3 kPa) ↑ in P_{CO_2}
	Failure of the $[HCO_3]$ to increase to the expected value = complicating metabolic acidosis; excessive increase in $[HCO_3]$ = complicating metabolic alkalosis
Respiratory alkalosis	Acute: 2.0 mEq/L (2.0 mmol/L) ↓ $[HCO_3]$ for each 10 mm Hg (1.3 kPa) ↓ in P_{CO_2}
	Chronic: 4.0-5.0 mEq/L (4.0-5.0 mmol/L) ↓ $[HCO_3]$ for each 10 mm Hg (1.3 kPa) ↓ in P_{CO_2}
	Failure of the $[HCO_3]$ to decrease to the expected value = complicating metabolic alkalosis; excessive decrease in $[HCO_3]$ = complicating metabolic acidosis

The overall effect of one or more acid-base disorders is reflected in the blood pH, which may be near normal (due to appropriate compensation), acidemic (indicated by a pH below the normal range), or alkalemic (indicated by a pH above the normal range).

Although the most accurate measurement of pH and P_{CO_2} is obtained from arterial blood, in many cases, venous blood gases can be used either diagnostically or to follow therapy. However, in patients in shock, there may be a significant discrepancy between arterial and venous blood gases, with lower pH and higher P_{CO_2} values in the latter. In other patients with critical illness, there is minimal difference between the acid-base parameters determined on venous versus arterial blood gas analysis.

Metabolic Acidosis
General Approach

A depressed serum bicarbonate level is the primary indicator of metabolic acidosis in patients without an additional acid-base disorder. Because respiratory alkalosis with renal compensation can also cause a depressed serum bicarbonate level, the diagnosis should be confirmed with measurement of the pH and P_{CO_2}. When metabolic acidosis is present, the anion gap is useful in assessing whether the decreased serum bicarbonate is due to an unmeasured organic anion such as lactate (increased anion gap metabolic acidosis) or to a loss of bicarbonate (normal anion gap metabolic acidosis). The anion gap is calculated from the following equation:

$$\text{Anion Gap} = \text{Serum Sodium (mEq/L)} - [\text{Serum Chloride (mEq/L)} + \text{Serum Bicarbonate (mEq/L)}]$$

The normal reference range for the anion gap is approximately 8 to 10 mEq/L ± 2 mEq/L (8-10 mmol/L ± 2 mmol/L). In normal subjects, albumin is the major unmeasured anion responsible for the anion gap. Changes in the serum albumin concentration can have a significant effect on the anion gap. Unless a correction is made for the change in the albumin concentration from normal, patients with hypoalbuminemia may seem to have a decreased anion gap, and patients with hyperalbuminemia may seem to have an increased anion gap. In patients with abnormalities in albumin concentration, an albumin-corrected anion gap should be calculated as follows:

$$\text{Albumin-Corrected Anion Gap} = \text{Anion Gap} + 2.5 \times [\text{Normal Albumin} - \text{Measured Albumin (g/dL)}]$$

When an increased anion gap metabolic acidosis is present, calculation of the corrected bicarbonate is helpful in assessing the possible presence of a coexisting normal anion gap metabolic acidosis and/or metabolic alkalosis:

$$\text{Corrected Bicarbonate} = 24 \text{ mEq/L} - \Delta \text{ Anion Gap (mEq/L)}$$

(in which Δ anion gap is the increase in the albumin-corrected anion gap above normal)

A measured bicarbonate less than the corrected bicarbonate suggests a concomitant normal anion gap metabolic acidosis. A measured bicarbonate greater than the corrected bicarbonate suggests a concomitant metabolic alkalosis.

Another method is to assess the ratio of the change in the anion gap (Δ anion gap) to the change in bicarbonate level (Δ bicarbonate), or the "Δ-Δ ratio." A ratio of <1 may reflect the presence of concurrent normal anion gap metabolic acidosis, whereas a ratio of >2 may indicate the presence of metabolic alkalosis.

In patients with an increased anion gap acidosis, calculation of the plasma osmolal gap is helpful in assessing the presence of unmeasured solutes, such as ingestion of certain toxins (for example, methanol or ethylene glycol). The plasma osmolal gap is the difference between the measured and calculated plasma osmolality. Plasma osmolality can be calculated using the following formula:

$$\text{Plasma Osmolality (mOsm/kg } H_2O) = 2 \times \text{Serum Sodium (mEq/L)} + \text{Plasma Glucose (mg/dL)}/18 + \text{BUN (mg/dL)}/2.8$$

When the measured osmolality exceeds the calculated osmolality by >10 mOsm/kg H_2O, the osmolal gap is considered elevated. Although an elevated osmolal gap usually reflects the presence of unmeasured solutes, an increased osmolal gap may also be seen in pseudohyponatremia, in which the plasma osmolality (and measured osmolality) is normal while the calculated osmolality is low (See Fluid and Electrolytes).

- A depressed serum bicarbonate level is the primary indicator of metabolic acidosis in patients without an additional acid-base disorder.
- When metabolic acidosis is present, the anion gap is useful in assessing whether the decreased serum bicarbonate is due to an unmeasured organic anion (increased anion gap metabolic acidosis) or to a loss of bicarbonate (normal anion gap metabolic acidosis).

Increased Anion Gap Metabolic Acidosis

An increased albumin-corrected anion gap metabolic acidosis occurs when unmeasured anions are present. These anions may be metabolic by-products (for example, lactate or ketoacids) or associated with ingested substances (for example, ethylene glycol or methanol); the plasma osmolal gap may be used to differentiate between these causes.

Lactic acidosis is a common cause of an increased anion gap metabolic acidosis. Types and causes of lactic acidosis are described in **Table 13**.

Diabetic ketoacidosis (DKA) and alcoholic ketoacidosis (AKA) are also common causes of increased anion gap metabolic acidosis. DKA usually presents with an increased anion gap metabolic acidosis but can present with a normal anion gap in the absence of hypovolemia due to excretion of ketoacids

in the urine. Symptoms include polyuria, polydipsia, dehydration, nausea, vomiting, abdominal pain, and hyperventilation. Insulin deficiency, increased catecholamines, and glucagon result in incomplete oxidation of fatty acids, which leads to the production of acetoacetate and β-hydroxybutyrate. The presence of acetoacetate or acetone can be measured using the nitroprusside assay in urine dipsticks or by directly measuring serum assays for specific ketone bodies. Because β-hydroxybutyrate is the dominant acid in DKA, the urine dipstick results can be falsely negative in the presence of severe DKA. Ketoacidosis will reverse with insulin and fluid administration; therefore, sodium bicarbonate therapy is generally reserved for patients with a pH <7.0 or metabolic instability due to acidosis (See MKSAP 17 Endocrinology and Metabolism).

AKA occurs in patients with chronic ethanol abuse. Patients present with abdominal pain and vomiting after abruptly stopping alcohol. Increased alanine and aspartate aminotransferase levels and hyperbilirubinemia are common due to concurrent alcoholic hepatitis. AKA typically responds to treatment with intravenous saline and intravenous glucose, with rapid clearance of the associated ketones due to a reduction in counter-regulatory hormones and the induction of endogenous insulin.

A number of other unmeasured anions, most often associated with medications or toxin ingestions, can also cause increases in the anion gap (**Table 14**). Although a single organic

TABLE 13. Causes of Lactic Acidosis

Condition	Cause	Clinical and Laboratory Manifestations	Treatment	Comments
Lactic acidosis		Serum lactate level >4.0 mEq/L (4.0 mmol/L)	Treat underlying cause; sodium bicarbonate when arterial pH is <7.1 to raise pH to 7.2	Most common cause of increased AG metabolic acidosis
Type A lactic acidosis	Tissue hypoperfusion	Evidence of multi-system organ dysfunction typically present	Correct cause of hypoperfusion	—
Type B lactic acidosis				
Propofol	Propofol >4 mg/kg/h for >24 h	Rhabdomyolysis; hyperlipidemia; cardiogenic shock	Discontinue propofol; HD	—
Metformin	Metformin use in patients with S_{Cr} >1.4-1.5 mg/dL (123.8-132.6 μmol/L)	—	HD	Rare complication; mortality 30%-50%
Hematologic malignancy	Thought to be due to anaerobic metabolism in cancer cells	Severe type B lactic acidosis; hypoglycemia	Treat underlying malignancy	Portends very poor prognosis; seen in high-grade B-cell lymphomas
D-Lactic acidosis	Short-bowel syndrome[a]; undigested carbohydrates in the colon are metabolized to D-lactate	Intermittent confusion; slurred speech; ataxia; increased AG metabolic acidosis with normal serum lactate level	Antibiotics (e.g., metronidazole or neomycin) directed toward bowel flora; restriction of dietary carbohydrates	Diagnosis requires measurement of D-lactate because D-isomer is not measured by specific assays

AG = anion gap; HD = hemodialysis; S_{Cr} = serum creatinine.

[a]After jejunoileal bypass or small-bowel resection.

TABLE 14. Selected Causes of Increased Anion Gap Metabolic Acidosis

Condition	Cause	Clinical and Laboratory Manifestations	Treatment	Comments
Ethylene glycol ingestion	Glycolic acid accumulation; calcium oxalate precipitation in renal tubules and crystals in the urine	Flank pain; AKI; hypocalcemia; nephrocalcinosis; cardiovascular collapse; neurotoxicity; pulmonary edema	HD Fomepizole Sodium bicarbonate Pyridoxine and thiamine in suspected ethylene glycol toxicity	Suspect ingestion with increased AG acidosis and a serum bicarbonate level <10 mEq/L (10 mmol/L) and a plasma osmolal gap >10 mOsm/kg H_2O May be difficult to differentiate from methanol ingestion
Methanol ingestion	Formic acid accumulation	Impaired vision/blindness mediated by formic acid; papilledema; mydriasis; afferent pupillary defect; abdominal pain; pancreatitis	Fomepizole HD Sodium bicarbonate Folic acid in suspected methanol toxicity	Suspect ingestion with increased AG acidosis and a serum bicarbonate level <10 mEq/L (10 mmol/L) and a plasma osmolal gap >10 mOsm/kg H_2O May be difficult to differentiate from ethylene glycol ingestion 80%-90% mortality rate with methanol ingestion; permanent blindness may occur
Propylene glycol toxicity	Large doses of propylene glycol (a solvent used for IV medications), most commonly lorazepam diluted in propylene glycol (80%)	AKI; AG metabolic acidosis with increased plasma osmolal gap; toxicity when propylene glycol levels >25 mg/dL or plasma osmolal gap >10 mOsm/kg H_2O	Discontinue the IV infusion HD	Monitor acid-base status and plasma osmolality when lorazepam doses >1 mg/kg/d; unlikely to develop if 24-h lorazepam dose is limited to <166 mg/d
Salicylate toxicity	Salicylate anion accumulation; ingestion of as little as 10 grams of aspirin in adults	Tinnitus; tachypnea; low-grade fever; nausea/vomiting; impaired mental status; cerebral edema and fatal brainstem herniation; acute lung injury; noncardiogenic pulmonary edema; hepatic injury; respiratory alkalosis; with severe intoxication, AG metabolic acidosis, lactic acidosis, ketoacidosis	IV glucose (100 mL of 50% dextrose) in adults when mental status changes are present, irrespective of the plasma glucose level HD for AKI, impaired mental status, cerebral edema, serum salicylate levels >80 mg/dL, severe AG metabolic acidosis, pulmonary edema Vitamin K for increased INR	Toxicity can develop from ingestion or mucocutaneous exposure to salicylate preparations such as methyl salicylate (oil of wintergreen)
Acetaminophen toxicity	Pyroglutamic acidosis; most common in critically ill patients, those with poor nutrition, liver disease, CKD, and in vegetarians	Impaired mental status; on urine testing for organic anions, high concentrations of urine pyroglutamate	Discontinue acetaminophen Sodium bicarbonate Possibly N-acetylcysteine to regenerate depleted glutathione stores	Female preponderance (80%); genetic factors may play a role

AG = anion gap; AKI = acute kidney injury; CKD = chronic kidney disease; HD = hemodialysis; IV = intravenous.

CONT.

anion may be primarily responsible for each condition, multiple metabolic products may also contribute to the anion gap. For example, an elevated lactate may accompany many of the disorders discussed in Table 14. ▣

KEY POINTS

- Lactic acidosis is defined as a serum lactate level >4.0 mEq/L (4.0 mmol/L); management includes treatment of the underlying cause and sodium bicarbonate when arterial pH is <7.1.
- Ethylene glycol or methanol ingestion should be suspected in patients with an increased anion gap acidosis associated with a serum bicarbonate level <10 mEq/L (10 mmol/L) and a plasma osmolal gap >10 mOsm/kg H$_2$O.

Normal Anion Gap Metabolic Acidosis

The normal physiologic response to systemic acidosis is an increase in urine acid excretion. Therefore, an initial diagnostic step in normal anion gap metabolic acidosis is to determine whether the kidney is appropriately excreting acid or whether impaired kidney acid excretion is the cause of the metabolic acidosis. Increased acid excretion by the kidney is reflected as a marked increase in urine ammonium. However, urine ammonium is difficult to measure directly. Because ammonium carries a positive charge, chloride is excreted into the urine in equal amounts with ammonium to maintain electrical neutrality. Therefore, the amount of chloride in the urine reflects the amount of ammonium present, and the urine anion gap can be used as an indicator of the ability of the kidney to excrete acid:

Urine Anion Gap = Urine Sodium + Urine Potassium – Urine Chloride

If the kidney is able to appropriately excrete acid, the urine anion gap is negative, and if there is a defect in kidney acid excretion, the urine anion gap is positive. For example, in patients with normal anion gap metabolic acidosis due to extrarenal bicarbonate loss (for example, laxative abuse or diarrhea) or an acid load, the kidney should excrete increased urine ammonium (and chloride), resulting in a markedly negative

(-20 to -25 mEq/L [-20 to -25 mmol/L]) urine anion gap. In contrast, in patients with impaired urine acidification due to kidney disease or a defect in the distal renal tubule, urine ammonium (and chloride) levels are low, with the urine anion gap being markedly positive (20 to 40 mEq/L [20 to 40 mmol/L]). Along with serum potassium and urine pH, determination of the urine anion gap can help differentiate between common causes of normal anion gap metabolic acidosis (**Table 15**).

Type 2 (Proximal) Renal Tubular Acidosis

Metabolic acidosis in type 2 (proximal) renal tubular acidosis (RTA) is caused by a defect in the proximal tubule resulting in a diminished ability to reabsorb filtered bicarbonate (**Table 16**). Type 2 (proximal) RTA is usually not an isolated phenomenon but rather part of Fanconi syndrome, a generalized defect in proximal tubular function. Bicarbonate will be lost in the urine until the resorptive threshold for bicarbonate is reached, causing a normal anion gap metabolic acidosis. The impaired reabsorption of bicarbonate is also associated with decreased sodium chloride reabsorption and increased sodium delivery to the distal tubule and sodium loss, causing hypovolemia and triggering secondary hyperaldosteronism; this leads to a tendency for salt wasting and hypokalemia.

Because distal urine acidification capability is preserved, the urine pH in patients with type 2 (proximal) RTA is variable. When bicarbonate intake exceeds the resorptive threshold, the proximal tubule does not reabsorb the normal amount of filtered bicarbonate and the urine pH is alkalotic. If bicarbonate intake is below the resorptive threshold, the filtered bicarbonate can be reabsorbed normally, and the intact distal tubule can acidify the urine to a pH <5.5. Treatment of type 2 (proximal) RTA consists of alkali replacement with the addition of a thiazide diuretic, which causes mild volume depletion that enhances the proximal reabsorption of sodium and bicarbonate.

Type 1 (Hypokalemic Distal) Renal Tubular Acidosis

Type 1 (hypokalemic distal) RTA results from a defect in urine acidification in the distal tubule with impaired excretion of hydrogen ions (**Table 17**). Patients with type 1 (hypokalemic distal) RTA are unable to acidify their urine below a pH of 6.0, even after an acid load. Because proximal reabsorption of

TABLE 15. Diagnostic Approach to Normal Anion Gap Metabolic Acidosis			
Diagnosis	**Serum Potassium**	**Urine AG**	**Urine pH**
Ammonium chloride ingestion (acid load)	Normal	Negative	<5.5
Diarrhea and acidosis	Normal	Negative	<5.5
Type 2 (proximal) RTA	Decreased	Negative	Variable[a]
Type 1 (hypokalemic distal) RTA	Decreased	Positive	>5.5
Type 4 (hyperkalemic distal) RTA	Increased	Positive	<5.5

AG = anion gap; RTA = renal tubular acidosis.

[a]Patients with type 2 (proximal) RTA have normal distal renal tubular function and can acidify the urine once the serum bicarbonate drops to a point at which the filtered load of bicarbonate can be normally reabsorbed.

TABLE 16. Causes of Type 2 (Proximal) Renal Tubular Acidosis
Isolated Type 2 (Proximal) Renal Tubular Acidosis
Primary: hereditary (Na-Hco₃ cotransporter); sporadic (often transient)
Hereditary carbonic anhydrase deficiency: carbonic anhydrase inhibitors
Fanconi Syndrome (associated glycosuria, phosphaturia, aminoaciduria, hypouricemia)
Primary: hereditary Fanconi syndrome
Genetic: cystinosis; Wilson disease
Acquired: Sjögren syndrome; paraproteinemias; vitamin D deficiency
Drugs/toxins: ifosfamide; tacrolimus; cyclosporine; toluene; outdated tetracycline; lead; mercury; cidofovir; tenofovir

TABLE 17. Causes of Type 1 (Hypokalemic Distal) Renal Tubular Acidosis
Primary: hereditary
Genetic: sickle cell disease; Fabry disease; Wilson disease; elliptocytosis
Medullary cystic kidney disease
Autoimmune disorders: Sjögren syndrome; systemic lupus erythematosus
Nephrocalcinosis/hypercalciuria
Dysproteinemias: amyloidosis; cryoglobulinemia; hypergammaglobulinemia
Drugs/toxins: amphotericin B; lithium; analgesic abuse
Tubulointerstitial disease: reflux nephropathy; obstructive uropathy; kidney transplant rejection

CONT.

filtered citrate increases in acidosis, hypocitraturia is also present, which results in calcium phosphate kidney stones and nephrocalcinosis. Treatment consists of potassium citrate at a dose of 1 mEq/kg/d.

Type 4 (Hyperkalemic Distal) Renal Tubular Acidosis

Type 4 (hyperkalemic distal) RTA is caused by aldosterone deficiency or resistance. Primary aldosterone deficiency is seen in primary adrenal deficiency (Addison disease). Hyporeninemic hypoaldosteronism occurs in patients with various kidney diseases (including acute glomerulonephritis) and chronic nephropathies (such as diabetes mellitus, systemic lupus erythematosus, or AIDS). Patients with conditions that cause tubulointerstitial disease, including urinary obstruction, sickle cell disease, medullary cystic kidney disease, and kidney transplant rejection, may demonstrate resistance to aldosterone. Drug-induced type 4 (hyperkalemic distal) RTA can be caused by numerous drugs that reduce aldosterone production, including ACE inhibitors, cyclooxygenase inhibitors, trimethoprim, and heparin.

Initial treatment includes correction of the underlying cause if possible, with discontinuation of offending medications. In most cases, treatment of hyperkalemia with sodium bicarbonate or sodium polystyrene sulfonate results in improvement of the acidosis. Replacement of mineralocorticoids with fludrocortisone is indicated for patients with Addison disease and should be considered for those with hyporeninemic hypoaldosteronism unless hypertension or heart failure is present. Management should also include dietary potassium restriction to approximately 2000 mg/d.

Mixed Forms of Renal Tubular Acidosis

Genetic defects in carbonic anhydrase result in combined proximal and distal RTA. An acquired form can develop in patients treated with topiramate, which inhibits carbonic anhydrase in both the proximal and distal tubule. Topiramate is associated with an increased risk of calcium phosphate stones because of the high urine pH (>6.0 despite acidemia) and hypocitraturia.

Acidosis in Acute and Chronic Kidney Disease

In patients with acute and chronic kidney disease, metabolic acidosis is mediated by two mechanisms: 1) decreased urine ammonium excretion with hyperkalemia when the glomerular filtration rate (GFR) decreases to <45 mL/min/1.73 m², causing normal anion gap metabolic acidosis, and 2) retention of sulfates, phosphates, and organic acids when the GFR decreases to <15 mL/min/1.73 m², resulting in an increased anion gap metabolic acidosis. **H**

KEY POINTS

- Treatment of type 2 (proximal) renal tubular acidosis consists of alkali replacement with the addition of a thiazide diuretic.

- Treatment of type 1 (hypokalemic distal) renal tubular acidosis consists of potassium citrate at a dose of 1 mEq/kg/d.

- Treatment of type 4 (hyperkalemic distal) renal tubular acidosis includes correction of the underlying cause, treatment of hyperkalemia, discontinuation of offending medications, and dietary potassium restriction.

Metabolic Alkalosis

Metabolic alkalosis is defined by the retention of excess alkali and is diagnosed by an elevation in serum bicarbonate concentration. This disorder is caused by either a loss of acid or administration or retention of bicarbonate. The organ systems responsible for the initial metabolic alkalosis include the gastrointestinal (GI) tract (in vomiting-induced acid loss), the kidney (typically a mineralocorticoid effect, either as a primary disorder or in response to other causes of intravascular volume depletion, with resulting sodium and bicarbonate retention at the expense of acid and potassium secretion), and, rarely, the skin (from excessive sweating in patients with cystic fibrosis, resulting in chloride depletion and bicarbonate retention).

Metabolic alkalosis occurs in two phases: a generation phase in which the primary disorder (such as vomiting or the accumulation of alkali) occurs, and a maintenance phase in which the typical renal compensation of excreting excess bicarbonate in the distal tubule is ineffective. Conditions that contribute to the maintenance of metabolic alkalosis include volume contraction, ineffective arterial blood volume, hypokalemia, chloride depletion, and decreased glomerular filtration.

Symptoms of metabolic alkalosis are typically related to the underlying disorder itself rather than the alkalosis. The concomitant hypokalemia poses far greater risk due to the potential for cardiac arrhythmias. When severe (serum bicarbonate >50 mEq/L [50 mmol/L]), metabolic alkalosis

leads to hypocalcemia, hypoventilation, and hypoxemia, with potential neurologic consequences (seizures, delirium, stupor).

The first diagnostic step is a thorough history and physical examination. The assessment of blood pressure and volume status is critical to identify the likely etiology of the metabolic alkalosis (**Figure 8**). Laboratory evaluation of metabolic alkalosis to determine volume status and etiology is based on urine chloride rather than urine sodium. The urine sodium can be artificially high during periods of appropriate compensatory urine bicarbonate excretion because sodium is the primary cation excreted together with the bicarbonate. Urine sodium may also be misleading with diuretic use. Metabolic alkalosis is considered saline-resistant when associated with increased extracellular fluid volume and hypertension. Metabolic alkalosis is considered saline-responsive when associated with true

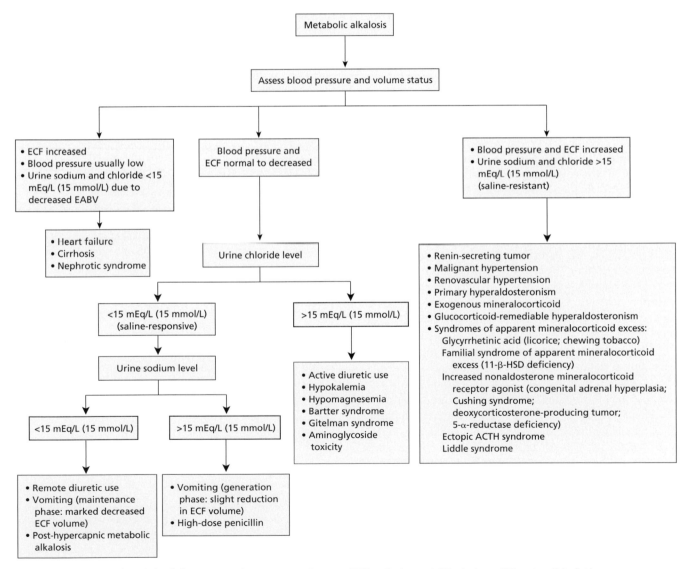

FIGURE 8. Evaluation of metabolic alkalosis. ACTH = adrenocorticotropic hormone; EABV = effective arterial blood volume; ECF = extracellular fluid; HSD = hydroxysteroid dehydrogenase.

hypovolemia and responds to correction of the volume deficit with isotonic saline.

The most common conditions that cause metabolic alkalosis are associated with chloride depletion (vomiting, nasogastric suction, and diuretic use). Although upper GI disorders (such as vomiting) are the most common GI source for the generation of metabolic alkalosis, rare lower GI disorders that cause chloride depletion include forms of chloride-secretory diarrhea such as villous adenoma and congenital chloridorrhea that lead to an increase in bicarbonate retention. A "contraction alkalosis" results from loss of extracellular fluid containing low amounts of bicarbonate that contract the extracellular volume around a constant amount of existing circulating bicarbonate.

In patients with low urine chloride (<15 mEq/L [15 mmol/L]), normal/low intravascular volume, and normal/low extracellular volume, treatment consists of administration of saline together with repletion of potassium (saline-responsive metabolic alkalosis) while addressing the primary cause of the alkalosis. In contrast, those with a low urine chloride (<15 mEq/L [15 mmol/L]) and normal/low intravascular volume but with an increased extravascular volume have a disorder of effective arterial blood volume such as heart failure, cirrhosis, or hypoalbuminemia from the nephrotic syndrome that results in secondary hyperaldosteronism, sodium and bicarbonate retention, and an increase in extracellular volume manifested by edema. Treatment is tailored to improving effective arterial blood volume and diuresis. For those who have a high urine chloride (>15 mEq/L [15 mmol/L]) with elevated blood pressure, hypokalemia, and do not appear to be overtly volume overloaded, a mineralocorticoid excess disorder must be considered (saline-resistant metabolic alkalosis). The lack of an overt increase in extravascular volume in the latter condition is often described as "aldosterone escape," in which sodium balance is attained through spontaneous diuresis that occurs after initial sodium retention that returns the vascular volume toward normal. This condition is treated with potassium repletion and treatment of the underlying condition.

Rarely, patients with metabolic alkalosis may appear to have clinical features consistent with saline-responsive metabolic alkalosis (normal/low extracellular fluid status, normal/low blood pressure) but have a urine chloride of >15 mEq/L (15 mmol/L). Diuretic use and inherited kidney disorders of sodium and chloride handling such as Bartter and Gitelman syndromes can mimic this presentation. These are two autosomal recessive genetic disorders of renal sodium and chloride transporters that clinically mimic loop diuretic and thiazide diuretic use, respectively. These diagnoses should be considered only after urine diuretic screening. Treatment focuses on the correction of volume and potassium depletion, and, in the case of Bartter syndrome, inhibition of prostaglandin production with indomethacin or ibuprofen to reduce sodium and chloride delivery to the distal tubule.

KEY POINTS

- The assessment of blood pressure and volume status is critical to identify the likely etiology of metabolic alkalosis.
- Treatment of metabolic alkalosis is based upon urine chloride and both extracellular and intravascular volume assessment.

Respiratory Acidosis

Respiratory acidosis is the result of inadequate CO_2 exchange from the pulmonary capillaries to the alveoli; the resultant arterial CO_2 retention (hypercapnia) is initially buffered by water, leading to formation of excess hydrogen ions and bicarbonate. Thus, the typical arterial blood gas in this setting demonstrates an elevation in P_{CO_2}, a decrease in pH, and a slight increase in bicarbonate (see Table 12).

The most common causes of respiratory acidosis are inadequate ventilation, interference with arterial-alveolar gas exchange, and airway obstruction (**Table 18**).

Clinical manifestations of respiratory acidosis are difficult to ascribe specifically to hypercapnia itself given the associated hypoxemia. Neurologic symptoms include headache, anxiety,

TABLE 18. Causes of Respiratory Acidosis
Inadequate Ventilation
Decreased respiratory drive: head trauma; cerebrovascular accident; obesity-hypoventilation syndrome; central sleep apnea; CNS tumor; edema; infection; medications (anesthetics, sedatives, opiates)
Neuromuscular dysfunction: spinal cord injury; Guillain-Barré syndrome; amyotrophic lateral sclerosis; periodic paralysis
Musculoskeletal dysfunction: kyphoscoliosis; severe obesity; polymyositis; severe hypokalemia or hypophosphatemia
Impaired Arterial-Alveolar Gas Exchange
Pneumonia
Acute lung injury/acute respiratory distress syndrome
Cardiogenic pulmonary edema
Pneumothorax
Hemothorax
Emphysema
Interstitial lung disease
Pulmonary fibrosis
Pulmonary embolism
Airway Obstruction
Upper airway: tonsillar hypertrophy; vocal cord paralysis; foreign body aspiration; laryngospasm; tracheal stenosis; angioedema
Lower airway: status asthmaticus; COPD
CNS = central nervous system.

CONT.
blurred vision, and tremor. When severe, symptoms can progress to confusion, somnolence, or seizures. Chronic respiratory acidosis may have milder neurologic effects such as memory loss, inattentiveness, or irritability. Additional symptoms of respiratory acidosis include cardiovascular effects such as vasodilation and tachycardia that may evolve to cardiac arrhythmias and decreased cardiac output. When respiratory acidosis is severe, renal vasoconstriction with enhanced sodium retention occurs, typically seen in those with severe lung disease and cor pulmonale.

Treatment entails oxygen supplementation and mechanical ventilation to decrease CO_2 if necessary while treating the underlying disease. **H**

KEY POINT

- Respiratory acidosis is associated with hypercapnia, with an elevation in P_{CO_2}, a decrease in pH, and a slight increase in bicarbonate.

Respiratory Alkalosis

Respiratory alkalosis is the result of enhanced CO_2 exchange from the pulmonary capillaries to the alveoli and to the expired air. Without compensatory mechanisms, the fall in arterial CO_2 (hypocapnia) leads to a rapid increase in arterial pH. However, immediate diffusion of hydrogen ions from intracellular stores (from hemoglobulin, phosphate, and other protein buffers) binds with bicarbonate, causing a reduction in serum bicarbonate, thus limiting this consequence. The typical arterial blood gas in this setting demonstrates a decrease in P_{CO_2}, an increase in pH, and a slight decrease in bicarbonate (see Table 12). Other electrolyte abnormalities may result from respiratory alkalosis, including an increase in cellular lactic acid production, an increase in the anion gap in part from an increase in negatively charged albumin, and a decrease in ionized calcium from enhanced binding to negatively charged albumin. Finally, severe hypophosphatemia can occur due to a shift of phosphate from extracellular to intracellular fluid.

The most common causes of respiratory alkalosis are an enhanced respiratory drive, hypoxemia, and pulmonary disease with stimulation of thoracic stretch receptors (**Table 19**). Symptoms include tachypnea and related neurologic findings such as lightheadedness, numbness and paresthesias, cramps, confusion, and, rarely, seizures. An important consideration when evaluating a patient with respiratory alkalosis is the potential for salicylate intoxication, which in its early phases presents with mental status changes, respiratory alkalosis, and an anion gap metabolic acidosis.

Treatment of respiratory alkalosis is directed at correction of the primary disorder. For salicylate intoxication, forced diuresis, urine alkalinization, or hemodialysis should be considered. For anxiety-induced or psychogenic hyperventilation, increasing the inspired P_{CO_2} by closed bag rebreathing may increase the P_{CO_2} and improve

TABLE 19. Causes of Respiratory Alkalosis
Enhanced Respiratory Drive
Sepsis
Hepatic failure
Anxiety
Psychosis
Subarachnoid hemorrhage
Pregnancy
Nicotine
Medications: salicylates; theophylline/aminophylline
Hormones: progesterone; medroxyprogesterone; epinephrine; norepinephrine; angiotensin II
Hypoxemia
High altitude
Severe anemia
Hypotension
Chronic heart failure
Pulmonary parenchymal disease
Pulmonary Disease with Thoracic Stretch Receptor Stimulation
Pneumonia
Acute respiratory distress syndrome
Pulmonary embolism
Hemothorax
Pneumothorax
Pulmonary edema

symptoms. In rare circumstances when there is severe alkalemia (for example, pH >7.55) with hemodynamic instability, arrhythmias, or altered mental status, strategies to reduce bicarbonate via acetazolamide or controlled hypoventilation with mechanical ventilation to increase P_{CO_2} may be considered. **H**

KEY POINT

- Respiratory alkalosis is associated with hypocapnia, with a decrease in P_{CO_2}, an increase in pH, and a slight decrease in bicarbonate.

Hypertension
Epidemiology

Hypertension prevalence in the United States is increasing, albeit more slowly over the past decade, and is estimated to be 29%. Efforts to effectively treat hypertension have slightly improved over time, but only approximately 50% of patients with hypertension are controlled to a blood pressure goal of <140/90 mm Hg.

Consequences of Sustained Hypertension

End-Organ Injury

In the brain and central nervous system, elevated blood pressure can lead to cerebral aneurysms, which may rupture (subarachnoid hemorrhage), and retinal hemorrhage. Longstanding hypertension can lead to arteriolosclerosis, resulting in arteriolar narrowing and distal ischemia. Clinical consequences include lacunar infarction and dementia.

In the heart, increased blood pressure leads to a compensatory myocardial hypertrophy that results in impaired relaxation (diastolic dysfunction) over time, which ultimately can lead to heart failure.

In the medium to large blood vessels, hypertension may cause pressure-related injury (aortic aneurysms and dissection) and contribute to the development of atherosclerosis through disruption of the vascular endothelium. When combined with elevated cholesterol, diabetes mellitus, and proinflammatory cytokines, this results in plaque formation. Plaque formation may result in thrombotic and embolic complications such as myocardial infarction, renal artery stenosis, embolic stroke, and atheroembolic peripheral arterial disease.

In the kidneys, hypertension has adverse effects on the renal vasculature, which may ultimately lead to kidney dysfunction. Chronic hypertension is associated with the development of both arteriolosclerosis and atherosclerosis. With severe hypertension, arteriolar injury with proliferation ("onion skin" lesions) and fibrinoid necrosis can occur, clinically manifesting as acute kidney injury with features of thrombotic microangiopathy and hematuria. Although debate exists as to whether hypertension as an isolated condition causes end-stage kidney disease, it clearly contributes to an accelerated progression to kidney failure in susceptible persons.

Clinical Impact

Hypertension is considered a primary cardiovascular risk factor that contributes to the development of stroke, coronary heart disease, peripheral vascular disease, and heart failure. In particular, hypertension is the strongest risk factor for hemorrhagic and ischemic stroke. Epidemiologic studies indicate that systolic blood pressures >115 mm Hg and diastolic blood pressures >75 mm Hg are associated in a linear fashion with cardiovascular events (**Figure 9**). Nearly 54% of stroke events and 47% of ischemic heart disease worldwide can be attributable

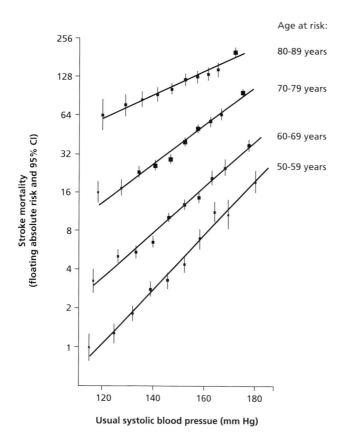
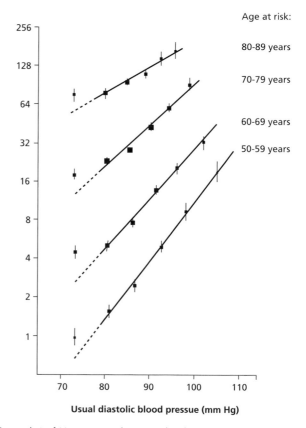

FIGURE 9. Stroke mortality rate by systolic and diastolic blood pressure, stratified by age. Meta-analysis of 61 prospective observational studies in adults with no previous vascular disease. "Usual" is defined as the long-term average blood pressure, accounting for blood pressure as a time-dependent variable in the studies included for meta-analysis.

to high blood pressure, which equates to 7.6 million premature deaths (13.5% of total) and 92 million disability-adjusted life years (6% of total). Despite these epidemiologic studies, treatment of hypertension to 115/75 mm Hg has not been demonstrated to correlate with equivalent reductions in cardiovascular risk.

KEY POINTS

- Only approximately 50% of patients with hypertension are controlled to a blood pressure goal of <140/90 mm Hg.
- Nearly 54% of stroke events and 47% of ischemic heart disease worldwide can be attributable to high blood pressure, which equates to 7.6 million premature deaths (13.5% of total) and 92 million disability-adjusted life years (6% of total).

Blood Pressure Measurement

Proper Technique

The current standard of care for blood pressure measurement employs the oscillometric method using either a properly calibrated automated device or manual measurement. This can be performed in the office or home, but the technique follows the same guidelines:

- a quiet environment with the patient in a seated position, with the back supported and feet on the floor following 5 minutes of rest
- the arm supported with the cuff at heart level; measurement should not be taken through clothes
- the cuff is placed on the upper arm, and the bladder portion should be large enough to encircle at least 80% of the arm to ensure that there is uniform compression of the brachial artery; proper cuff size is estimated by aligning the cuff parallel to the arm and wrapping the arm with the bladder; the bladder width should be large enough to encircle half the upper arm; the cuff should be inflated to a high enough pressure to exclude an auscultatory gap
- at least two measurements should be taken at least 30 seconds apart on each assessment, with repeated measurements as needed until two values are within 5 mm Hg of each other

Manual (Auscultatory) Blood Pressure Monitoring

The manual method for measuring blood pressure involves a cuff-based sphygmomanometer and stethoscope. The blood pressure is measured with the lower end of the cuff 2 to 3 cm above the antecubital fossa and the stethoscope over the brachial artery in the antecubital fossa. The cuff should be inflated at least 30 mm Hg above the estimated systolic blood pressure (indicated by disappearance of the palpated brachial pulse) to avoid error in blood pressure measurement by misinterpreting the auscultatory gap.

Electronic Blood Pressure Monitoring

Electronic blood pressure monitors are now extremely common in the office setting as well as at home due to the convenience and the relative standardization of measurement (through the elimination of user variation/error). These devices measure blood pressure through similar oscillometric methodology as manual blood pressure cuff assessment. Sensors detect the disappearance of the brachial pulse upon inflation and the increasing amplitude of the pulse upon deflation. In general, the systolic blood pressure is slightly lower and the diastolic blood pressure slightly higher than an intra-arterial measurement. Electronic devices should be properly calibrated and inspected, and patients should be encouraged to bring their devices to the office to compare readings obtained on personal versus office devices.

Ambulatory Blood Pressure Monitoring

Ambulatory blood pressure monitoring (ABPM) uses a continuously worn device that can be programmed to measure blood pressure every 15 to 20 minutes during the day and every 30 to 60 minutes at night. ABPM-ascertained hypertension is associated with a higher risk of cardiovascular death compared with hypertension determined in the office or at home (**Figure 10**). There is evidence supporting use of ABPM to confirm office-based blood pressure screening results to avoid misdiagnosis and overtreatment of individuals who may have elevated blood pressure readings only in the clinic. Beyond the benefits of accurate diagnosis of hypertension, there are numerous clinical circumstances under which ABPM provides valuable additional information over office-based measurements, including the evaluation of white coat hypertension, apparent resistant hypertension, masked hypertension, and suspected episodic hypertension.

Normal ranges for ABPM depend on the time frame of monitoring. Normal average daytime blood pressure by ABPM should be <140/90 mm Hg, with a normal nighttime average blood pressure of <125/75 mm Hg; the overall 24-hour average blood pressure should be <135/85 mm Hg. ABPM also can be used to determine if dipping is present, which is defined as the normal decrease in blood pressure at night by approximately 15% compared with daytime values. Failure of nighttime dipping is associated with an increased incidence of left ventricular hypertrophy. Additionally, elevated nighttime blood pressure by ABPM is strongly associated with an increased risk of cardiovascular death (see Figure 10).

Home Blood Pressure Monitoring

Patients can be instructed to perform frequent home blood pressure measurements, with readings at various times during the day totaling at least 12 measurements over 1 week. For a given systolic or diastolic blood pressure value, a home blood pressure average is associated with a risk of cardiovascular death higher than an office-based reading but lower than an ABPM average (see Figure 10). Home blood pressure monitoring

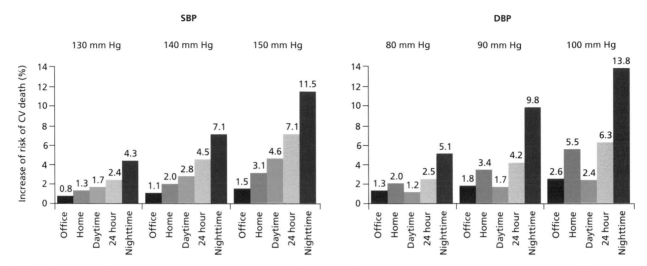

FIGURE 10. Increase in 11-year risk of cardiovascular mortality for 10 mm Hg increase in office, home, and ambulatory blood pressure at various initial blood pressure values. There were 2051 subjects. Office blood pressure at initial visit and after ambulatory blood pressure were averaged and pooled, two home blood pressure measurements (7 AM and 7 PM) concurrent with ambulatory blood pressure on the contralateral arm were averaged, and ambulatory blood pressure values were averaged over 24 hours, day (7 AM-11 PM), and night (11 PM-7 AM). CV = cardiovascular; DBP = diastolic blood pressure; SBP = systolic blood pressure.

is beneficial in monitoring blood pressure response to treatment, including lifestyle modifications. Patients should be instructed on appropriate technique and counseled on the frequency and timing of measurements to avoid very frequent blood pressure monitoring and the potential for medication self-adjustment. Whenever possible, upper-arm cuffs should be used unless medical conditions (such as trauma or surgery to the upper arm) require alternative sites; in these circumstances, wrist measurements are an alternative. Systolic pressure is higher and diastolic pressure is lower in the distal arteries, and calibration is critical in interpreting these values. Finger measurements lack accuracy and validation and thus should be discouraged.

KEY POINT

- Hypertension ascertained by ambulatory blood pressure monitoring is associated with a higher risk of cardiovascular death compared with hypertension determined in the office or at home.

Evaluation of the Patient with Newly Diagnosed Hypertension

The assessment of hypertension begins with proper determination of blood pressure, followed by evaluation of the patient's history, physical examination, screening laboratory data with a focus on the identification of specific causes (secondary hypertension), additional cardiovascular risk factors, and potential end-organ targets.

For the initial diagnosis of hypertension, most guidelines define hypertension as a systolic blood pressure ≥140 mm Hg and/or a diastolic blood pressure ≥90 mm Hg for office blood pressure readings (**Table 20**); however, exceptions exist for some subgroups, and guidelines continue to evolve. Importantly, a diagnosis should not be made in the office setting until the threshold blood pressure has been documented on at least three visits over a period of at least 1 week or longer. There is evidence that confirming clinic-based blood pressure elevations with ABPM is effective at avoiding overdiagnosis

BP Category	Office-Based Readings (mm Hg)	24-Hour Ambulatory Readings (mm Hg)	Self-Recorded BP (mm Hg)
Normal	SBP <120 and DBP <80	<130/80	<135/85
Prehypertension	SBP 120-139 or DBP 80-89	—	—
Hypertension, Stage 1	SBP 140-159 or DBP 90-99	≥135/85	≥135/85
Hypertension, Stage 2	SBP ≥160 or DBP ≥100	—	—
White Coat Hypertension	≥140/90	<135/85	<135/85
Masked Hypertension	<140/90	>135/85	>135/85

TABLE 20. Classification of Blood Pressure for Adults

BP = blood pressure; DBP = diastolic blood pressure; SBP = systolic blood pressure.

and overtreatment for patients in whom elevated blood pressures are detected only in the clinic.

History

The history of a patient with newly diagnosed hypertension should consider the potential for a familial pattern of hypertension as well as a family history of heart disease, kidney disease, and stroke. Questions should also focus on related symptoms, including episodic (such as headache or palpitations) and persistent (such as vision changes or foamy urine) symptoms, as well as risk factors for hypertension and cardiovascular disease (obesity, smoking, alcohol, caffeine, diet, diabetes, emotional stress, sleep apnea). A review of medications, including over-the-counter and herbal medications, is important because a number of these agents can contribute to elevated blood pressure (**Table 21**).

Physical Examination

The physical examination of a patient with newly diagnosed hypertension should focus on the following:

- accurate blood pressure measurement in both arms

- potential causes of hypertension such as the presence of an abdominal bruit suggestive of renovascular hypertension or an enlarged/palpable thyroid suggestive of hyperthyroidism

- potential end-organ targets, including an eye examination to assess for arteriovenous nicking and papilledema as well as a cardiovascular examination to assess for volume status, pulses in all extremities, bruits, and left ventricular hypertrophy (left ventricular heave, S_4 gallop)

Testing

A patient with newly diagnosed hypertension should undergo laboratory testing for kidney function, fasting plasma glucose, fasting serum lipid panel, serum potassium, and serum calcium. Electrocardiography (ECG) should be obtained to assess for the presence of left ventricular hypertrophy (LVH) or silent myocardial injury. Although echocardiography is a more sensitive test for LVH, in general, echocardiography is not indicated in the assessment of hypertension except in patients with known heart disease; the presence of left bundle branch block on ECG, given its association with sudden death; or suspected white coat hypertension.

A urinalysis should be performed to assess for albuminuria and hematuria. Standard urine dipsticks do not detect moderately increased albuminuria (formerly known as microalbuminuria), which is an increasingly recognized marker of microvascular injury and is independently associated with an increased risk of cardiovascular events in hypertensive individuals with or without diabetes. Albumin generally comprises approximately 50% of the total protein excreted in the urine, with the remainder comprised of proteins of smaller molecular weight that are secreted into the urine. Because albuminuria, and not total proteinuria, has been associated with cardiovascular events, testing should be directed in this fashion. Measurement of a first morning urine sample for albumin and creatinine can permit calculation of an albumin-creatinine ratio, which is a good estimate for moderately increased albuminuria (30-300 mg/g).

The use of plasma renin activity to risk-stratify patients with hypertension or to predict response to specific interventions is of unclear value and is not recommended for routine use.

TABLE 21. Over-the-Counter and Prescription Agents that Increase Blood Pressure

Type	Agent	Mechanism(s)
OTC	Black licorice (European)	Mineralocorticoid activity enhancement; sodium retention
OTC	Ethanol	Adrenergic stimulation
OTC	NSAIDs	Sodium retention
OTC/Rx	Sympathomimetics; appetite suppressants; decongestants; vigilance enhancers (e.g., amphetamines)	Vasoconstriction; sodium retention
Rx	Selective serotonin or serotonin-norepinephrine reuptake inhibitors	Adrenergic stimulation
Rx	Erythrocyte stimulation agents (e.g., erythropoietins)	Vasoconstriction
Rx	Antiretroviral therapies	Not clear
Rx	Vascular endothelial growth factor antagonists (e.g., bevacizumab)	Vasoconstriction (endothelial dysfunction)
Rx	Glucocorticoids (e.g., prednisone)	Sodium retention; weight gain
Rx	Oral contraceptives	Increased renin-angiotensin system activity; sodium retention
—	Caffeine	Adrenergic stimulation
—	Cocaine; 3,4-methylenedioxymethamphetamine (also known as ecstasy); recreational drugs	Adrenergic stimulation

OTC = over the counter; Rx = prescription.

However, there are circumstances in which the plasma aldosterone-plasma renin ratio may be used to screen for primary hyperaldosteronism. The 2008 Endocrine Society recommendations include screening patients with hypokalemia and hypertension as well as patients with moderate to severe hypertension even without significant hypokalemia (>160/100 mm Hg) and those with resistant hypertension. See Hypokalemia and Hypertension for more information.

KEY POINTS

HVC
- Echocardiography is not routinely indicated in the assessment of hypertension except in patients with known heart disease; the presence of left bundle branch block on electrocardiogram, given its association with sudden death; or suspected white coat hypertension.
- Plasma aldosterone-plasma renin ratio determination is recommended for patients with hypokalemia and hypertension as well as patients with moderate to severe hypertension even without significant hypokalemia and those with resistant hypertension.

Classification of Hypertension

Overview
The eighth report of the Joint National Committee (JNC 8), along with the European Society of Hypertension and the Canadian Hypertension Education Program, all currently define hypertension for non-elderly patients without chronic kidney disease (CKD) or diabetes as ≥140/90 mm Hg.

Prehypertension
JNC 8 did not address the concept of prehypertension. However, JNC 7 defined prehypertension as a systolic blood pressure of 120-139 mm Hg or a diastolic blood pressure of 80-89 mm Hg. This definition arose from the epidemiologic associations of "high normal" blood pressure and increased cardiovascular risk (see Figure 9), and the observed progression of many to overt hypertension. It is reasonable to identify and educate persons with prehypertension regarding their risk; however, data supporting the use of pharmacologic treatment to prevent complications or progression are lacking. Thus, treatment should focus on lifestyle modification and close monitoring, described later.

Stage 1 and 2 Hypertension
Hypertension is often classified by severity to bring awareness to the strong relationship of increasing blood pressure and cardiovascular morbidity and mortality (see Figure 9). The JNC 7 defines stage 1 hypertension as a systolic blood pressure of 140-159 mm Hg or a diastolic blood pressure of 90-99 mm Hg; stage 2 hypertension is defined as a systolic blood pressure of ≥160 mm Hg or a diastolic blood pressure of ≥100 mm Hg (see Table 20). These classifications have treatment implications, as those with stage 1 with average

blood pressure values just above the defined threshold may be amenable to lifestyle modification with close monitoring, whereas those with stage 2 typically require combination therapy to achieve adequate blood pressure control. See Management for more information.

KEY POINTS
- Several guidelines define hypertension for non-elderly patients without chronic kidney disease or diabetes mellitus as ≥140/90 mm Hg.
- Treatment of prehypertension should focus on lifestyle modification and close monitoring.

Primary Hypertension

Pathogenesis
Approximately 90% of patients diagnosed with hypertension have primary hypertension (formerly known as essential hypertension), in which there is no identifiable anatomic or screening laboratory finding that provides insight as to the cause of hypertension. For most patients, the pathogenesis remains unclear. A number of potential mechanisms have been proposed, with experimental data supporting all of the following theories: abnormal sodium handling by the kidney, increased sympathetic tone, and increased activity of the renin-angiotensin-aldosterone axis.

Genetic Factors
Increasingly, genetic studies have identified gene mutations or polymorphisms that may explain up to 20% to 30% of cases of primary hypertension. The best described mutations are those directly affecting sodium channels of the distal renal tubule and collecting duct as well as those that lead to excess mineralocorticoid effect upon the distal tubule. These defects lead to excess sodium reabsorption and hypertension. Other genetic polymorphisms that may predispose to hypertension involve oxidative stress mechanisms, mediators of vascular smooth muscle tone, and vasoactive mediators.

Societal Factors
The increased prevalence of hypertension is a result of worldwide changes in diet and lifestyle over time. The adoption of a Western diet and an increase in sodium intake has resulted in prevalence rates of 20% to 30% in geographic regions that previously had virtually no prior prevalence of hypertension. Age, race, obesity, insulin resistance, and hyperuricemia have all emerged as significant risk factors for hypertension.

Management
General Approach
The JNC 8 hypertension management recommendations are summarized as follows:
- Lifestyle modifications: implement in all patients with prehypertension and hypertension. Continue even if

pharmacologic treatment becomes necessary. Modifiable risk factors should be treated.

- General adult population <60 years of age: pharmacologic treatment is recommended if the systolic blood pressure is ≥140 mm Hg or the diastolic blood pressure is ≥90 mm Hg. The goal of therapy is <140/90 mm Hg.

- Patients ≥60 years of age: pharmacologic treatment is recommended if the systolic blood pressure is ≥150 mm Hg or the diastolic blood pressure is ≥90 mm Hg. The goal of therapy is <150/90 mm Hg, although patients with a blood pressure of <140/90 mm Hg on well-tolerated therapy do not need to have their treatment changed.

- Patients ≥18 years of age with diabetes or CKD: the initiation threshold and goal for pharmacologic treatment is 140/90 mm Hg.

- General non-black population, including those with diabetes: thiazide diuretics, ACE inhibitors, angiotensin receptor blockers (ARBs), and calcium channel blockers (CCBs) all may be considered for initial treatment.

- Black patients, including those with diabetes: initial therapy should be a thiazide diuretic or CCB. As a group, black patients have less blood pressure reduction with equivalent ACE inhibitor dosing compared with non-black patients. Furthermore, black patients initially treated with ACE inhibitors rather than CCBs have about a 50% higher rate of stroke, and combined cardiovascular outcomes are better with a thiazide diuretic than with an ACE inhibitor.

- All patients (regardless of race or the presence/absence of diabetes) >18 years of age with CKD (including those with and those without proteinuria): initial therapy should be an ACE inhibitor or ARB because these agents are renoprotective and improve renal outcomes.

- Black patients with CKD but without proteinuria: the initial agent can be a CCB, thiazide diuretic, ACE inhibitor, or ARB. If the initial choice is not an ACE inhibitor or ARB, then one of these should be the second drug added if necessary to lower the blood pressure to target (<140/90 mm Hg).

Visit http://jama.jamanetwork.com/article.aspx?articleid=1791497 for more information on the JNC 8 recommendations.

Lifestyle Modifications

A critical component of blood pressure treatment is modification of diet and activity. Lifestyle interventions should be stressed to patients not only with sustained hypertension but also to those with prehypertension to reduce future hypertension and cardiovascular disease. Examples of nonpharmacologic measures include the following: 1) a low sodium diet; 2) a diet such as DASH (Dietary Approaches to Stop Hypertension) that emphasizes vegetables, fruits, whole grains, legumes, and low-fat dairy products and limits sweets, red meat, and saturated/total fat; 3) weight loss; and 4) exercise, which can be of significant benefit for blood pressure control and management.

All interventions produce a reduction in blood pressure, even in normotensive individuals, but their effects are magnified in those who are hypertensive. In adults up to age 75 to 80 years with a blood pressure of 120-159/80-95 mm Hg, reducing sodium intake from 3300 mg/d to 1500 mg/d lowers blood pressure by an average of 7/3 mm Hg. A more modest reduction of approximately 1150 mg/d reduces blood pressure by an average of 3 to 4/1 to 2 mm Hg. Combining a reduced sodium intake with a DASH dietary pattern has an additive effect on lowering blood pressure. Weight loss of 5.0 kg (11 lb) may be expected to lead to a reduction of 4/3 mm Hg, although this effect may be higher in those who are hypertensive. Independent of weight loss or dietary intervention, aerobic exercise for 40 minutes 3 to 4 times per week lowers blood pressure by 2 to 5/1 to 4 mm Hg. Thus, implementing lifestyle interventions can produce reductions in blood pressure equivalent to antihypertensive agents and should be recommended for all patients with hypertension. Other interventions such as moderating alcohol intake and increasing potassium and calcium in the diet have more modest and less reproducible effects in lowering blood pressure. Tobacco cessation strategies should be encouraged. Although tobacco use has variable effects upon blood pressure, the strong synergistic relationship between hypertension, tobacco use, and the development of atherosclerotic disease over time should be addressed at each visit.

Pharmacologic Therapy

In patients who are unresponsive to an adequate trial of lifestyle modification, pharmacologic therapy is indicated. Timing of initiation of medications should be dictated by the severity of hypertension. For example, a non-elderly patient with a systolic blood pressure of 140-150 mm Hg may benefit from a 3- to 6-month trial of lifestyle modification alone with close monitoring, whereas an individual with stage 2 hypertension or with evidence of end-organ disease should be started on medications together with lifestyle modification. The selection of initial antihypertensive therapy has been extensively reviewed for potential individual benefits in efficacy, overall mortality, cardiovascular-related mortality, and cardiovascular and renal events. In multiple reviews and meta-analyses, the attained blood pressure is far more critical than the agent used to achieve blood pressure control and prevent cardiovascular events. For this reason, the JNC 8 recommends the use of any one of four drug classes, thiazide diuretics (thiazides), CCBs, ACE inhibitors, and ARBs, as initial therapy in the general nonblack population (elderly and non-elderly). All performed similarly in preventing cardiovascular mortality and morbidity end points with the exception of heart failure, in which a slight advantage of thiazides over CCBs and ACE inhibitors and a slight advantage of ACE inhibitors over CCBs were noted in two trials. However, these differences were not considered by JNC 8 to be compelling.

In the general black population, initial therapy with a thiazide diuretic or CCB is recommended.

Specific non-recommended initial agents by JNC 8 include β-blockers (due to higher cardiovascular-related events and mortality compared with ARBs) and α-blockers (due to higher cardiovascular-related events and mortality compared with thiazides), although clinical conditions such as atrial fibrillation or benign prostatic hyperplasia may supersede these recommendations (**Table 22**).

See **Table 23** for a list of frequently used antihypertensive medications and their side effects.

Choice of Diuretic

Thiazide diuretics remain as a first-line option for the treatment of hypertension. Most large randomized clinical trials have been performed with either hydrochlorothiazide or chlorthalidone, medications with similar primary mechanism of action (inhibition of the Na^+Cl^- cotransporter in the distal renal tubule) but with differing potency. The maximal recommended doses are 25 mg of chlorthalidone and 50 mg of hydrochlorothiazide; side effects increase beyond these doses with little further antihypertensive effect.

Loop diuretics are short-acting agents and as such do not have a role in the management of hypertension aside from use in patients with clinically significant fluid retention. In the setting of CKD stage 4 and greater (glomerular filtration rate [GFR] <30 mL/min/1.73 m^2), thiazides lose potency, and loop diuretics may often be required.

Agents that act at the distal Na^+ channel in the renal tubule ("potassium-sparing diuretics" such as spironolactone, eplerenone, and amiloride) are weaker diuretics than thiazides and are often reserved for treatment of aldosterone-mediated hypertension or resistant hypertension. Because the mechanism of action of these agents predisposes to hyperkalemia, use of these agents in combination with other drugs that act on the renin-angiotensin system (ACE inhibitors, ARBs, and direct renin inhibitors) must be cautiously considered and closely monitored.

Choice of Calcium Channel Blocker

There are no evidence-based recommendations regarding selection of a dihydropyridine (amlodipine, felodipine, nifedipine) CCB versus a non-dihydropyridine (diltiazem, verapamil) CCB for the treatment of hypertension; therefore, the mechanisms of action and side-effect profiles typically dictate their utilization. Non-dihydropyridine CCBs act upon calcium channels in the heart and may lead to increased relaxation and decreased atrioventricular node conduction, whereas dihydropyridine CCBs act upon calcium channels of the vasculature, increasing vasodilation.

Of note, there is an FDA safety alert regarding the use of statins together with CCBs. Specifically, the use of simvastatin at doses 10 mg and above and lovastatin at doses 20 mg and above is contraindicated with verapamil or diltiazem, and simvastatin at doses 20 mg and above is contraindicated with amlodipine due to an increased risk of myopathy.

Choice of Renin-Angiotensin System Agent

ACE inhibitors and ARBs have comparable effects upon blood pressure reduction and similar efficacy in reducing proteinuria, slowing CKD progression, and preventing cardiovascular events. The direct renin inhibitor aliskiren has similar antihypertensive efficacy but has not been extensively studied in head-to-head trials compared with other renin-angiotensin system (RAS) agents. Beyond cost considerations, the primary rationale for selecting one versus another lies in side-effect profiles. ACE inhibitors are associated with a 15% to 20% incidence of dry cough not seen with ARBs. ACE inhibitors also carry a higher rate of angioedema, a rare but life-threatening side effect. Angioedema can occur with direct renin inhibitors at rates similar to ACE inhibitors, whereas the risk of angioedema with ARBs is only slightly higher than with the use of β-blockers. Individuals with a history of angioedema or who develop angioedema on an ACE inhibitor or a direct renin inhibitor may (with great caution) be tried on ARBs, with a small risk of recurrence. All RAS agents are contraindicated in pregnancy due to fetal urogenital developmental abnormalities.

TABLE 22. Potential Factors that Influence the Selection of an Initial Antihypertensive Agent

Agent	Potential Clinical Indications	Potential Clinical Contraindications
Thiazide diuretic	Isolated systolic hypertension in elderly; hypertension in black patients; heart failure	Gout; hyponatremia; glucose intolerance; concomitant lithium use
ACE inhibitor/ARB	Heart failure; post-MI; CKD; proteinuria; diabetes mellitus/metabolic syndrome	Pregnancy[a]; hyperkalemia; bilateral renal artery stenosis
CCB	Isolated systolic hypertension in elderly; hypertension in black patients	Heart failure (non-dihydropyridines)
β-Blocker	Post-MI; heart failure; tachyarrhythmia; pregnancy; angina (NOT recommended for initial use except under these conditions)	Peripheral arterial disease; COPD; glucose intolerance

ARB = angiotensin receptor blocker; CCB = calcium channel blocker; CKD = chronic kidney disease; MI = myocardial infarction.

[a]Absolute contraindication.

TABLE 23. Frequently Used Antihypertensive Medications

Class/Agent	Dose/Frequency	Common Side Effects
Thiazide Diuretics		**Hypokalemia; hyponatremia; hyperlipidemia; hyperuricemia; hyperglycemia**
Hydrochlorothiazide	12.5-50 mg daily	
Chlorthalidone	12.5-25 mg daily	
ACE Inhibitors		**Hyperkalemia; cough**
Captopril	25-75 mg three times daily	
Lisinopril	5-40 mg daily	
Enalapril	5-20 mg twice daily	
Benazepril	10-40 mg daily	
Angiotensin Receptor Blockers		**Hyperkalemia**
Candesartan	4-32 mg daily	
Losartan	25-100 mg daily	
Valsartan	40-320 mg daily	
Irbesartan	75-300 mg daily	
Calcium Channel Blockers		
Dihydropyridines		
Amlodipine	2.5-10 mg daily	Pedal edema
Felodipine	2.5-10 mg daily	Headache
Nifedipine (extended release)	30-180 mg daily	
Non-dihydropyridines		
Diltiazem (extended release)	120-360 mg daily	Constipation
Verapamil (extended release)	120-480 mg daily	
β-Blockers		**Fatigue; bronchospasm; sexual dysfunction; hyperglycemia**
Atenolol	25-100 mg daily	
Metoprolol tartrate	25-100 mg twice daily	
Metoprolol succinate	25-200 mg daily	
Labetalol	100-600 mg three times daily	
Potassium Channel Openers (Vasodilators)		**Edema**
Hydralazine	25-75 mg three times daily	Lupus-like syndrome
Minoxidil	2.5-10 mg twice daily	Hypertrichosis
α-Blocker		**Orthostatic hypotension; dizziness**
Prazosin	1-10 mg twice daily	
Central α-Agonists		**Fatigue; depression; rebound hypertension**
Clonidine, oral	0.1-0.4 mg twice daily	
Clonidine, patch	0.1-0.3 mg/24 h applied once every 7 days	
Potassium-Sparing Diuretics		**Hyperkalemia**
Spironolactone	25-50 mg daily	Gynecomastia
Amiloride	5 mg daily or twice daily	
Eplerenone	50 mg daily or twice daily	

The use of dual RAS agents (ACE inhibitor, ARB, or the direct renin inhibitor aliskiren) is not recommended (see next section).

Combination Therapy

There is general agreement that a single antihypertensive agent or lifestyle modification alone is unlikely to control blood pressure in patients who are >20/10 mm Hg above target blood pressure. In this circumstance, initial therapy may include lifestyle modification with a combination of agents either separately or in a fixed-dose pill. A thiazide diuretic in combination with an ACE inhibitor or ARB is commonly employed, as is the combination of an ACE inhibitor or ARB with a CCB. These combinations have been supported by both the JNC 8 and European Society of Hypertension as reasonable approaches to management. Although no definitive recommendations exist regarding the best combination of agents to employ, there is some evidence that an ACE inhibitor/CCB combination may be more effective than an ACE inhibitor/ thiazide combination. Combination of a thiazide and CCB is also an effective strategy, although there have not been large clinical trials comparing this combination to other combination therapies. Conversely, the use of dual RAS agents (ACE inhibitor, ARB, or the direct renin inhibitor aliskiren) is not recommended because of lack of benefit in renal or cardiovascular end points and increased adverse events.

Assessment of Efficacy and Medication Titration

After lifestyle modification and a pharmacologic treatment regimen have been implemented, patients should be assessed monthly until blood pressure goals have been achieved.

As antihypertensive agents are titrated or added when there is inadequate blood pressure control, it is important to recognize that there is a nonlinear and diminishing blood pressure–lowering effect when titrating from 50% maximal dose to 100% maximal dose of any agent. A general rule of thumb is that 75% of an agent's blood pressure–lowering effect may be achieved with 50% of its maximal dose. If blood pressure control requires an additional >5 mm Hg reduction, it is unlikely to be achieved by increasing the single agent from 50% to 100% maximal dose. A combination of two agents at moderate dose is often more successful at achieving blood pressure goals than one agent at maximal dose. This strategy also minimizes the side effects that are more commonly noted at higher doses.

KEY POINTS

HVC
- Modification of diet and activity can produce blood pressure reductions that are equivalent to antihypertensive agents.

- The eighth report of the Joint National Committee recommends a blood pressure goal of <140/90 mm Hg in adult patients <60 years of age and a goal of <150/ 90 mm Hg for those ≥60 years of age.

(Continued)

KEY POINTS *(continued)*

- The eighth report of the Joint National Committee recommends as initial therapy of hypertension in the general nonblack population the use of any one of four drug classes: thiazide diuretics, calcium channel blockers, ACE inhibitors, and angiotensin receptor blockers.

- For patients whose blood pressure is >20/10 mm Hg above target blood pressure, initial treatment may include combination therapy.

- A combination of two hypertensive agents at moderate   HVC dose is often more successful at achieving blood pressure goals than one agent at maximal dose, which can help minimize the side effects more commonly noted at higher doses.

White Coat Hypertension

The term *white coat hypertension* (also known as isolated clinic hypertension or office hypertension) is applied to patients with average blood pressure readings in the office ≥140/90 mm Hg and out-of-office readings <135/85 mm Hg as determined by home measurements or ABPM. Prevalence may be as high as 10% to 20% of patients diagnosed with hypertension. Whenever possible, ABPM should be employed to confirm the diagnosis. Although small reports suggest an increased risk of stroke in patients with white coat hypertension compared with normotensive individuals, there does not appear to be increased cardiovascular risk when studies are pooled in meta-analyses. However, white coat hypertension is associated with an increased likelihood of progressing to hypertension, therefore justifying evaluation for other risk factors, lifestyle modification, and close monitoring. In addition to the evaluation of hypertension (see Testing), screening echocardiography may be beneficial in this setting to determine early end-organ manifestations of hypertension that might guide therapy.

Masked Hypertension

Patients with masked hypertension have normal office blood pressure measurements but elevated blood pressure (>135/85 mm Hg) in the ambulatory setting. ABPM should be considered in such patients, especially in the presence of other cardiovascular risk factors or target organ damage. Although prospective trials are lacking, treatment of masked hypertension with lifestyle modification, and pharmacologic agents if necessary, should be considered to achieve ambulatory blood pressure <135/85 mm Hg.

Resistant Hypertension

Treatment-resistant hypertension is defined as blood pressure that remains above goal despite concurrent use of three antihypertensive agents of different classes, one of which is a diuretic. Prevalence can be as high as 10%. The approach to this condition begins with the elimination of "pseudoresistance" (inappropriate blood pressure measurement techniques, sclerotic noncompressible arteries, the presence of white coat hypertension, or poor patient medication adherence). After these factors have been eliminated, a search for identifiable causes of hypertension should be undertaken (**Table 24**). Screening for significant alcohol intake should also be performed.

The addition of a diuretic is critical before diagnosing a patient as having resistant hypertension. The combination of a calcium channel blocker, RAS agent, and diuretic is synergistic. Adding a low-dose aldosterone antagonist (such as spironolactone or eplerenone) may improve blood pressure control. Chronotherapy (moving at least one long-acting medication to nighttime) has been shown to restore dipping, which is associated with lower cardiovascular events. Although other vasodilators (such as hydralazine or minoxidil) and centrally acting agents (such as clonidine or guanfacine) have been used, side effects are common; these drugs are reserved for patients with the most resistant hypertension.

TABLE 24. Identifiable Causes of Hypertension and Associated Diagnostic Tests[a]

Diagnosis	Diagnostic Test
Chronic kidney disease	Estimated GFR
Coarctation of the aorta	CT angiography
Cushing syndrome (most commonly due to chronic exogenous glucocorticoid therapy)	Overnight dexamethasone suppression test (not necessary if the patient is on chronic glucocorticoid therapy) or 24-hour urine free cortisol; late evening salivary cortisol
Drug-induced/related	Drug screening
Pheochromocytoma	24-Hour urine metanephrines and 24-hour urine catecholamines; if preclinical suspicion is high, measure plasma free metanephrines instead
Hyperaldosteronism	Plasma aldosterone-plasma renin activity ratio, measured midmorning in an ambulatory patient who is euvolemic and normokalemic
Renovascular hypertension	Doppler flow study; MR or CT angiography
Sleep apnea	Polysomnography
Thyroid dysfunction	TSH level
Primary hyperparathyroidism	Serum calcium level

GFR = glomerular filtration rate; TSH = thyroid-stimulating hormone.

[a]Diagnostic testing for causes of secondary hypertension should be guided by history and physical examination findings consistent with the secondary cause being considered.

KEY POINT

- Resistant hypertension is defined as blood pressure that remains above goal despite concurrent use of three antihypertensive agents of different classes, one of which is a diuretic.

Secondary Hypertension

Identifiable (secondary) causes of hypertension are discovered in 2% to 10% of patients with hypertension; consequently, all patients with hypertension do not need to be screened unless a potential cause is suggested based on the history, physical examination, or the recommended initial laboratory testing for patients with newly diagnosed hypertension. Possible situations in which screening for identifiable causes should be considered include the following: young age of onset (in childhood or adult serum), especially in the absence of family history; severe or resistant hypertension; abrupt worsening of blood pressure in a previously well-controlled patient; or clinical features of an underlying disorder associated with hypertension (see Table 24).

Kidney Disease
Pathophysiology and Epidemiology
Both acute and chronic kidney disease are the most common identifiable conditions associated with hypertension. More than 80% of patients with late-stage CKD are hypertensive. The pathophysiology of hypertension in kidney disease is complex, but sodium retention is the predominant mechanism and is related to a reduction in GFR, resistance to natriuretic peptides, and increased activity of the renin-angiotensin-aldosterone system. Impaired nitric oxide availability and sympathetic overactivity are also thought to play significant roles in causing hypertension. Uncontrolled hypertension is an important correctable factor associated with CKD progression.

Clinical Manifestations
The prevalence of hypertension increases with progressive reduction in GFR. Patients may have edema, but hypervolemia may be present despite the absence of edema.

Diagnosis
Because of the strong association of hypertension with kidney disease, measurement of renal indices, including serum creatinine and urine albumin, is recommended during the initial evaluation of all patients diagnosed with hypertension. Kidney ultrasonography is recommended if kidney function is impaired, if there is suspicion for fibromuscular dysplasia, or if there is a family history of polycystic kidney disease. Additional diagnostic testing is based on urinalysis and imaging results.

Management
The JNC 8 recommends a blood pressure goal of <140/90 mm Hg for patients with CKD, with or without diabetes. The Kidney

Disease: Improving Global Outcomes (KDIGO) guidelines suggest a lower blood pressure goal of <130/80 mm Hg in patients with proteinuria >500 mg/g.

In patients with CKD and hypertension, JNC 8 recommends use of an ACE inhibitor or ARB as initial or add-on therapy if not contraindicated, regardless of race, although special considerations may apply to black patients (see Special Populations). An increase in the serum creatinine of up to 30% is acceptable with the use of ACE inhibitors or ARBs, but if a more severe decline in kidney function occurs, overdiuresis or the presence of bilateral renal artery stenosis should be considered.

Control of sodium balance is an essential component of blood pressure management in patients with kidney disease. Dietary sodium restriction to <2000 mg/d combined with appropriate use of diuretics is advised. As the GFR declines (especially <30 mL/min/1.73 m^2), thiazide diuretics become less effective. Loop diuretics should be employed in such patients, with doses titrated to clinical response. Other drugs effective in kidney disease are CCBs. Nocturnal administration of at least one long-acting antihypertensive medication is recommended to restore the normal fall in blood pressure at night (chronotherapy), which is frequently absent in patients with CKD and hypertension. In patients with a GFR <15 mL/min/1.73 m^2, blood pressure may improve with better volume control associated with initiation of dialysis.

Renovascular Hypertension

Pathophysiology and Epidemiology

Renovascular disease is not invariably associated with renovascular hypertension. Although renovascular disease may be seen in a significant proportion of patients with hypertension, the true incidence of renovascular hypertension is unknown. The pathogenesis of hypertension in the acute stage of renal artery stenosis relates to hypoperfusion of the kidney, leading to release of renin and angiotensin and subsequent systemic vasoconstriction and hypertension. Renin and aldosterone levels are typically high at this stage. With damage to the contralateral kidney or with bilateral renal artery stenosis, the pathogenesis switches to a volume-dependent hypertension with normal or low renin levels. Correcting the stenosis at this stage may not lead to improvement in blood pressure because there may be irreversible parenchymal damage in the affected kidney from chronic ischemia or the contralateral kidney from the effects of hypertension.

Most patients with renovascular disease (>90%) have atherosclerosis. In younger patients, especially women, fibromuscular dysplasia may be seen (**Figure 11**).

Clinical Manifestations

Recurrent episodes of "flash" pulmonary edema or a marked elevation in serum creatinine with control of blood pressure, especially with the use of an ACE inhibitor or ARB, suggests renovascular disease. The presence of a renal bruit is insensitive in the diagnosis of renal artery stenosis, but hypertension

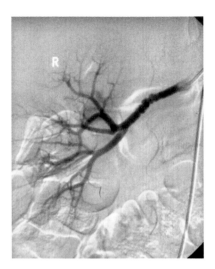

FIGURE 11. Renal angiogram showing typical fibromuscular dysplasia. This noninflammatory, nonatherosclerotic disorder of unclear etiology most commonly affects the arterial media, causing distortion of the arterial wall ("string of beads" sign) that may result in renal artery stenosis.

and a systolic/diastolic abdominal bruit is associated with a positive likelihood ratio of 4.8.

Diagnosis

Duplex Doppler of the renal arteries is an effective screening test when performed in an experienced vascular laboratory. However, MR or CT angiography may be required to confirm the anatomic diagnosis. The gold standard is renal arteriography, but in view of significant side effects, this is undertaken only if an intervention to correct a discovered stenosis is planned. Peripheral renin and aldosterone profiling are generally not helpful in later stages of renovascular disease.

Management

No clinical trials have demonstrated that percutaneous intervention (angioplasty or stenting) to improve blood flow to the stenotic kidney results in improvement of hypertension or a lessening of kidney deterioration. Thus, medical management, including correction of modifiable cardiovascular risk factors, is the primary therapeutic intervention in most patients with renal artery stenosis. Percutaneous intervention may be considered in select patients such as those with a short duration of hypertension, recurrent flash pulmonary edema with bilateral renal artery stenosis, and in young women with fibromuscular dysplasia.

Hypokalemia and Hypertension

Hyperaldosteronism, usually from an aldosterone-producing adenoma or bilateral idiopathic hyperaldosteronism, may be present in up to 10% of patients with hypertension. Hypokalemia in the absence of diuretic therapy or in response to low-dose thiazide therapy is an important clue to the presence of this disorder, although not all patients with hyperaldosteronism have hypokalemia. The plasma aldosterone-plasma

CONT.

renin activity ratio (ARR) is used to evaluate for this condition if suspected (see Table 24). Many medications can interfere with interpretation of the ARR; testing can therefore be challenging because discontinuing hypertensive medications in patients with refractory hypertension can be difficult. Spironolactone and diuretics should be stopped before testing for 4 to 6 weeks and several days, respectively. See MKSAP 17 Endocrinology and Metabolism for details on primary hyperaldosteronism.

An important differential diagnosis in patients with hypokalemia and hypertension are disorders associated with mutation of sodium channels in the distal nephron and other disorders of adrenal steroid synthesis. This group of disorders includes Liddle syndrome, syndrome of apparent mineralocorticoid excess, and familial hyperaldosteronism type 1 (also known as glucocorticoid-remediable hyperaldosteronism). In these disorders, severe early-onset hypertension associated with hypokalemia is present, but renin and aldosterone levels are suppressed because of primary sodium absorption.

Pheochromocytoma

Catecholamine-secreting tumors of chromaffin cells of the adrenal medulla (pheochromocytomas) and the sympathetic ganglia (extra-adrenal pheochromocytomas or paragangliomas) cause hypersecretion of norepinephrine and epinephrine, leading to hypertension. Patients present with symptoms of sympathetic overactivity. Screening tests for urine catecholamines and metanephrines should be performed, followed by imaging to localize the suspected tumor. Surgical removal is the only definitive treatment. See MKSAP 17 Endocrinology and Metabolism for details on pheochromocytoma.

KEY POINTS

- The eighth report of the Joint National Committee recommends a blood pressure goal of <140/90 mm Hg in patients of all ages who have chronic kidney disease with or without diabetes mellitus.

- Blood pressure management in patients with kidney disease includes the use of an ACE inhibitor or angiotensin receptor blocker as well as control of sodium balance.

- **HVC** • Medical management is the primary therapeutic intervention in most patients with renal artery stenosis.

Special Populations

Women

Although the prevalence of hypertension in women is lower before the age of 50 years, the eventual prevalence is similar to men. Hypertensive complications are lower in women (especially coronary artery disease). The response to hypertensive therapy is similar to men, but women derive much better cardiovascular benefit.

Oral contraceptives may be associated with overt hypertension in up to 5% of women. Stopping the drug usually leads to return of the blood pressure to baseline.

ACE inhibitors, ARBs, and aldosterone blockers should be avoided in women who are likely to become pregnant and are contraindicated in pregnant women.

Patients with Diabetes Mellitus

The JNC 8 and the American Diabetes Association both recommend a goal blood pressure of <140/90 mm Hg in patients with diabetes who are hypertensive. More aggressive lowering of the systolic blood pressure to <120 mm Hg in patients with type 2 diabetes at increased cardiovascular risk resulted in no significant cardiovascular benefit (except for a reduction in stroke) in the ACCORD study. In patients with moderately increased albuminuria or overt nephropathy (proteinuria >500 mg/g) a goal blood pressure of <130/80 mm Hg is suggested per the KDIGO guidelines.

In the absence of CKD, first-line therapy in nonblack patients with diabetes is similar to treatment of patients without diabetes: a thiazide diuretic, CCB, ACE inhibitor, or ARB. In black patients with diabetes, a thiazide diuretic or CCB is recommended for initial therapy. β-Blockers and α-blockers are not recommended as initial therapy for either group. Combination therapy of ACE inhibitors, ARBs, and direct renin inhibitors should not be used in patients with diabetes because of the increased risk of acute kidney injury and hyperkalemia without demonstrated benefit in long-term renal and cardiovascular outcomes. See Table 22 for more information.

Black Patients

Hypertension is more prevalent in black patients and associated with higher cardiovascular and renal complications than in other racial groups. The JNC 8 recommends a blood pressure goal for black patients of <140/90 mm Hg (for age ≥60 years, the target is <150/90 mm Hg, regardless of race).

A thiazide diuretic or a CCB alone or in combination is recommended as initial therapy. A potential conflict may occur with this recommendation and the guidance to use either an ACE or ARB in patients with CKD. To address this, the JNC 8 recommends that initial therapy in black patients with CKD and proteinuria be with an ACE inhibitor or ARB; in black patients without proteinuria, treatment options include a thiazide diuretic, CCB, ACE inhibitor, or ARB. See Table 22 for more information.

Older Patients

The prevalence of hypertension can be as high as 60% to 80% in patients >65 years. Frailty, sluggish baroceptor reflexes, and orthostasis are frequently seen in the elderly population. Isolated systolic hypertension (systolic >160 mm Hg and diastolic <90 mm Hg) is more common in such patients. A lower diastolic blood pressure may be associated with worse cardiovascular outcomes in epidemiologic studies, but this has not been seen in clinical trials; thus, there are no firm recommendations for the optimal level of diastolic blood pressure below which organ perfusion (especially coronary) is impaired. The JNC 8 treatment goal for patients ≥60 years is <150/90 mm Hg. For older patients being treated for isolated systolic hypertension, the Systolic Hypertension in the Elderly Program recommends that the diastolic blood pressure be maintained above 60 mm Hg.

The choice of antihypertensive agents is similar to the general population, but a thiazide diuretic or a long-acting CCB may be more effective. ACE inhibitors or ARBs can also be used (see Table 22). Older patients are more prone to develop hyponatremia from thiazides, and the dose of medications to control blood pressure may be lower than in younger patients. Orthostasis and subsequent falls are common in older persons, and drugs that are associated with worsening or causing orthostasis (such as α-blockers, vasodilators, and centrally acting agents) should be avoided if possible.

A recent study defining frailty as the inability to walk 6 meters in less than 8 seconds demonstrated no association with hypertension and mortality, and, in those who were unable to complete the walk test, a reduction in mortality was noted with increased blood pressure. This suggests that the risk of complications, morbidity, and mortality related to lower blood pressure in frail individuals may supersede the potential benefit of lower blood pressure goals.

KEY POINTS

- ACE inhibitors, angiotensin receptor blockers, and aldosterone blockers should be avoided in women who are likely to become pregnant and are contraindicated in women who are pregnant.

- In the absence of chronic kidney disease, first-line therapy of hypertension in nonblack patients with diabetes mellitus is similar to treatment of patients without diabetes: a thiazide diuretic, calcium channel blocker, ACE inhibitor, or angiotensin receptor blocker.

- In black patients with hypertension, a thiazide diuretic or calcium channel blocker alone or in combination is recommended as initial therapy.

- The treatment goal for patients with hypertension who are ≥60 years is <150/90 mm Hg.

Chronic Tubulointerstitial Diseases

Pathophysiology and Epidemiology

Tubulointerstitial diseases primarily affect the tubules and/or interstitium of the kidney. Acute interstitial nephritis is an inflammatory process affecting the kidney interstitium and is associated with acute kidney injury (AKI) over the course of days to weeks, whereas chronic tubulointerstitial diseases develop over months to years and are a cause of slowly declining kidney function. Chronic tubulointerstitial diseases most commonly result from previous injury due to acute interstitial nephritis, but can also result from other glomerular, vascular, or obstructive diseases that may cause irreversible injury to the tubules and interstitium, even with treatment and resolution of the initial disease process. They are difficult to manage because of the diverse causes, an insidious presentation typically occurring over months to years, and often indeterminate findings on examination and laboratory testing; careful and meticulous evaluation is therefore essential. See **Table 25** for causes of tubulointerstitial diseases. See Acute Kidney Injury for more information on acute interstitial nephritis.

KEY POINT

- Chronic tubulointerstitial diseases most commonly result from previous injury due to acute interstitial nephritis, develop over months to years, and result in slowly declining kidney function.

Diagnosis and Evaluation

Symptoms and physical findings in patients with tubulointerstitial disease can be minimal or absent unless an active associated disease is present. Thus, the diagnosis is often triggered by abnormalities detected on laboratory testing performed for other purposes. History and physical examination should focus on conditions associated with tubulointerstitial disease and potential treatable causes. A careful review of medications is particularly important (see Table 25).

Many patients with chronic tubulointerstitial disease already have advanced kidney disease at the time of detection. Laboratory studies reflect the consequences of tubular dysfunction associated with these diseases. Urinalysis may be bland, often without the sterile pyuria and leukocyte casts associated with acute interstitial nephritis. Proteinuria may be present but is typically <2000 mg/24 h. Abnormal handling of glucose, amino acids, uric acid, phosphate, and bicarbonate (termed *Fanconi syndrome*) may be present, and renal tubular acidosis (RTA) is common. Patients often have concentrating defects and may present with nocturia and polyuria. With more advanced disease, anemia may be present due to the destruction of erythropoietin-producing cells in the kidney. Ultrasound can show atrophic kidneys consistent with chronicity. The role of kidney biopsy in diagnosing chronic tubulointerstitial disease is uncertain but may be appropriate in selected patients.

See **Table 26** for more information on the clinical manifestations of chronic tubulointerstitial disease.

KEY POINT

- Chronic tubulointerstitial disease should be considered in patients with slowly progressive or stable chronic kidney disease of unclear cause associated with bland urine sediment, proteinuria <2000 mg/24 h, and atrophic kidneys on ultrasound.

TABLE 25. Causes of Chronic Tubulointerstitial Diseases

Autoimmune Disorders

Anti-tubular basement membrane antibody-mediated tubulointerstitial nephritis

Sarcoidosis

Sjögren syndrome

Systemic lupus erythematosus

IgG4-related disease

Tubulointerstitial nephritis with uveitis (TINU)[a]

Toxic Causes

Balkan endemic nephropathy/aristolochic acid nephropathy (with increased risk of transitional cell carcinoma)

Heavy metal nephropathy (e.g., lead, cadmium, mercury)

Hereditary Tubulointerstitial Nephritis

Medullary cystic kidney disease

Mitochondrial disorders

Nephronophthisis

Infection-Related Causes

Polyoma BK virus (most commonly post-kidney transplantation)

Brucellosis

Cytomegalovirus

Epstein-Barr virus

Fungal infections

Legionella species

Mycobacterium tuberculosis

Toxoplasmosis

Chronic pyelonephritis

Malignancy-Related Causes

Leukemia

Lymphoma

Malignancy-associated monoclonal gammopathies (e.g., multiple myeloma, plasmacytoma)

Medication-Induced Causes

Analgesic nephropathy

Phosphate nephropathy

Oxalate nephropathy

Calcineurin inhibitors

Cyclooxygenase-2 inhibitors

Lithium

NSAIDs

Prolonged exposure to any medication that can cause acute interstitial nephritis: 5-aminosalicylates (e.g., mesalamine); allopurinol; cephalosporins; fluoroquinolones; H_2 blockers; indinavir; penicillins; proton pump inhibitors; rifampin; sulfonamides

Secondary Tubulointerstitial Injury Due to Glomerular and Vascular Disorders (e.g., hypertensive nephrosclerosis)

Urinary Tract Obstruction

[a]TINU is an uncommon immune-mediated syndrome with the combination of tubulointerstitial nephritis and uveitis associated with autoimmune disorders, including hypoparathyroidism, thyroid disease, IgG4-related disease, and rheumatoid arthritis.

TABLE 26. Clinical Manifestations of Chronic Tubulointerstitial Diseases

Abnormality[a]	Cause
Decline in GFR	Obstruction of tubules; damage to microvasculature; interstitial fibrosis and sclerosis of glomeruli
Proximal tubular damage (Fanconi syndrome)	Incomplete absorption and kidney wasting of glucose, phosphate, uric acid, bicarbonate, and amino acids
Normal anion gap metabolic acidosis	Proximal and distal RTA; decreased ammonia production
Polyuria and isosthenuria	Decreased concentrating and diluting ability
Proteinuria	Decreased tubular protein reabsorption (usually <2000 mg/24 h)
Hyperkalemia	Defect in potassium secretion (type 4 [hyperkalemic] distal RTA)
Hypokalemia	Defect in potassium reabsorption (type 1 [hypokalemic] distal RTA)
Anemia	Injury to erythropoietin-producing cells in the kidney

GFR = glomerular filtration rate; RTA = renal tubular acidosis.

[a]The degree of these abnormalities depends on the extent and location of injury.

Causes

See Table 25 for a list of causes of chronic tubulointerstitial disease.

Immunologic Diseases

Various immunologic diseases are associated with tubulointerstitial disease, including Sjögren syndrome, sarcoidosis, IgG4-related disease, and systemic lupus erythematosus (SLE). The incidence and severity of kidney involvement vary with the activity of the disease and treatment of the underlying process, typically with immunosuppressive therapy.

Sjögren Syndrome

Characterized by lymphocytic and plasmacytic infiltration of the parotid, salivary, and lacrimal glands, Sjögren syndrome can produce a similar injury in other nonexocrine glands and in the kidneys. Interstitial disease is the most common kidney manifestation of Sjögren syndrome; glomerular involvement is uncommon. Diagnosis is usually made by identifying tubulointerstitial disease in the context of confirmed Sjögren syndrome, although kidney biopsy will demonstrate granuloma formation.

Sarcoidosis

The tubulointerstitial disease of sarcoidosis typically presents at the time of initial diagnosis of the disease and may be advanced; severe tubulointerstitial disease is uncommon in patients with long-standing disease. Because sarcoidosis can cause kidney damage through other mechanisms, including direct ureteral involvement, retroperitoneal fibrosis, and hypercalcemia, hypercalciuria, nephrolithiasis, and nephrocalcinosis via excessive production of 1,25-dihydroxy vitamin D in granulomas, tubulointerstitial disease usually requires confirmation by kidney biopsy showing the presence of noncaseating granulomas and interstitial nephritis.

IgG4-Related Disease

IgG4-related disease is a group of diseases characterized by infiltration of different organs by lymphoplasmacytic infiltrates of IgG4-positive plasma cells with resultant fibrosis and is often associated with elevated serum IgG4 levels. There is often other organ involvement and occasionally associated glomerular lesions, including membranous and membranoproliferative glomerulonephritis.

Systemic Lupus Erythematosus

The tubulointerstitial disease of SLE typically occurs with concomitant glomerulonephritis. The degree of tubulointerstitial involvement in SLE is a poor prognostic sign with an associated increased risk for hypertension, progressive kidney dysfunction, and end-stage kidney disease.

Infections

Numerous infections, including those caused by bacteria, mycobacteria, viruses, parasites, and fungi, are associated with acute interstitial nephritis and chronic tubulointerstitial nephritis (see Acute Kidney Injury). The pathophysiology of infection-related interstitial nephritis may be direct infiltration of the kidney or an inflammatory response triggered by the infecting agent.

Malignancy

Kidney infiltration by lymphoma and leukemia may occur and present with non–nephrotic-range proteinuria, sterile pyuria, and enlarged kidneys on imaging studies. Diagnosis may be confirmed by biopsy. Gammopathies associated with lymphoproliferative disorders or multiple myeloma may also cause tubulointerstitial disease (see Kidney Manifestations of Gammopathies).

Numerous antineoplastic agents have been associated with tubulointerstitial disease, including carboplatin, cisplatin, cyclophosphamide, ifosfamide, nitrosoureas (such as carmustine, lomustine, semustine, and streptozocin), and panitumumab. Clinical features may include chronic kidney disease (CKD), mild proteinuria, and evidence of tubular dysfunction manifested as Fanconi syndrome and electrolyte abnormalities.

Medications
Analgesics

Long-term use of analgesic agents, particularly combinations of potentially nephrotoxic medications, is associated with chronic tubulointerstitial disease. However, the types and doses of medications leading to CKD have not been clearly defined. NSAIDs can cause AKI and may accelerate progression of underlying CKD, but it is controversial whether NSAIDs can cause de novo chronic disease. There is some evidence that acetaminophen may increase the risk of CKD with prolonged exposure. Clinical manifestations are nonspecific and may include slowly progressive CKD, varying degrees of usually mild proteinuria, hypertension, and anemia.

Calcineurin Inhibitors

The calcineurin inhibitors cyclosporine and tacrolimus can cause reversible AKI and a usually irreversible chronic tubulointerstitial disease. Duration of exposure and cumulative dose are risk factors, and laboratory features may include kidney dysfunction, hyperkalemia, hypomagnesemia, hypophosphatemia, hyperuricemia, and type 4 (hyperkalemic distal) RTA. Kidney biopsy shows patchy tubular atrophy and interstitial fibrosis. Therapy includes calcineurin dose reduction or non-calcineurin alternatives, if possible.

Lithium

Chronic lithium therapy can cause chronic tubulointerstitial disease, CKD, and nephrogenic diabetes insipidus. Prolonged duration of therapy and the cumulative dose are risk factors, but serum lithium levels do not correlate well with the risk of nephrotoxicity (patients can develop CKD with consistently therapeutic levels). Clinical features include polyuria and nocturia due to the loss of concentrating ability in the kidney (diabetes insipidus), and type 1 (hypokalemic distal) RTA can occur.

Diagnosis is often clinical based on history of lithium exposure, inappropriately dilute urine following water restriction, and variable degrees of CKD. Therapies include stopping lithium if possible to prevent further injury or concomitant use of amiloride to prevent entry of lithium into tubular cells if stopping lithium is not possible. Following lithium discontinuation, the prognosis of CKD is variable; mild improvement, stabilization, or progressive loss of kidney function can occur.

Lead

Prolonged lead exposure over years can cause lead nephropathy. Clinical features include CKD, bland urine sediment, subnephrotic proteinuria, and hyperuricemia. Kidney biopsy reveals a nonspecific chronic interstitial nephritis. The diagnosis should be considered in patients with current or past exposure to lead, extrarenal manifestations of lead toxicity, and elevated blood lead levels (although lead levels may have normalized if exposure has been reduced or stopped).

Hyperuricemia

Hyperuricemia is associated with chronic uric acid nephropathy due to deposition of sodium urate crystals in the interstitium. The inflammatory response causes interstitial fibrosis and CKD. Clinical features include hyperuricemia, CKD, bland urine sediment, subnephrotic proteinuria, and unremarkable kidney imaging. Kidney biopsy is required to make the diagnosis because clinical features are nonspecific.

Obstruction

Urinary obstruction can result in AKI and CKD. Clinical features may include hypertension, CKD, and changes in urinary habits such as incontinence, nocturia, and polyuria. Flank pain and renal or ureteral colic are usually not features of chronic obstruction given its insidious course. Imaging (typically ultrasonography) may reveal hydronephrosis and renal cortical thinning. Type 4 (hyperkalemic distal) RTA may occur, consistent with the tubular atrophy and injury on pathology. Treatment includes relief of the obstruction, and prognosis depends on the duration and severity of the obstruction. Recovery is usually diminished with obstruction of longer than 6 to 12 weeks.

KEY POINT

- Causes of chronic tubulointerstitial disease include various immunologic diseases, infections, malignancy, medications, lead exposure, hyperuricemia, and obstruction.

Management

Rapid determination and treatment of underlying causes of chronic tubulointerstitial disease may result in slower progression or slight reversal of kidney dysfunction, but significant improvement is unlikely with long-standing disease and chronic tubulointerstitial fibrosis. Practical steps include discontinuation of potentially offending drugs and toxins and treatment of underlying immunologic, infectious, obstructive, malignant, or other disease. Blood pressure control, use of ACE inhibitors or angiotensin receptor blockers when significant detectable proteinuria is present, and metabolic control of calcium and phosphate should be undertaken. Immunosuppressive therapy should be considered (in consultation with a nephrologist) in selected patients with an inflammatory cause and evidence of active disease.

KEY POINT

- Chronic tubulointerstitial diseases typically have limited improvement with therapy, even with rapid assessment and treatment of underlying causes.

Glomerular Diseases
Pathophysiology and Epidemiology

The glomerulus is the basic filtering unit of the kidney (**Figure 12**). Anatomically, each glomerulus consists of a tuft of capillaries formed by the branching of the afferent arteriole supported by

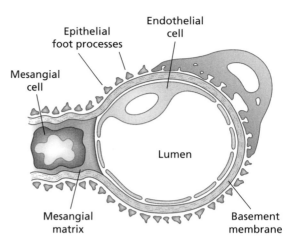

FIGURE 12. A normal glomerular capillary and surrounding structures. Each capillary consists of a layer of endothelial cells surrounded by a basement membrane on which sit specialized epithelial cells called *podocytes*. These layers constitute a barrier to plasma proteins and cells, which prevent their passage into the urine.

a structural matrix (the mesangium) produced and maintained by specialized (mesangial) cells. Each kidney has approximately 1 million glomeruli providing 2 m² of glomerular capillary filtering surface. The glomerular basement membrane (GBM) provides both a size- and charge-selective barrier to the passage of circulating macromolecules. On the urinary side of the GBM lies a layer of podocytes, which are specialized epithelial cells that provide another barrier to plasma proteins via a specialized intercellular junction (the slit diaphragm). The glomerular capillary tufts are surrounded by Bowman's capsule, a single layer of parietal epithelial cells that form a cup-like sac that is continuous with the renal tubule and into which the filtrate from the glomerular capillaries is collected and passed to the renal tubule.

From a histologic standpoint, glomerular disease can be *diffuse* (all glomeruli are involved) or *focal* (only some glomeruli are involved). At the level of the individual glomerulus, a process is *global* if the whole glomerular tuft is involved or *segmental* if only a part is involved. To describe the pathologic process, the terms *proliferative* (an increase in the number of cells in the glomerulus), *sclerosing* (presence of scarring), and *necrotizing* (areas of cell death) are often used (for example, focal and segmental necrotizing glomerulonephritis; diffuse global proliferative lupus nephritis). Extracapillary proliferation or *crescentic* lesions are associated with accumulations of macrophages, fibroblasts, proliferating epithelial cells, and fibrin within Bowman's space; represent rupture of the glomerular membrane; and signify severe injury to the glomerular capillary wall. Interstitial fibrosis, which accompanies uncontrolled glomerular disease, is a poor prognostic sign.

Several mechanisms lead to glomerular dysfunction. Podocyte dysfunction can occur in genetic disease affecting key basement membrane proteins such as hereditary nephritis (also known as Alport syndrome). In diseases such as minimal change glomerulopathy and focal segmental glomerulosclerosis (FSGS), circulating factors directly affect podocyte function and lead to proteinuria. In diabetes mellitus and amyloidosis, there is mechanical disruption of the glomerulus due to accumulation of normal or abnormal protein both in the capillary loops of the glomerulus and the mesangium. Immune mechanisms include in situ formation of immune complexes in membranous glomerulopathy or the localized effects of anti-GBM antibodies in Goodpasture syndrome; in conditions such as postinfectious glomerulonephritis and systemic lupus erythematosus, immune-mediated kidney injury is caused by deposition of circulating immune complexes.

Presently, more than 10% of the U.S. population has proteinuria or kidney dysfunction, often caused by glomerular disease. Diabetic kidney disease affects millions of people and is the major cause of end-stage kidney disease (ESKD) in the United States. Glomerular diseases associated with infections such as malaria, schistosomiasis, HIV, and hepatitis B and C are major worldwide health issues.

Clinical Manifestations of Glomerular Disease

Glomerular disease syndromes are typically classified by their characteristic features, including the pattern of abnormalities on urinalysis, any systemic features present, and the degree of kidney failure. The most common distinction is usually made between the nephrotic syndromes, in which leakage of plasma proteins is a predominant feature, and the nephritic syndromes (which reflect inflammation of the glomerulus and are also referred to as glomerulonephritis [GN]), in which there is passage of plasma proteins, erythrocytes, and leukocytes through the glomerulus into the renal tubule. These classifications, however, are not exclusive because some conditions may present with either or both patterns, and some disorders may progress from one pattern to the other. Therefore, kidney biopsy may be required to establish a diagnosis and guide appropriate therapy.

Glomerular disease may be limited primarily to the kidney but frequently occurs secondary to other systemic conditions, including infectious and autoimmune disorders. Infectious diseases linked to glomerular disease include poststreptococcal GN, HIV-associated glomerulopathy, and hepatitis C–associated cryoglobulinemic GN. Systemic lupus erythematosus is a classic example of a systemic immune complex disease associated with GN. IgA vasculitis and pauci-immune small-vessel vasculitis can also cause GN.

Glomerular disease should be suspected when proteinuria and/or hematuria are seen on urinalysis. The findings of nephrotic-range proteinuria or dysmorphic erythrocytes and erythrocyte casts in the urine sediment are also more specific for a glomerular origin. See Clinical Evaluation of Kidney Function for more details.

The Nephrotic Syndrome

The nephrotic syndrome is characterized by a urine protein excretion of >3500 mg/24 h or a urine protein-creatinine ratio of >3500 mg/g (termed *nephrotic-range proteinuria*) that may be accompanied by hypoalbuminemia, edema, and hyperlipidemia. However, many patients with high levels of proteinuria may not have the full syndrome.

The pathogenesis of the nephrotic syndrome is not completely understood. Hypoalbuminemia is thought to occur from urinary loss of albumin and increased catabolism (including uptake and catabolism of albumin by the proximal tubule). Edema results predominantly from increased sodium absorption by the distal nephron and increased capillary permeability. Elevated lipids occur from a combination of increased hepatic apolipoprotein synthesis in response to a low plasma oncotic pressure and decreased activity of key enzymes such as lipoprotein lipase and lecithin-cholesterol acyltransferase. Other complications include hypercoagulability, possibly related to loss of natural anticoagulants such as protein C and antithrombin III and upregulation of coagulation factors produced by the liver in response to a low oncotic pressure. Patients with untreated nephrotic syndrome also have a propensity for infection (possibly related to urinary loss of immunoglobulin). Urinary loss of binding proteins may be associated with deficiencies of vitamin D, thyroxine, and iron.

The nephrotic syndrome may be idiopathic (primary) or secondary to systemic diseases such as diabetes, infection, or autoimmune diseases. Although minimal change glomerulopathy is the most common cause of the nephrotic syndrome in children, membranous glomerulopathy and FSGS are the most common causes of idiopathic nephrotic syndrome in adults. Membranous glomerulopathy is the most common cause in white persons and FSGS in black persons. Diabetes is not only the most common secondary cause of the nephrotic syndrome but also the most common cause of the nephrotic syndrome in adults.

Initial evaluation begins by excluding secondary causes related to systemic disease, infection, malignancy, or medication. Screening includes testing for diabetes as well as antinuclear antibody and complement measurements for connective tissue disease. In some patients, cryoglobulins, hepatitis B and C serologies, HIV testing, serum protein and immunoelectrophoresis, and serum free light chains may be useful. Most adult patients with the nephrotic syndrome require a kidney biopsy to obtain a definitive diagnosis.

Treatment of the consequences of the nephrotic syndrome should occur simultaneously with treatment of the specific cause. Elevated lipid levels are typically treated with statin medications, with additional drugs added as needed for control of triglycerides. Anticoagulation may be needed if thrombotic complications occur. Prophylactic anticoagulation is not routinely provided to all patients with the nephrotic syndrome but is suggested in patients who have an additional risk factor for thrombosis. Prophylactic anticoagulation may also be considered in patients who are nephrotic with a serum albumin level ≤2.0 g/dL (20 g/L) with low bleeding risk regardless of cause. In patients with membranous glomerulopathy, the serum albumin threshold to anticoagulate in patients with low risk for bleeding has been suggested to be ≤2.8 g/dL (28 g/L). Edema is treated with a low salt diet and loop diuretics (alone or in combination with a thiazide and potassium-sparing diuretics).

The Nephritic Syndrome

The nephritic syndrome is associated with glomerular inflammation resulting in hematuria, proteinuria, and leukocytes in the urine sediment. The hallmark of hematuria in the nephritic syndrome is the presence of dysmorphic erythrocytes, with or without erythrocyte casts, that reflects a proliferative lesion in the glomeruli (which can be focal or diffuse). Proteinuria in the nephritic syndrome may be highly variable (from a few hundred milligrams to nephrotic levels). Systemic findings may include edema, hypertension, and kidney failure.

Three pathophysiologic mechanisms are associated with the nephritic syndrome: anti-GBM antibodies, pauci-immune GN (defined by necrotizing GN with few or no immune deposits), and immune complex deposition. Three different clinical syndromes may result from these mechanisms based on their time course: acute GN, rapidly progressive GN (RPGN), or chronic GN.

Serum complement levels may be useful in differentiating the underlying etiology of GN; levels are typically normal in anti-GBM antibody disease and pauci-immune GN but are low in immune complex GN (with the exception of IgA nephropathy). Additionally, crescentic lesions on pathologic examination of the kidney in a patient with the nephritic syndrome are associated with RPGN and a poor prognosis without treatment.

KEY POINTS

- The nephrotic syndrome is characterized by a urine protein excretion of >3500 mg/24 h or a urine protein-creatinine ratio of >3500 mg/g that may be accompanied by hypoalbuminemia, edema, and hyperlipidemia.
- Diabetes mellitus is the most common cause of the nephrotic syndrome in adults; membranous glomerulopathy and focal segmental glomerulosclerosis are the most common causes of idiopathic nephrotic syndrome in adults.
- The nephritic syndrome is associated with glomerular inflammation with evidence of hematuria, variable proteinuria, and sometimes leukocytes in the urine sediment; it may be associated with edema, hypertension, and kidney failure.
- Serum complement levels help differentiate the underlying etiology of glomerulonephritis (GN); levels are typically normal in anti–glomerular basement membrane antibody disease and pauci-immune GN but are low in immune-complex GN (with the exception of IgA nephropathy).

Conditions Associated With the Nephrotic Syndrome

See **Table 27** for details on nondiabetic conditions associated with the nephrotic syndrome.

Focal Segmental Glomerulosclerosis
Epidemiology and Pathophysiology
Approximately 25% of adults with idiopathic nephrotic syndrome have focal segmental glomerulosclerosis (FSGS) on biopsy. Incidence is increasing in all races, but it is especially common in black persons.

FSGS may result from genetic mutations to podocyte proteins, may be idiopathic, or may be secondary to another process. Some cases of idiopathic FSGS are thought to be related to a circulating plasma factor because a significant number of patients show recurrence after kidney transplantation. Secondary causes of FSGS include hyperfiltration injury to the glomerulus as in chronic hypertension, diabetes, and instances when kidney mass is reduced (progressive kidney disease, obesity, sickle cell disease, reflux nephropathy, congenital small kidneys, and after nephrectomy). Finally, direct podocyte injury can cause FSGS as seen in infections (HIV) and drugs (pamidronate, interferon).

Clinical Manifestations
Patients with idiopathic FSGS present with either asymptomatic proteinuria or edema. More than two thirds of patients are fully nephrotic at presentation; subnephrotic proteinuria may occur, especially with secondary FSGS from hyperfiltration injury. Hypertension, microscopic hematuria, and varying degrees of kidney failure are common. Serologic tests for systemic disease are typically negative, and complement activation is normal.

Diagnosis
The hallmark of FSGS is the presence of segmental scars in some glomeruli. Electron microscopy shows visceral epithelial cell foot process effacement but no immune deposits. There are several variants of FSGS, but the "collapsing" form is diagnosed when there is severe podocyte hyperplasia leading to collapse of the glomerular tuft. HIV infection is typically associated with collapsing FSGS.

Treatment and Prognosis
In idiopathic FSGS, only a minority of patients experience a spontaneous remission. Therefore, treatment is indicated in most patients. Therapy is usually with glucocorticoids or calcineurin inhibitors, both at the time of initial presentation and for relapsing disease. A complete or partial remission may be seen in up to 40% to 60% of patients using these treatments. Patients who enter remission (even partial) have a good prognosis compared with patients who have refractory disease. FSGS recurs in the transplanted kidney in 30% or more of cases.

TABLE 27. Nondiabetic Conditions Associated With the Nephrotic Syndrome

Condition	Frequency as a Cause of the Nephrotic Syndrome	Comments
Focal segmental glomerulosclerosis	36%-80%	Most common cause of primary nephrotic syndrome in the United States
		Predilection for black persons
		Five subtypes: not otherwise specified; perihilar variant; tip variant; cellular variant; collapsing variant (may be associated with HIV infection, heroin use, parvovirus infection, or pamidronate exposure)
		May be associated with or secondary to:
		Genetic mutations of podocyte proteins
		Direct podocyte injury (e.g., permeability factor), viral infections (e.g., HIV), drugs (e.g., pamidronate)
		Hyperfiltration (e.g., morbid obesity) and decreased kidney mass (congenital kidney dysplasia, reflux nephropathy)
Membranous glomerulopathy	18%-41%	Primary form (most common worldwide): antiphospholipase A_2 receptor autoantibodies can be found in 75% of cases
		May be associated with or secondary to:
		Systemic lupus erythematosus
		Infections: hepatitis B and C virus infections; syphilis; malaria
		Medication exposure: penicillamine; NSAIDs; TNF-α inhibitors; tiopronin
		Mercury or gold exposure
		Malignancies: bladder, breast, colon, lung, pancreas, prostate, stomach carcinoma; carcinoid; sarcomas; lymphomas; leukemias
		Thyroid disease
		Highest predilection for renal vein thrombosis among all causes of the nephrotic syndrome
Minimal change glomerulopathy	9%-16%	Most common cause of primary nephrotic syndrome in children
		May be associated with or secondary to:
		Atopic diseases
		Mononucleosis
		Malignancies: Hodgkin lymphoma and carcinomas
		Medication exposure: NSAIDs; interferon; pamidronate; lithium; rifampin

TNF = tumor necrosis factor.

In secondary FSGS caused by infection or drugs, treatment of the infection or removal of the offending agent may halt progression of the disease and improve symptoms. In obese patients with likely secondary FSGS, weight loss is sometimes associated with a drop in proteinuria, as is the use of ACE inhibitors or angiotensin receptor blockers (ARBs), and is the preferred initial therapy.

Membranous Glomerulopathy
Epidemiology and Pathophysiology
Membranous glomerulopathy (MG) is the most common cause of idiopathic nephrotic syndrome in adult white persons. MG may also be associated with infections (hepatitis B and C, malaria, syphilis), systemic lupus erythematosus, medications (gold salts, NSAIDs), and malignancies (solid tumors, lymphomas). In most patients with idiopathic MG, circulating antibodies directed to podocyte surface antigens

(phospholipase A_2 receptor [PLA_2R]) activate complement and damage the GBM.

Clinical Manifestations
Pathological changes of MG may precede clinical manifestations by months. The clinical presentation of MG is indistinguishable from other causes of the nephrotic syndrome (edema, hypertension, microhematuria), but the propensity to thromboembolic events (particularly renal vein thrombosis) is much higher. Secondary causes should be sought, particularly occult malignancy in older patients.

Diagnosis
Diagnosis of MG is made by kidney biopsy. Light microscopy shows glomerular capillary loops that often appear thickened without any proliferative lesions. Immunofluorescence and electron microscopy show subepithelial immune dense

deposits. Where available, PLA$_2$R antibodies should be measured.

Treatment and Prognosis

Up to one third of patients with idiopathic MG remit spontaneously in 6 to 12 months. Conservative management is appropriate during this period. In patients with idiopathic MG who have persistent disease after 6 to 12 months or who have worsening kidney function or a thromboembolic event, regimens containing alternating glucocorticoids with cyclophosphamide or calcineurin inhibitors (cyclosporine or tacrolimus) may be employed. Other options for relapsing or refractory disease include mycophenolate mofetil, adrenocorticotropic hormone, and the anti–B-cell antibody rituximab. Renal survival is excellent if patients enter remission. In general, older patients, men, and those with heavy, persistent proteinuria and kidney dysfunction are at risk of progression.

Among the secondary causes of MG, treatment of hepatitis B virus infection with antiviral agents has been associated with improvement of proteinuria; glucocorticoids are not of benefit. Similarly, remission of proteinuria may occur with treatment of an associated malignancy or withdrawal of drugs, without needing immunosuppression. Treatment of lupus MG employs immunosuppressive regimens similar to primary MG.

Minimal Change Glomerulopathy

Epidemiology and Pathophysiology

Minimal change glomerulopathy (MCG; also known as minimal change disease) is the most common cause of idiopathic nephrotic syndrome in children and accounts for approximately 10% of cases in adults. Secondary causes of MCG include medications (such as NSAIDs, lithium, pamidronate, and the interferons) and malignancies (such as Hodgkin lymphoma and thymoma). A history of viral respiratory infection, atopy, or immunization preceding the onset of edema may be present. The pathogenesis of MCG is not fully understood but is thought to be related to production of cytokines by immune cells that lead to podocyte dysfunction.

Clinical Manifestations

Patients with MCG typically present with acute onset of edema and weight gain due to fluid retention. Urine protein levels tend to be significantly elevated (urine protein-creatinine ratio typically 5000-10,000 mg/g). Azotemia may occur, especially in older adults. The urine sediment is typically benign with few erythrocytes or erythrocyte casts. Complement levels are normal and serologic test results for systemic disease are negative.

Diagnosis

Diagnosis of MCG is confirmed with kidney biopsy, which shows normal glomeruli on both light and immunofluorescence microscopy. The tubules may show lipid accumulation. On electron microscopy, the GBM is normal with extensive effacement of visceral epithelial foot processes.

Treatment and Prognosis

Patients typically respond to glucocorticoids within 8 to 16 weeks. However, relapse is common, and in up to 40% of patients, the course of MCG is one of remission followed by relapse. For frequently relapsing or glucocorticoid-dependent disease, treatment options include cyclophosphamide, calcineurin inhibitors (tacrolimus or cyclosporine), mycophenolate mofetil, and rituximab. Although uncommon, progressive kidney failure may occur.

Diabetic Nephropathy

Epidemiology and Pathophysiology

Diabetic nephropathy (DN) is the leading cause of ESKD in the United States, accounting for approximately 40% of new patients presenting with kidney failure. Risk factors for developing DN include older age, race (American Indian, Mexican American, and black), poor glycemic control, hypertension, cigarette smoking, and a family history of kidney disease. The strongest clinical indicator for progressive kidney disease is the level of urine albumin. The pathogenesis of DN involves an early phase of hyperfiltration, which is mediated by hyperglycemia-associated elevation of angiotensin levels. This (reversible) phase is followed by a general activation of inflammatory and profibrotic pathways, resulting in laying down of extracellular matrix in all compartments of the kidney, followed by fibrosis and, eventually, ESKD.

From a pathologic standpoint, DN affects every compartment of the kidney. In the glomerulus, there is expansion of the mesangium and thickening of the basement membrane, followed by focal (nodular) sclerosis (the Kimmelstiel-Wilson lesion) then global sclerosis of the glomerulus. Interstitial fibrosis, tubular atrophy with thickened tubular basement membranes, and arteriolosclerosis are also seen.

Clinical Manifestations

Moderately increased albuminuria (formerly known as micro-albuminuria), defined as a urine albumin-creatinine ratio of 30 to 300 mg/g, is typically the first abnormality seen in patients with type 1 and type 2 diabetes. It occurs in approximately 30% of patients after a mean of 5 to 15 years from diagnosis in type 1 and at less predictable intervals in type 2. Overt nephropathy (urine protein-creatinine ratio >300 mg/g) occurs around 10 to 15 years from disease onset in approximately 50% of patients with moderately increased albuminuria and progresses to ESKD in most patients.

Diagnosis

Annual testing for moderately increased albuminuria should begin at the time of diagnosis in type 2 diabetes and 5 years after diagnosis in type 1 diabetes. Kidney biopsy is not indicated unless there is a suspicion of another glomerular disease. However, the presence of findings of another systemic disease, abnormal serologies, acute onset of the nephrotic syndrome or short duration from onset of diabetes to onset of proteinuria, and rapid rate of progression of kidney dysfunction suggest an alternative diagnosis and are indications for kidney biopsy.

Treatment and Prognosis

Achieving targets of glycemic control (hemoglobin A_{1c} <7%) and blood pressure (<140/90 mm Hg, according to the eighth report of the Joint National Committee) has been shown to prevent or delay progression of DN. The use of tighter glycemic (hemoglobin A_{1c} <6.5%) and blood pressure (<130/80 mm Hg) targets is controversial.

In patients who have diabetes with moderately increased albuminuria or severely increased albuminuria (formerly known as macroalbuminuria or overt proteinuria), ACE inhibitors or ARBs have been shown to slow progression. However, overly aggressive inhibition of the renin-angiotensin system, particularly with a combination of direct renin inhibitors/ACE inhibitors/ARBs, has not been shown to improve kidney outcomes and may be associated with hyperkalemia and episodes of acute kidney injury. Because of this, combination therapy is not recommended.

KEY POINTS

- Treatment of idiopathic focal segmental glomerulosclerosis includes glucocorticoids or calcineurin inhibitors, both at the time of initial presentation and for relapsing disease.
- Up to one third of patients with idiopathic membranous glomerulopathy remit spontaneously in 6 to 12 months; conservative management is appropriate during this period.

(Continued)

KEY POINTS *(continued)*

- Patients with minimal change glomerulopathy typically respond to glucocorticoids; for frequently relapsing or glucocorticoid-dependent disease, treatment options include cyclophosphamide, calcineurin inhibitors, mycophenolate mofetil, and rituximab.
- Achieving targets of glycemic control (hemoglobin A_{1c} <7%) and blood pressure (<140/90 mm Hg) has been shown to prevent or delay progression of diabetic nephropathy.
- ACE inhibitors or angiotensin receptor blockers have been shown to slow progression of diabetic nephropathy.

Conditions Associated With the Nephritic Syndrome

See **Table 28** for details on conditions associated with the nephritic syndrome.

Rapidly Progressive Glomerulonephritis
Epidemiology and Pathophysiology

Rapidly progressive glomerulonephritis (RPGN) is a clinical syndrome characterized by evidence of GN with progression to kidney failure within weeks. It represents a clinical pattern of disease that may be associated with any etiology of GN or may be idiopathic. However, RPGN is particularly common with anti-GBM antibody disease (in younger patients) and pauci-immune small-vessel vasculitis (in older patients).

TABLE 28. Conditions Associated With the Nephritic Syndrome		
Condition	**Frequency as a Cause of the Nephritic Syndrome**	**Comments**
Anti–glomerular basement membrane antibody disease	3%	Frequent cause of RPGN
Pauci-immune glomerulonephritis	15%-25%	Frequent cause of RPGN
Immune complex–mediated glomerulonephritis		
IgA nephropathy	25%-30%	Often asymptomatic; rarely causes RPGN
Henoch-Schönlein purpura	—	Often acute onset, occasionally with RPGN
Lupus nephritis[a]	20%	Variably associated with RPGN
Infection-related glomerulonephritis[a]	4%-8%	—
Membranoproliferative glomerulonephritis[a]	6%-10%	Rarely causes RPGN
Cryoglobulinemia[a]	—	Frequent cause of RPGN
Thin basement membrane disease	—	Asymptomatic microhematuria; good prognosis
Hereditary nephritis (also known as Alport syndrome)	—	Chronic and slowly progressive; extrarenal abnormalities involving the eye and cochlea

RPGN = rapidly progressive glomerulonephritis.

[a]Typically associated with low serum complement levels.

CONT.

Clinical Manifestations

Patients with RPGN typically present with the nephritic syndrome and may sometimes be in advanced kidney failure at the time of presentation. Other symptoms and clinical findings related to an underlying cause may also be present, such as systemic signs of vasculitis (arthritis, epistaxis, hemoptysis) or lung hemorrhage (Goodpasture syndrome). Kidney function usually deteriorates rapidly unless treatment is instituted.

Diagnosis

The diagnostic approach to RPGN is similar to that in patients with GN. Testing may indicate the underlying condition. For example, serologic tests may show positivity to ANCA in patients with systemic vasculitis or to anti-GBM antibodies in patients with anti-GBM antibody disease. Chest imaging may show diffuse infiltrates in a patient with pulmonary hemorrhage or nodules in the presence of granulomatosis with polyangiitis (formerly known as Wegener granulomatosis). Definitive diagnosis is made with kidney biopsy, which typically shows glomerular crescents associated with inflammation of glomerular capillaries. The specific diagnosis is made with immunofluorescence microscopy (immune complexes, linear anti-GBM antibody staining, or pauci-immune GN).

Treatment and Prognosis

All patients with RPGN (except those with infection-related GN who are actively infected) should be treated with high-dose intravenous (pulse) glucocorticoids, followed by oral glucocorticoid therapy. Most patients with RPGN also receive cyclophosphamide (oral or intravenous) or rituximab in cases of pauci-immune GN. Plasmapheresis is indicated in the presence of pulmonary hemorrhage or severe kidney failure to remove circulating antibody. Rapid diagnosis is critical; a delay may result in irreversible kidney failure or death from pulmonary hemorrhage. See Anti–Glomerular Basement Membrane Antibody Disease and Pauci-Immune Glomerulonephritis for further details.

Anti-Glomerular Basement Membrane Antibody Disease

Epidemiology and Pathophysiology

Anti-GBM antibody disease is an autoimmune disease caused by antibodies directed against the noncollagenous domain of type IV collagen. These antibodies bind to the GBM, inciting an inflammatory response, damage to the GBM, and the formation of a proliferative and often crescentic glomerulonephritis. The same process can occur with the basement membrane of pulmonary capillaries, leading to pulmonary hemorrhage (known as *Goodpasture syndrome*). Anti-GBM antibody disease accounts for <15% of cases of RPGN.

Clinical Manifestations

Patients with anti-GBM antibody disease present with a nephritic picture. Kidney function may rapidly deteriorate over days to weeks. Patients with pulmonary hemorrhage may have life-threatening respiratory failure with diffuse alveolar infiltrates on chest radiograph.

Diagnosis

In anti-GBM antibody disease, all of the classic features of the nephritic syndrome are usually present at the time of diagnosis. Serologies show normal complement levels and elevated anti-GBM antibody levels. On kidney biopsy, there is a proliferative GN, often with many crescents. There is linear deposition of immunoglobulin (usually IgG) along the GBM by immunofluorescence, but electron microscopy does not show electron-dense deposits.

Treatment and Prognosis

In patients with anti-GBM antibody disease, immunosuppressive therapy with cyclophosphamide and glucocorticoids, combined with daily plasmapheresis to remove circulating anti-GBM antibodies, leads to stabilization or improvement if treated early. The renal prognosis is poor in patients who require dialysis at the time of presentation. Relapses are rare.

Pauci-Immune Glomerulonephritis

See Systemic Vasculitis in MKSAP 17 Rheumatology for more information.

Epidemiology and Pathophysiology

Pauci-immune GN is caused by microscopic vessel vasculitis affecting the kidney, resulting in necrotizing lesions in the glomeruli with few or no immune deposits. The renal lesion may occur with or without systemic vasculitis and is the most common cause of RPGN. Most patients have circulating ANCA directed against neutrophils. Three forms of systemic vasculitis are associated with pauci-immune GN: granulomatosis with polyangiitis (GPA; formerly known as Wegener granulomatosis), with granulomas associated with necrotizing vasculitis; microscopic polyangiitis (MPA), which is similar to GPA but without granulomas; and eosinophilic granulomatosis with polyangiitis (EGPA; formerly known as Churg-Strauss syndrome).

Clinical Manifestations

Kidney manifestations of pauci-immune GN may range from minimal disease with only hematuria to RPGN. Systemic symptoms may be nonspecific, including low-grade fever, myalgia, fatigue, and arthritis. Other clinical manifestations may include leukocytoclastic vasculitis resulting in palpable purpura, as well as pulmonary disease (the spectrum can vary from a nonresolving pulmonary infiltrate to fulminant pulmonary hemorrhage.) Compared with MPA, GPA may manifest with more prominent upper and lower respiratory tract involvement with granulomatous lesions on biopsy, often associated with tissue destruction (saddle nose, tracheal stenosis, hearing loss). Patients with EGPA usually have a history of asthma, pulmonary infiltrates, and eosinophilia.

Diagnosis

More than 80% of patients with MPA or GPA are ANCA positive. GPA is closely associated with proteinase 3 (PR3)-ANCA, whereas MPA is primarily associated with myeloperoxidase (MPO)-ANCA. Up to 10% of patients with GPA and MPA are ANCA negative. Complement levels are normal. Tissue biopsy is required to make the diagnosis, but an empiric decision to begin treatment should be considered in rapidly deteriorating disease. Kidney biopsy shows absent or minimal staining with immunoglobulin (hence the term *pauci-immune*). The spectrum of abnormalities may range from mild focal and segmental GN to a diffuse necrotizing and crescentic GN. There is variable interstitial inflammation (granulomas imply a diagnosis of GPA) and vasculitis of arterioles and venules. Glomerular and interstitial fibrosis accompanies chronic disease.

Treatment and Prognosis

For induction, combination therapy with glucocorticoids and cyclophosphamide, with or without plasmapheresis, has markedly improved kidney and patient survival rates in those with ANCA vasculitis. The anti–B-cell antibody rituximab is equally effective and safer compared with cyclophosphamide in patients with mild-moderate disease. Maintenance regimens using azathioprine, mycophenolate mofetil, or methotrexate have been employed after patients have achieved remission.

Adverse prognostic signs include older age, severe pulmonary involvement, and severe kidney failure at time of presentation.

KEY POINTS

- Rapidly progressive glomerulonephritis is a clinical syndrome characterized by evidence of glomerulonephritis with progression to kidney failure within weeks.
- In patients with anti–glomerular basement membrane antibody disease, cyclophosphamide and glucocorticoids combined with daily plasmapheresis leads to stabilization or improvement if treated early.
- Kidney manifestations of pauci-immune glomerulonephritis may range from minimal disease with only hematuria to rapidly progressive glomerulonephritis; kidney biopsy shows absent or minimal staining with immunoglobulin.

Immune Complex-Mediated Glomerulonephritis
IgA Nephropathy
Epidemiology and Pathophysiology

IgA nephropathy (IgAN) is the most frequent cause of chronic GN, particularly in Asia and Northern Europe, and is rare in people of African descent. IgAN occurs more commonly in men, with a peak occurrence in the second to third decades of life. The pathogenesis of IgAN is thought to involve several sequential events beginning with genetic predisposition to the disease, the occurrence of IgA molecules that are galactose

deficient at the hinge region of the immunoglobulin molecule, and the formation of autoantibodies against the abnormal IgA leading to immune complex formation. Immune complexes with associated inflammatory lesions are seen in the glomeruli in IgAN or in multiple extrarenal sites in IgA vasculitis (Henoch Schönlein purpura).

Clinical Manifestations

In adults, asymptomatic microscopic hematuria with or without proteinuria is the most common presentation of IgAN. Episodic gross hematuria following an upper respiratory tract infection (also known as *synpharyngitic nephritis*) is another classic presentation. Other features of nephritis such as hypertension, edema, and kidney failure with RPGN may occur in the acute phase or in patients with chronic disease.

Diagnosis

No serologic tests are diagnostic of IgAN. Serologic tests for systemic diseases and complement levels are usually normal. Kidney biopsy is required to make the diagnosis. On light microscopy, the most common finding is mesangial proliferation. Occasionally, endocapillary proliferation and crescents may be seen. The finding of IgA deposits as either the dominant or the codominant immunoglobulin on immunofluorescence is the diagnostic criterion for this condition.

Treatment and Prognosis

IgAN is a chronic condition, and many patients have a benign course with a 20-year kidney survival of approximately 75%. Low-risk patients are usually not actively treated and are followed with continued observation. Proteinuria >1000 mg/g, hypertension, kidney dysfunction, and mesangial and endothelial proliferation with tubulointerstitial damage are associated with a worse outcome. Patients with proteinuria and risk factors for progression may benefit from ACE inhibitors or ARBs. A 6-month course of glucocorticoids has also shown benefit in such patients.

IgA Vasculitis (Henoch-Schönlein Purpura)

Henoch-Schönlein purpura (HSP) is an IgA-associated small-vessel vasculitis seen predominantly in children but may occur in adults (see MKSAP 17 Rheumatology, Systemic Vasculitis). Kidney involvement is similar to IgAN, with the typical manifestations of the nephritic syndrome, often with acute kidney injury. Organ involvement may occur concurrently or sequentially. Recurrences, especially during the first year, are common. Diagnosis is confirmed either by finding an IgA-dominant leukocytoclastic vasculitis or by kidney biopsy, which shows lesions similar to IgAN. HSP is typically self-limiting. Some patients with severe abdominal findings are treated with short courses of high-dose glucocorticoids. Patients with severe GN are occasionally treated with immunosuppressive drugs; however, there are no reliable data to gauge efficacy.

Lupus Nephritis

See Systemic Lupus Erythematosus in MKSAP 17 Rheumatology for more information.

Epidemiology and Pathophysiology

Kidney involvement in systemic lupus erythematosus (SLE) is common, and lupus nephritis (LN) is a major source of morbidity. SLE/LN is the archetypal immune complex disease with immune deposits in all areas of the glomerulus. This leads to distinct patterns of histology, which are classified by the International Society of Nephrology into six classes (**Table 29**).

Clinical Manifestations

Patients typically present with extrarenal symptoms of SLE at the time of diagnosis of LN, with active lupus serologies and low complement levels. Occasionally, LN may be the initial manifestation. Patients with class I or II LN may have minimal or no renal findings, and those with classes III and IV present with varying degrees of the nephritic syndrome. Patients with class V LN present predominantly with proteinuria. Class VI is the end stage of long-standing LN. A kidney biopsy is indicated when clinically manifest kidney disease is present (typically proteinuria >500 mg/g and hematuria).

Diagnosis

Serologic tests for SLE, including antinuclear antibodies and anti–double-stranded DNA antibodies, are typically positive. C3 and C4 complement levels are depressed, signifying activation of the classical complement pathway. Kidney biopsy is required to make the diagnosis and classify the lesions of LN (see Table 29). The histologic class and degree of activity and chronicity on biopsy are helpful in guiding therapy.

Treatment and Prognosis

Patients with class I and II lesions require no specific therapy directed at the kidney. Most patients with class III LN and all patients with class IV LN benefit from aggressive combination immunosuppressive therapy. In class V (membranous) LN, the clinical course is generally more benign, and therapy is similar to idiopathic membranous glomerulopathy. Induction therapy for severe proliferative LN (active class III or class IV) includes glucocorticoids with either cyclophosphamide or mycophenolate mofetil. The addition of plasmapheresis has not been shown to improve outcomes. Maintenance therapy with mycophenolate mofetil or azathioprine may be used after the 6-month induction period.

See **Table 30** for more information on the treatment of the specific LN classes.

Infection-Related Glomerulonephritis

Epidemiology and Pathophysiology

In the past, streptococcal infection with nephritogenic strains followed by GN led to the term *postinfectious* or *poststreptococcal GN* (PSGN) being employed. Over the past three decades, however, there has been a shift in the epidemiology of this group of diseases, especially in developed countries. Older adults and immunocompromised patients now constitute a significant proportion of such patients. The sites of infection can be widespread (not just the upper respiratory tract and skin as in PSGN). Nonstreptococcal infection, particularly with *Staphylococcus*, is as or more common than streptococcal infection. Finally, GN can be present at the time of infection (rather than a delay of at least a week after the infection, as in PSGN). The term *infection-related glomerulonephritis* (IRGN), therefore, is more appropriate. Diabetes is a major risk factor for staphylococcal-associated GN, with methicillin-resistant strains more common in such patients. Rarely, coagulase-negative *Staphylococcus* and gram-negative organisms (*Escherichia coli* being the most common) may be associated with GN.

IRGN is an immune complex–mediated disease. The antigen in the immune complex is derived from the infectious agent. After depositing in the subepithelial area (either within preformed immune complexes or as in-situ immune complex formation), complement activation and subsequent recruitment of inflammatory cells occur, leading to a proliferative GN.

Clinical Manifestations

Patients with IRGN clinically present with acute nephritic syndrome. In PSGN, the clinical manifestations typically occur

TABLE 29.	Classification of Lupus Nephritis
Classification	**Comments**
I. Minimal mesangial LN	No renal findings
II. Mesangial proliferative LN	Mild clinical kidney disease; minimally active urine sediment; mild to moderate proteinuria (never nephrotic) but may have active serology
III. Focal proliferative LN, <50% glomeruli involved (active; active and chronic; or chronic)	More active urine sediment changes; often active serology; increased proteinuria (about 25% nephrotic); hypertension may be present; some evolve into class IV pattern; active lesions require treatment, chronic lesions do not
IV. Diffuse proliferative LN (>50% glomeruli involved); all may be with segmental or global involvement (active; active and chronic; or chronic)	Most severe kidney involvement with active urine sediment, hypertension, heavy proteinuria (frequent nephrotic syndrome), and often reduced GFR; serology very active; active lesions require treatment
V. Membranous LN glomerulonephritis	Significant proteinuria (often nephrotic) with less active serology
VI. Advanced sclerosing LN	More than 90% glomerulosclerosis; no treatment prevents kidney failure

GFR = glomerular filtration rate; LN = lupus nephritis.

TABLE 30.   Treatment of Lupus Nephritis

Class/Group	Treatment Recommendation
Class I	Treat as dictated by the extrarenal clinical manifestations of lupus
Class II	Proteinuria <1000 mg/24 h: as dictated by the extrarenal clinical manifestations of lupus
	Proteinuria >3000 mg/24 h with glucocorticoids or calcineurin inhibitors (CNIs)
Class III and IV	For remission induction:
	Initial therapy with glucocorticoids, combined with either cyclophosphamide or mycophenolate mofetil (MMF)
	For maintenance therapy:
	Azathioprine or MMF and low-dose oral glucocorticoids
	CNI with low-dose glucocorticoids in patients who are intolerant of MMF and azathioprine
Class V	For normal kidney function and non-nephrotic-range proteinuria: treat with antiproteinuric and antihypertensive medications, and only treat with glucocorticoids and immunosuppressives as dictated by the extrarenal manifestations of lupus
	For persistent nephrotic proteinuria, glucocorticoids plus an additional immunosuppressive agent: cyclophosphamide, or CNI, or MMF, or azathioprine
Class VI	Glucocorticoids and immunosuppressives only as dictated by the extrarenal manifestations of lupus
Pregnant patients with active disease	Hydroxychloroquine and prednisone are first-line therapy; azathioprine for more serious disease (azathioprine is inactivated by the placenta)

Recommendations from Kidney Disease: Improving Global Outcomes (KDIGO) Glomerulonephritis Work Group. KDIGO Clinical Practice Guideline for Glomerulonephritis. Kidney Inter Suppl. 2012;2:139-274. Copyright, 2012. With permission from Macmillan Publishers, Ltd.

CONT.

after a latent period of 1 to 6 weeks. Staphylococcal GN typically is associated with ongoing infection at the time of development of nephritis. New-onset heart failure can occur in 25% of older patients.

Diagnosis

The diagnosis of IRGN is made on clinical grounds in patients who are nephritic and have an ongoing or preceding infection. A search for infection using microbiologic cultures usually shows the inciting organism in nonstreptococcal GN.

Most patients (especially those with PSGN) show depressed complement levels (usually C3, signifying activation of the alternative complement pathway). In PSGN, antibodies to streptococcal antigens (antistreptolysin-O, anti-DNAse B) are detected in almost all cases.

Adults may need a kidney biopsy to differentiate IRGN from other causes of kidney failure, notably acute interstitial nephritis from antibiotics or toxic acute kidney injury. Kidney biopsy typically shows a diffuse endocapillary proliferative and exudative glomerulonephritis, and, rarely, crescents on light microscopy. Immunofluorescence microscopy reveals C3-dominant or C3-codominant (with IgA or IgG) glomerular staining, which shows large "humps" of immune deposits in a predominant subepithelial distribution on electron microscopy. **H**

Treatment and Prognosis

Treatment of the underlying infection is usually all that is necessary. There are no data to show that immunosuppressive therapy has a role in the treatment of IRGN. Up to 50% of adult patients (especially those with diabetes, older patients, and those with preexisting chronic kidney disease) may have persistent kidney dysfunction or even progress to ESKD.

Membranoproliferative Glomerulonephritis
Epidemiology and Pathophysiology
Membranoproliferative glomerulonephritis (MPGN) refers to the histologic findings of mesangial and endocapillary proliferation combined with the thickening of the GBM. There are two distinct pathophysiologic mechanisms: immune complex deposition (with or without complement staining) and activation of the alternative complement pathway with complement deposition (with minimal immunoglobulin staining) of the glomeruli. Immunoglobulin-mediated MPGN is associated with immune complex disease such as SLE, infections such as hepatitis C, and monoclonal gammopathy. Complement-mediated MPGN includes dense deposit disease (DDD) and C3 glomerulonephritis (C3GN); DDD and C3GN are rare diseases associated with uncontrolled activation of the alternative complement pathway.

Clinical Manifestations
Most patients with idiopathic MPGN are children or young adults who present with proteinuria or the nephrotic syndrome; they may also present with chronic nephritis.

Diagnosis
MPGN is a descriptive diagnosis of the kidney biopsy findings. Unless obvious, a search for the underlying cause should be undertaken. The findings of immunoglobulin (with or without complement staining) on biopsy should prompt a search for infections, autoimmune disease, or monoclonal gammopathy. Serologic tests may show evidence of an underlying infection (such as hepatitis C) or autoimmune disease (such as SLE). Complement levels may be depressed in MPGN, with an intermittently low serum complement level in immunoglobulin-associated MPGN and a reduced C3 level in C3GN and DDD; MPGN with predominant complement staining on biopsy should lead to an investigation of alternative complement pathway disorders.

Treatment and Prognosis

Treatment of the causative infection, autoimmune disease, or monoclonal gammopathy is the primary therapy in patients with MPGN. There is no specific treatment available for the C3 glomerulopathies; immunosuppressive regimens, typically involving tapering doses of glucocorticoids, have been employed with varying results. There is a significant recurrence rate of MPGN in patients with kidney transplants.

Cryoglobulinemia

Cryoglobulins are immune-related proteins that precipitate at temperatures below 37.0 °C (98.6 °F) in vitro that may be associated with a systemic inflammatory syndrome involving small- to medium-vessel vasculitis. There is wide variation in the type of kidney disease associated with cryoglobulinemia depending on the underlying etiology, including glomerulonephritis. See Kidney Manifestations of Gammopathies for more information.

Collagen Type IV-Related Nephropathies

Type IV collagen is an essential component of the GBM. Two genetic diseases affecting type IV collagen, hereditary nephritis (Alport syndrome) and thin basement membrane disease, cause glomerular disease. See Genetic Disorders and Kidney Disease for more information.

KEY POINTS

- Kidney biopsy is required for diagnosis of IgA nephropathy, with the most common finding being mesangial proliferation on light microscopy.
- Kidney biopsy is required to make the diagnosis and classify the lesions of lupus nephritis.
- Most patients with class III lupus nephritis (LN) and all patients with class IV LN benefit from aggressive combination immunosuppressive therapy.
- The diagnosis of infection-related glomerulonephritis is made on clinical grounds in nephritic patients who have an ongoing or preceding infection.
- Immunoglobulin-mediated membranoproliferative glomerulonephritis (MPGN) is associated with immune complex disease; complement-mediated MPGN includes dense deposit disease and C3 glomerulonephritis.

Kidney Manifestations of Gammopathies

Overview

Monoclonal production of protein by lymphocytes or plasma cells is associated with specific kidney disorders that may predominantly involve the glomerular or tubular compartments. There is increasing recognition of kidney diseases associated with clonal disorders that do not fulfill criteria for lymphoma or overt myeloma; these conditions are known as *monoclonal disorders of renal significance*. Kidney manifestations of monoclonal gammopathies may include variable degrees of proteinuria (sometimes the full nephrotic syndrome), tubular dysfunction, hypertension, and kidney failure.

A monoclonal gammopathy is present when serum or urine electrophoresis shows a monoclonal band or if there are abnormalities in the serum free light chain ratio. Diagnosis of kidney involvement in monoclonal gammopathy usually requires biopsy, which shows evidence of immune deposits in glomeruli, the tubulointerstitial compartment, or blood vessels. The pattern of deposition on biopsy, either organized or non-organized, may be diagnostically helpful (**Table 31**).

Management of monoclonal gammopathies with kidney involvement is focused on treatment of the underlying monoclonal disorder to prevent further kidney injury. Therapy for the associated kidney disease is primarily supportive and based on the nature and degree of kidney involvement. Management of other potentially nephrotoxic complications associated with monoclonal gammopathies, including hypercalcemia, hyperuricemia, and volume contraction in patients with multiple myeloma, is an essential component of treatment.

See Multiple Myeloma and Related Disorders in MKSAP 17 Hematology and Oncology for more information.

Amyloidosis

Amyloid consists of randomly oriented fibrils composed of various proteins that form organized β-pleated sheets within the tissues; amyloid resulting from monoclonal lambda or kappa light chains is termed *AL amyloid* (*AA amyloid* results from AA protein, an acute phase reactant seen in chronic inflammatory diseases). In amyloidosis involving the kidney, glomerular lesions tend to be prominent and present with proteinuria, often in the nephrotic range. However, amyloid deposits may also be found in tubular basement membranes, interstitial space, and blood vessels. Findings on biopsy show deposits that stain apple green on Congo red staining under a polarizing microscope; these deposits are also visible on electron microscopy. Primary treatment depends on the type of

TABLE 31. Causes and Patterns of Immune Deposition in Monoclonal Gammopathy

Organized Deposits
AL amyloid
Immunotactoid glomerulonephritis
Fibrillary glomerulonephritis
Cryoglobulinemic glomerulonephritis
Non-Organized Deposits
Monoclonal deposition disease (light chain/heavy chain/both)

amyloidosis, with elimination of the monoclonal protein in AL amyloidosis and treatment of chronic inflammation in AA amyloidosis.

Monoclonal Immunoglobulin Deposition Disease

Monoclonal immunoglobulin deposition disease (MIDD) includes either light chain (kappa in 80% of cases) deposition, heavy chain deposition, or, rarely, both. MIDD is similar to AL amyloidosis as both entities are related to the overproduction and extracellular deposition of monoclonal immunoglobulins. However, the deposits in MIDD are not organized into β-pleated sheets, are Congo red negative, and are granular rather than fibrillar on microscopy.

In the kidney, light or heavy chains may be deposited in the glomerulus, tubule, or both, with the clinical presentation dependent on the sites of involvement. Albuminuria, sometimes with the full nephrotic syndrome, may be accompanied by hypertension and kidney failure.

Multiple Myeloma

Multiple myeloma may present with a variety of kidney manifestations depending on the nature of the monoclonal protein. Most commonly, nephrotoxic light chains are filtered and accumulate in the renal tubule, causing tubular injury and forming casts within the tubules (known as *cast nephropathy* or *myeloma nephropathy*). The risk of tubular injury and cast formation is increased with volume contraction and dehydration.

In some patients, particularly those with "smoldering" myeloma, light chains may be absorbed and crystallize in proximal tubular cells, leading to tubular dysfunction and a secondary Fanconi syndrome. Patients present with chronic kidney disease or acute kidney injury and are found to have renal glycosuria, proximal renal tubular acidosis, and phosphate wasting. Kidney biopsy shows monoclonal proteins in the proximal tubules with a crystalline structure.

Patients with multiple myeloma may also present with AL amyloidosis, which typically presents with significant proteinuria and often normal tubular function. However, other patients may also manifest MIDD with significant proteinuria but also tubular dysfunction and kidney failure.

[H] Cryoglobulinemia

Cryoglobulins are proteins that contain immunoglobulins that precipitate in vitro at temperatures below 37.0 °C (98.6 °F). There are three types: type I (only monoclonal Ig, typically IgM), associated with Waldenström macroglobulinemia or myeloma; type II (usually polyclonal IgG associated with monoclonal IgM), associated with hepatitis C virus infection; and type III (polyclonal IgG and IgM), associated with connective tissue disease and infections, including hepatitis C. Kidney involvement typically occurs more often with type II

cryoglobulins, which form immune complexes leading to a systemic vasculitic syndrome, associated with glomerulonephritis typically with membranoproliferative features.

Patients with cryoglobulinemia may manifest a spectrum of kidney abnormalities, including mild proteinuria and hematuria, the nephrotic syndrome, and rapidly progressive glomerulonephritis with rapid deterioration of kidney function. C4 (and sometimes C3) complement levels are typically low, and rheumatoid factor is positive.

See Systemic Vasculitis in MKSAP 17 Rheumatology for more information. [H]

Fibrillary and Immunotactoid Glomerulonephritis

Fibrillary glomerulonephritis (FGN) and immunotactoid glomerulopathy (ITG) are rare kidney-limited disorders associated with deposition of nonamyloid fibrils in the glomerulus. FGN and ITG may be associated with malignancies, and ITG is more typically associated with a B-cell neoplasm. Treatment of these disorders has not been well investigated due to their rarity.

KEY POINTS

- In amyloidosis involving the kidney, glomerular lesions tend to be prominent and present with proteinuria, often in the nephrotic range.
- Cast nephropathy occurs when nephrotoxic light chains are filtered and accumulate in the renal tubule, causing tubular injury and forming casts within the tubules.
- Patients with cryoglobulinemia may manifest a spectrum of kidney abnormalities, including mild proteinuria and hematuria, the nephrotic syndrome, and rapidly progressive glomerulonephritis with rapid deterioration of kidney function.

Genetic Disorders and Kidney Disease

Cystic Kidney Disorders

Table 32 provides details on cystic kidney disorders, including autosomal dominant polycystic kidney disease, autosomal recessive polycystic kidney disease, tuberous sclerosis complex, and nephronophthisis.

Autosomal Dominant Polycystic Kidney Disease

The hallmark of autosomal dominant polycystic kidney disease (ADPKD) is large kidneys with multiple kidney cysts, with most cysts originating in the renal collecting duct (**Figure 13**). Genetic mutations in *PKD1* and *PKD2* account for approximately 85% and 15% of cases, respectively. These genes code for proteins that regulate differentiation and proliferation of renal

TABLE 32. Cystic Kidney Disorders

Disorder	Inheritance	Gene(s)	Features/Comments
ADPKD	AD	PKD1 PKD2	Most common inherited kidney disorder (5% of ESKD cases); intracranial cerebral aneurysm; mitral valve prolapse; hepatic cysts; diverticulosis
ARPKD	AR	PKHD1	Pediatric; ESKD; hepatic fibrosis; portal hypertension; homozygous mutations cause complete loss of function: severe cystic kidney disease, oligohydramnios, pulmonary hypoplasia, Potter syndrome; no specific therapies
Tuberous sclerosis complex	AD	TSC1 TSC2	Characterized by benign hamartomas (kidney, brain, skin, other organs); epilepsy, brain tumors, developmental delay, autism, and lung disease may also occur; renal angiomyolipomas are common; kidney cysts may develop
Nephronophthisis	AR	Multiple (13)	Most common genetic cause of ESKD in childhood/adolescence; interstitial fibrosis; renal medullary cysts; a renal concentrating defect and/or salt wasting; retinitis pigmentosa; no specific therapies

AD = autosomal dominant; ADPKD = autosomal dominant polycystic kidney disease; AR = autosomal recessive; ARPKD = autosomal recessive polycystic kidney disease; ESKD = end-stage kidney disease.

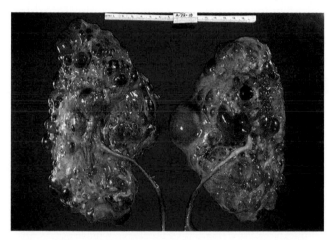

FIGURE 13. Autosomal dominant polycystic kidney disease with multiple bilateral cysts with replacement of the normal smooth architecture of the kidneys.

Image from the CDC Public Health Image Library.

tubular epithelial cells. More than 90% of the inheritance is as an autosomal dominant trait, with spontaneous germline mutations in the remaining cases.

Screening and Diagnosis

Screening for and diagnosis of ADPKD is usually performed by kidney ultrasonography with age-specific criteria. In 15- to 29-year-old at-risk individuals with a family history of ADPKD, the presence of at least two kidney cysts (unilateral or bilateral) is sufficient for diagnosis. Acquired kidney cysts are a common ultrasound finding in older patients without ADPKD, particularly those with chronic kidney disease (CKD). Therefore, in at-risk individuals 30 to 59 years of age, the presence of at least two cysts in each kidney is required for diagnosis; this increases to four cysts in each kidney for those older than 60 years. Conversely, the absence of at least two cysts in each kidney excludes the diagnosis of ADPKD in at-risk individuals between the ages of 30 and 59 years.

Direct mutational analysis of the PKD1 and PKD2 genes is reserved for equivocal cases and/or cases in which a definitive diagnosis is required, such as in living related donors for an affected family member.

Clinical Manifestations

Clinical manifestations of ADPKD include gradual kidney enlargement, which may cause persistent abdominal pain and/or early satiety. ESKD occurs on average at age 54 years in patients with PKD1 mutations and at age 74 years in those with PKD2 mutations. The total kidney volume as measured by MRI and the rate of increase in total kidney volume on serial MRI scans predict the development of ESKD.

Hypertension is common in patients with ADPKD, often preceding CKD. Kidney cyst enlargement leads to stimulation of the intrarenal and circulating renin-angiotensin-aldosterone system (RAAS).

More than 50% of patients with ADPKD develop recurrent flank or back pain; causes include kidney stones, cyst rupture or hemorrhage, or infection. Nephrolithiasis occurs in approximately 20% of patients. Hematuria usually indicates cyst rupture into the collecting system and is commonly self-limited. Hemorrhage into a cyst typically presents with pain rather than hematuria. Cyst infections can present with either positive or negative blood and urine cultures. Cardiovascular disease is the most common cause of death in patients with ADPKD.

Extrarenal manifestations include diverticulosis, hernias, valvular abnormalities (including mitral valve prolapse and aortic regurgitation), pancreatic cysts, and seminal vesicle cysts. Hepatic cysts can be detected by MRI in approximately 80% of patients but have rare clinical sequelae.

A ruptured intracranial cerebral aneurysm (ICA), resulting in a subarachnoid or intracerebral hemorrhage, is the most serious extrarenal complication of ADPKD. ICAs can be detected in 10% to 12% of patients with ADPKD. The prevalence is higher in ADPKD patients with a family history of hemorrhagic stroke or ICA; these patients should undergo screening MR angiography of the cerebral arteries if kidney function is normal, with follow-up scans at regular intervals.

Management

There are no specific therapies for ADPKD. The vasopressin antagonist tolvaptan has been shown to reduce the rate of increase in total kidney size and the rate of glomerular filtration rate loss in ADPKD, likely from blockade of intracellular adenosine monophosphate, which is overproduced in cysts; however, poor tolerance, hepatotoxicity, and expense are barriers to use. A generous fluid intake (>3 L/d) may reduce circulating antidiuretic hormone and thus forestall progression, in addition to reducing the risk of nephrolithiasis.

Patients with hypertension respond well to an ACE inhibitor or angiotensin receptor blocker (ARB), although dual therapy with an ACE inhibitor and ARB has not been shown to be beneficial compared to treatment with an ACE inhibitor alone. Clinical guidelines recommend treatment of patients with hypertension and CKD to a blood pressure <140/90 mm Hg, although some experts recommend <130/80 mm Hg. There is evidence that a lower blood pressure target may result in a slower increase in kidney volume and decreased albumin excretion, but without a definitive improvement of the rate of decline of the glomerular filtration rate. Therefore, the optimal blood pressure target in patients with ADPKD is unclear. Treatment of cyst infection and pyelonephritis requires antibiotics capable of penetrating the cysts, which include fluoroquinolones and trimethoprim-sulfamethoxazole. Finally, all cardiovascular risk factors should be treated.

Tuberous Sclerosis Complex

Tuberous sclerosis complex (TSC) results from mutations in the *TSC1* or *TSC2* genes. The *TSC* genes code for proteins that have a tumor suppressing effect, and disruption of these gene products allows for abnormal cell proliferation in different tissues. Although TSC is most frequently diagnosed in the pediatric patient population, it may be detected first in adulthood when disease is mild.

Renal angiomyolipomas (AMLs) occur in 75% of patients and are detected by CT (**Figure 14**), ultrasonography, or MRI. Renal cell carcinoma is much less common, occurring in 1% to 2% of adults with TSC. Patients with TSC can also develop single or multiple kidney cysts.

Therapy is rarely required for the kidney complications of TSC. Surgery or related interventions (radiofrequency ablation, selective arterial embolization) may be required for large AMLs or hemorrhagic AMLs. The mammalian target of rapamycin (mTOR) inhibitor everolimus is approved for the nonsurgical management of TSC-associated brain tumors and AMLs; however, the role of this and other mTOR

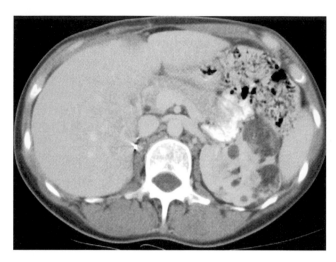

FIGURE 14. CT scan of multiple renal angiomyolipomas. In this CT scan, the kidney has multiple lesions with fat, vascular, and smooth muscle components. The lesions can be isolated lesions predominantly in women or multiple and bilateral in tuberous sclerosis complex with no gender predominance.

inhibitors in the prospective therapy of renal AMLs is unclear.

KEY POINTS

- The hallmark of autosomal dominant polycystic kidney disease is large kidneys with multiple kidney cysts; other manifestations include hypertension, flank or back pain, nephrolithiasis, hematuria, and infection.

- In patients with autosomal dominant polycystic kidney disease, treatment of hypertension using an ACE inhibitor or an angiotensin receptor blocker is appropriate, but the optimal blood pressure target is unclear.

- Kidney manifestations of tuberous sclerosis complex include renal angiomyolipomas and kidney cysts.

Noncystic Kidney Disorders

Table 33 provides details on noncystic kidney disorders, including autosomal dominant interstitial kidney disease, collagen type IV–related nephropathies, hereditary nephrotic syndromes, and Fabry disease.

Collagen Type IV-Related Nephropathies

These disorders involve mutations to the genes coding for type IV collagen. Type IV collagen is a key component of the glomerular basement membrane (GBM) but is also widely distributed in other organs.

Hereditary Nephritis

Hereditary nephritis (also known as Alport syndrome) is a rare cause of ESKD, with a prevalence of 0.4% among adult U.S. patients. There are three genetic variants: X-linked (80%), autosomal recessive (15%), and autosomal dominant (5%). Female carriers variably develop kidney disease

TABLE 33. Noncystic Kidney Disorders

Disorder	Inheritance	Gene(s)	Features/Comments
ADIKD (medullary cystic kidney disease)	AD	*UMOD; REN; MUC*	Rare; medullary cysts may or may not be present; slow progression to ESKD; bland urine sediment; may be associated with gout and anemia
Collagen type IV–related nephropathies			
Hereditary nephritis	X-linked	*COL4A5*	Sensorineural hearing loss; lenticonus (conical deformation of the lens)
	AD or AR	*COL4A3*	Similar phenotype as X-linked with some variability
	AD or AR	*COL4A4*	Similar to *COL4A3*
Thin glomerular basement membrane disease	Primarily AD	*COL4A3; COL4A4*	Also known as benign familial hematuria; microscopic or macroscopic hematuria
Hereditary nephrotic syndromes			
Congenital nephropathy (Finnish type)	AR	*NEPH1; NEPH2*	Severe perinatal nephrotic syndrome; ESKD; kidney transplantation is only treatment
Familial FSGS	AR or AD	*NEPH2; ACTN4; TRPC6*	Nephrotic syndrome; ESKD; should be considered in those with prednisone-resistant FSGS
Denys-Drash syndrome	AR	*WT1*	Cause of pediatric nephrotic syndrome; associated with urogenital abnormalities
Fabry disease	X-linked	*GLA*	Premature coronary artery disease; severe neuropathic pain; telangiectasias; angiokeratomas

AD= autosomal dominant; ADIKD = autosomal dominant interstitial kidney disease; AR = autosomal recessive; ESKD = end-stage kidney disease; FSGS = focal segmental glomerulosclerosis.

depending on activity of the X chromosome in somatic renal cells.

Hereditary nephritis is accompanied by sensorineural hearing loss and characteristic ocular findings. Proteinuria, hypertension, and CKD usually develop over time. ESKD occurs between the late teenage years and the fourth decade of life. Diagnosis is confirmed by kidney biopsy. There are no specific therapies for hereditary nephritis. Antiproteinuric therapy with RAAS inhibitors is a mainstay of management. Kidney transplantation is the optimal treatment for ESKD, with no recurrence in the transplanted kidney.

Thin Glomerular Basement Membrane Disease

Thin glomerular basement membrane disease is associated with type IV collagen abnormalities that cause thinning of the GBM, resulting in hematuria. Up to 5% of the population may

be affected; 30% to 50% of patients have a family history of hematuria. The disease is characterized by microscopic or macroscopic hematuria, which often initially occurs in childhood. Long-term prognosis is excellent, with rare progression to CKD. Blood pressure control with agents to decrease proteinuria is of benefit.

Fabry Disease

Fabry disease is a rare X-linked inherited disorder of α-galactosidase A deficiency, an enzyme deficiency in the glycosphingolipid pathway, leading to progressive deposit of globotriaosylceramide (Gb3) in lysosomes. Fabry disease should be considered as a cause of CKD of unknown etiology in young adulthood.

Diagnosis includes measurement of leukocyte enzymatic activity, with subsequent genetic confirmation. Screening for the disease is recommended for family members of affected patients. Enzyme replacement therapy with recombinant human α-galactosidase A is effective.

KEY POINTS

- Hereditary nephritis (also known as Alport syndrome) is associated with sensorineural hearing loss and lenticonus; proteinuria, hypertension, and chronic kidney disease usually develop over time.

- Thin glomerular basement membrane disease is characterized by microscopic or macroscopic hematuria, which often initially occurs in childhood.

- Fabry disease should be considered as a cause of chronic kidney disease of unknown etiology in young adulthood.

Acute Kidney Injury

Pathophysiology and Epidemiology

Acute kidney injury (AKI) is characterized by rapid loss of kidney function over hours to days, resulting in accumulation of creatinine, urea, and other waste products and/or decreased urine output. It may be associated with sodium and water retention and development of metabolic disturbances. AKI can occur in individuals with previously normal kidney function or in those with preexisting kidney disease.

AKI occurs in approximately 5% to 7% of hospital admissions and up to 30% of ICU admissions. It is associated with significant in-hospital morbidity and mortality. Risk factors include older age, diabetes mellitus, chronic kidney disease (CKD), and states of decreased effective arterial circulation.

Although often reversible, AKI can result in incomplete renal recovery with progression to CKD and end-stage kidney disease (ESKD).

Definition and Classification

The Acute Dialysis Quality Initiative (ADQI) developed the RIFLE (Risk, Injury, Failure, Loss, and ESKD) criteria to standardize the definition of AKI. The Acute Kidney Injury Network (AKIN) modified the RIFLE criteria to include less severe AKI (**Table 34**). Due to the need for a single definition for clinical practice and research, the Kidney Disease Improving Global Outcomes (KDIGO) AKI consensus guidelines combined both classification systems and define AKI as an increase in serum creatinine ≥0.3 mg/dL (26.5 µmol/L) within 48 hours, ≥1.5 times baseline (known to have occurred within the previous 7 days), or urine volume <0.5 mL/kg/h for 6 hours.

AKI can be categorized as prerenal, intrinsic, and postrenal (**Table 35**). Prerenal AKI is caused by hypoperfusion of an otherwise normal kidney; postrenal is caused by obstruction of the urinary tract. Intrinsic AKI is caused by disease of the renal parenchyma.

Clinical Manifestations

Clinical manifestations of AKI depend on the cause and severity. AKI is often asymptomatic until severe loss of kidney function occurs. As a result, mild or moderate AKI is often identified by laboratory studies only. Patients can present with oliguria (urine output <400-500 mL/24 h), anuria (urine output <100 mL/24 h), or no change in urine volume. Patients with severe AKI may present with uremic symptoms, including anorexia, nausea, vomiting, muscle cramps, restless legs syndrome, mental status changes, asterixis, seizures, and

---

TABLE 34. RIFLE and AKIN Criteria for Acute Kidney Injury

	RIFLE[a]		AKIN[a]		Both
Stage	Serum Creatinine Criteria	Stage	Serum Creatinine Criteria		Urine Output Criteria
R	Increase in S_{Cr} of 1.5-fold from baseline or GFR decrease >25%	1	Increase in S_{Cr} of 1.5-fold from baseline or increase in S_{Cr} of ≥0.3 mg/dL (26.5 µmol/L)		<0.5 mL/kg/h for 6 h
I	Increase in S_{Cr} of 2-fold from baseline or GFR decrease >50%	2	Increase in S_{Cr} of 2-fold from baseline		<0.5 mL/kg/h for 12 h
F	Increase in S_{Cr} >3-fold from baseline or GFR decrease >75% or S_{Cr} ≥4.0 mg/dL (353.6 µmol/L) with an acute rise of ≥0.5 mg/dL (44.2 µmol/L)	3	Increase in S_{Cr} >3-fold from baseline or S_{Cr} ≥4.0 mg/dL (353.6 µmol/L) with an acute rise of ≥0.5 mg/dL (44.2 µmol/L)		<0.3 mL/kg/h for 24 h or anuria for 12 h
L	Persistent kidney failure for >4 wk	—	—		—
E	Persistent kidney failure for >3 mo	—	—		—

AKIN = Acute Kidney Injury Network; GFR = glomerular filtration rate; RIFLE = risk (R), injury (I), failure (F), loss (L), end-stage kidney disease (E); S_{Cr} = serum creatinine.

[a]For AKIN, the increase in serum creatinine must occur in <48 hours. For RIFLE, acute kidney injury should be both abrupt (within 1 to 7 days) and sustained (>24 hours). For AKIN, those who receive dialysis are considered to have met the criteria for stage 3.

TABLE 35.	Causes of Acute Kidney Injury
Category	**Examples**
Prerenal	
Volume depletion	Kidney losses
	Gastrointestinal fluid losses
	Hemorrhage
	Burns
Decreased cardiac output (cardiopulmonary syndrome)	Heart failure
	Massive pulmonary embolus
	Acute coronary syndrome
Systemic vasodilation	Sepsis
	Anaphylaxis
	Anesthesia
	Cirrhosis
Intrarenal vasoconstriction	Hypercalcemia
	Drugs (NSAIDs, COX-2 inhibitors, amphotericin B, calcineurin inhibitors, contrast agents)
	Hepatorenal syndrome
Efferent arteriolar vasodilation	Renin inhibitors
	ACE inhibitors
	Angiotensin receptor blockers
Intrinsic	
Acute tubular necrosis	Ischemia (may result from prolonged prerenal AKI causes)
	Drugs (aminoglycosides, vancomycin, amphotericin B, pentamidine, cisplatin, foscarnet, tenofovir, carboplatin, ifosfamide, contrast agents, sucrose, immune globulins, mannitol, hydroxyethyl starch, dextran, NSAIDs)
	Pigment (rhabdomyolysis, intravascular hemolysis)
Acute interstitial nephritis	Drugs (β-lactams, penicillin, fluoroquinolones, sulfonamides, rifampin, NSAIDs, COX-2 inhibitors, proton pump inhibitors, 5-aminosalicylates, indinavir, abacavir, allopurinol, phenytoin, triamterene, Chinese herb nephropathy)
	Infection (pyelonephritis, viral nephritides, leptospiroses, *Legionella*)
	Autoimmune (Sjögren syndrome, sarcoidosis, SLE, IgG4-related disease)
	Malignancy (lymphoma, leukemia, multiple myeloma)
Rapidly progressive glomerulonephritis	ANCA-associated vasculitis
	Anti–glomerular basement membrane antibody disease
	Immune complex glomerulonephritis (SLE, endocarditis, postinfectious, cryoglobulinemia, IgA nephropathy, Henoch-Schönlein purpura)
Vascular	Macrovascular (bilateral renal artery stenosis, bilateral renal vein thrombosis, polyarteritis nodosa, abdominal compartment syndrome)
	Microvascular (atheroembolic disease, HUS, TTP, APLS, HELLP, systemic sclerosis, malignant hypertension, clopidogrel, cyclosporine, tacrolimus, mitomycin, sirolimus, ticlopidine, quinine, gemcitabine)
Intratubular obstruction	Monoclonal gammopathy (multiple myeloma)
Crystals	Tumor lysis syndrome
	Drugs (sulfonamides, triamterene, ciprofloxacin, acyclovir, indinavir, methotrexate, orlistat, large doses of vitamin C, sodium phosphate [oral and enemas])
	Toxins (ethylene glycol)

(Continued on the next page)

TABLE 35. Causes of Acute Kidney Injury *(Continued)*

Category	Examples
Postrenal	
Upper tract obstruction	Nephrolithiasis
	Blood clots
	External compression from tumor, fibrosis, and radiation
Lower tract obstruction	Benign prostatic hyperplasia
	Neurogenic bladder (often related to diabetes mellitus)
	Blood clots
	Cancer
	Urethral stricture

AKI = acute kidney injury; APLS = antiphospholipid antibody syndrome; COX = cyclooxygenase; HELLP = hemolysis, elevated liver enzymes, and low platelets; HUS = hemolytic uremic syndrome; SLE = systemic lupus erythematosus; TTP = thrombotic thrombocytopenic purpura.

CONT.

pericarditis. Patients may also develop symptoms from fluid overload, electrolyte disturbances, anemia, and platelet dysfunction. H

KEY POINTS

- Acute kidney injury occurs in approximately 5% to 7% of hospital admissions and up to 30% of ICU admissions.
- Kidney Disease Improving Global Outcomes acute kidney injury (AKI) consensus guidelines define AKI as an increase in serum creatinine ≥0.3 mg/dL (26.5 µmol/L) within 48 hours, ≥1.5 times baseline (known to have occurred within the previous 7 days), or urine volume <0.5 mL/kg/h for 6 hours.

Diagnosis

The diagnosis of AKI begins with a detailed history, physical examination, and laboratory/imaging studies to determine whether the cause is prerenal, postrenal, or intrinsic. The history includes a review of possible contributing factors of AKI such as the use of diuretics or nephrotoxic medications, predisposing conditions for AKI, and urinary obstructive symptoms. Drug history includes over-the-counter medications, herbal remedies, and recreational drugs. The physical examination focuses on volume status, signs of systemic disease, and evidence of urinary obstruction.

The diagnosis of AKI is primarily determined by increasing levels of blood urea nitrogen (BUN) and serum creatinine (knowledge of previous serum creatinine measurements can distinguish between AKI and CKD). Although useful, these variables can be influenced by nonrenal factors (**Table 36**). Urinalysis, microscopic evaluation of the urine sediment, and urine indices are extremely beneficial in determining the cause of AKI (**Table 37**).

In patients with oliguria, the fractional excretion of sodium (FE_{Na}) can help differentiate between prerenal AKI and acute tubular necrosis (ATN). FE_{Na} is calculated as $(U_{Sodium} \times P_{Cr})/(U_{Cr} \times P_{Sodium}) \times 100$. FE_{Na} <1% indicates prerenal AKI, whereas FE_{Na} >2% indicates ATN. Despite its usefulness, the FE_{Na} has significant limitations. For example, FE_{Na} <1% can be seen in contrast-induced nephropathy, acute interstitial nephritis, rhabdomyolysis, glomerulonephritis, and early obstruction because the tubular handling of sodium is intact in these conditions. Conversely, FE_{Na} may be >2% in patients who are prerenal and are on diuretics or have adrenal insufficiency, bicarbonaturia, or CKD; this is due to the increased distal tubular delivery of sodium in these conditions. In the setting of diuretics, the fractional excretion of urea (FE_{Urea}), calculated as $(U_{Urea} \times P_{Cr})/(U_{Cr} \times P_{Urea}) \times 100$, is more accurate because urea excretion is not promoted by diuretics and is still retained in volume-depleted states. FE_{Urea} <35% is suggestive of a prerenal state. Kidney biopsy should be considered when other causes of AKI are ruled out or when glomerulonephritis is suspected.

Kidney ultrasonography should be performed to rule out obstructive uropathy as the cause of AKI. Additional useful information includes kidney size, echotexture, and renal

TABLE 36. Causes of Elevated Blood Urea Nitrogen and Serum Creatinine Without Acute Kidney Injury

Elevated Blood Urea Nitrogen
Gastrointestinal bleeding
Protein loading, including albumin infusions
Catabolic steroids
Tetracycline antibiotics
Elevated Serum Creatinine
Medications that block creatinine secretion: cimetidine; trimethoprim
Creatine ethyl ester intake
Substances that interfere with creatinine assay: acetoacetate; cefoxitin; flucytosine

TABLE 37. Diagnostic Findings in Acute Kidney Injury

Condition	BUN-Creatinine Ratio	Urine Osmolality (mOsm/kg H_2O)	Urine Sodium (mEq/L)	FE_{Na}	Urinalysis and Microscopy
Prerenal	>20:1	>500	<20	<1%	Specific gravity >1.020; normal or hyaline casts
ATN	10:1	~300	>40	>2%[a]	Specific gravity ~1.010; pigmented granular (muddy brown) casts and tubular epithelial cells
AIN	Variable	Variable, ~300	Variable, >40	Variable, >2% or can be low	Mild proteinuria; leukocytes; erythrocytes; leukocyte casts; eosinophiluria
Acute GN	Variable	Variable, >500	Variable, <20	Variable, <1%	Proteinuria; dysmorphic erythrocytes; erythrocyte casts
Intratubular obstruction	Variable	Variable	Variable	Variable	Crystalluria or Bence-Jones proteinuria
Acute vascular syndromes	Variable	Variable	Variable, >20	Variable	Variable hematuria
Postrenal	>20:1	Variable	Variable, >20	Variable	Variable, bland

AIN = acute interstitial nephritis; ATN = acute tubular necrosis; BUN = blood urea nitrogen; FE_{Na} = fractional excretion of sodium; GN = glomerulonephritis.

[a]FE_{Na} can be low in contrast-induced nephropathy and pigment nephropathy.

vascular status. Decreased kidney size and cortical thickness are characteristic of CKD; however, kidney size can be preserved in patients with long-standing diabetic nephropathy, HIV nephropathy, or amyloidosis. Increased echogenicity is a nonspecific indicator suggestive of renal parenchymal disease that may be useful in differentiating an intrinsic kidney etiology from other potential causes. H

KEY POINTS

- In patients with oliguria, the fractional excretion of sodium (FE_{Na}) can help differentiate between prerenal acute kidney injury (AKI) and acute tubular necrosis (ATN); FE_{Na} <1% indicates prerenal AKI, whereas FE_{Na} >2% indicates ATN.

- In the setting of diuretics, a fractional excretion of urea (FE_{Urea}) <35% can be used to diagnose prerenal acute kidney injury.

- Kidney ultrasonography should be performed to rule out obstructive uropathy as the cause of acute kidney injury.

Causes

Prerenal Acute Kidney Injury

Prerenal AKI (also known as prerenal azotemia) is the most common form of AKI in the outpatient setting (see Table 35). Prerenal AKI results from decreased renal perfusion, leading to a reduction in glomerular filtration rate (GFR) with no structural damage to the kidney. Drugs with antiprostaglandin activity such as NSAIDs or those that block the renin-angiotensin system can interfere with the kidney's ability to autoregulate renal blood flow and can decrease GFR in the setting of volume depletion or decreased effective arterial circulation.

Patients with prerenal AKI may have a history of acute volume loss, heart failure, the nephrotic syndrome, liver disease, acute infection, or recent diuretic or NSAID use. Prerenal AKI laboratory findings are listed in Table 36.

Prerenal AKI and ATN lie along a continuum of renal hypoperfusion, and prolongation of the prerenal state can lead to ATN. Management includes discontinuation of nephrotoxins and treatment of the underlying cause.

KEY POINT

- Management of prerenal acute kidney injury includes discontinuation of nephrotoxins and treatment of the underlying cause.

Intrinsic Kidney Diseases

Intrinsic AKI is categorized by injury to the structural components of the kidney, including the tubules (including intratubular obstruction), glomeruli, and interstitium (see Table 35). The important distinction between intrinsic AKI and pre- and postrenal AKI is the presence of structural injury and the primary cause of kidney dysfunction.

Acute Tubular Necrosis

The most common cause of hospital-acquired AKI is ATN, which represents damage and destruction of the renal tubular epithelial cells, and is most commonly caused by ischemia or toxins. A careful evaluation of hemodynamics, volume status, and physical findings of associated illness can help determine the cause of ATN. Laboratory findings are listed in Table 37 (**Figure 15**).

Treatment of ATN is supportive, with elimination of predisposing factors. Pharmacologic therapies to prevent or treat ATN have been unsuccessful. Acute dialysis may be necessary to support patients through the course of AKI. Renal recovery is dependent upon the severity of the kidney injury and associated comorbid conditions. Nonoliguric ATN represents a lesser degree of injury than oliguric ATN and has a better prognosis. Complete or partial renal recovery of AKI usually occurs within 1 to 4 weeks. Although patients who require dialysis may recover kidney function, the likelihood decreases the longer they require dialysis.

Ischemic Acute Tubular Necrosis
Patients at risk for ischemic ATN include those with prolonged prerenal AKI (see Table 35). Unlike prerenal AKI, the GFR in ischemic ATN does not improve with restoration of renal blood flow. The loss of GFR is attributed to renal vasoconstriction, tubular obstruction from sloughed cellular material, and backleak of glomerular ultrafiltrate across the exposed tubular basement membrane. Ischemic ATN is frequently reversible, but if the ischemia is severe enough to cause cortical necrosis, irreversible injury can occur.

Renal hypoperfusion without hypotension can result in normotensive ischemic ATN when the normal adaptive responses of the kidney to maintain renal perfusion are impaired. Risk factors for impaired renal autoregulation include older age, atherosclerotic or renovascular disease, hypertension, diabetes, CKD, myeloma kidney, and medications such as ACE inhibitors, angiotensin receptor blockers (ARBs), or NSAIDs. Normotensive ischemic ATN should be suspected in high-risk patients who develop AKI when their blood pressures are lowered below their usual levels, even if the levels remain in the normal range.

Drug-Induced Acute Tubular Necrosis
Recognizing drug-induced ATN is important because eliminating the nephrotoxic agent often leads to renal recovery. Incidence increases in older patients and in patients with decreased effective blood volume, CKD, or concomitant nephrotoxin exposure. Drug-induced ATN can result from hemodynamic changes or direct tubular injury. Exposure to hyperosmolar substances such as intravenous immune globulin, mannitol, or hydroxyethyl starch can cause osmotic nephrosis, a form of ATN that is characterized by vacuolization and swelling of the renal proximal tubular cells.

Common causes of drug-induced ATN are listed in Table 35. Contrast agents and calcineurin inhibitors cause AKI through intrarenal vasoconstriction. Aminoglycosides and anticancer drugs such as cisplatin and carboplatin are directly toxic to the proximal tubular epithelial cells and cause nonoliguric ATN 5 to 10 days after therapy. Amphotericin B causes dose-related AKI through intrarenal vasoconstriction and direct toxicity to proximal tubule epithelium. Liposomal amphotericin B formulations may be associated with less nephrotoxicity. Vancomycin nephrotoxicity is associated with high trough vancomycin levels or high vancomycin dose, concomitant nephrotoxic agents, and prolonged therapy.

Pigment Nephropathy
Myoglobin and hemoglobin are heme pigment–containing proteins that can cause AKI. Causes include trauma, metabolic and electrolyte disorders, endocrinopathies, drugs, toxins, seizures, hyperthermia/hypothermia, compartment syndrome, infections, and excessive exercise. Laboratory findings of rhabdomyolysis-induced AKI include hyperkalemia, hyperphosphatemia, hyperuricemia, hypocalcemia, metabolic acidosis, elevated serum creatinine, and elevated muscle enzymes such as creatine kinase (typically >5000 U/L), lactate dehydrogenase (LDH), and aspartate and alanine aminotransferases. The urine dipstick is positive for blood in the absence of erythrocytes. Urine findings include a reddish-brown urine supernatant, myoglobinuria, pigmented granular casts, and FE_{Na} <1%.

Mechanisms of rhabdomyolysis-induced AKI include intravascular volume depletion from fluid sequestration within damaged muscle, renal vasoconstriction, direct and ischemic tubule injury from myoglobin, and tubular obstruction from intraluminal cast formation. Measures to prevent and treat early AKI include aggressive intravenous isotonic fluid resuscitation, correction of the underlying cause, and

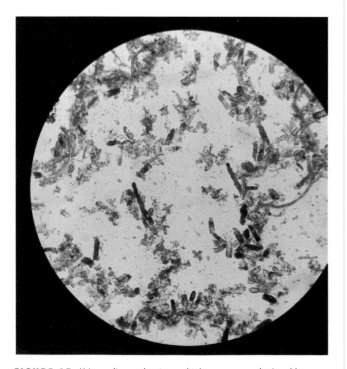

FIGURE 15. Urine sediment showing multiple, coarse granular (muddy brown) casts characteristic of acute tubular necrosis.

CONT.

maintenance of urine output >300 mL/h. Further studies are necessary to establish the effectiveness of bicarbonate and mannitol in AKI prevention. Acute dialysis may be indicated for severe AKI with electrolyte and acid-base abnormalities. Most patients recover kidney function.

Less commonly, heme pigment nephropathy occurs when large amounts of heme pigment are released into the circulation due to massive intravascular hemolysis. ATN associated with this form of pigment nephropathy also results from volume depletion, renal vasoconstriction, direct heme protein–mediated cytotoxicity, and intraluminal cast formation. Laboratory findings include anemia, increased LDH, decreased haptoglobin, and increased serum creatinine. The urine dipstick is positive for blood in the absence of erythrocytes. Other urine findings include pigmented granular casts and hemoglobinuria. Both myoglobinuria and hemoglobinuria can cause tea-colored urine and urine dipstick positive for blood; however, hemoglobin produces a reddish-brown color in centrifuged serum and myoglobin does not discolor the serum. Therapy is supportive, with intravenous isotonic fluids and treatment of the underlying cause.

Acute Interstitial Nephritis

Acute interstitial nephritis (AIN) may be associated with drugs, infection, autoimmune diseases, and malignancy (see Table 35). Only 10% to 30% of patients with AIN have the classic triad of fever, rash, and eosinophilia. Laboratory and urine findings for diagnosing AIN are listed in Table 37. Identification of eosinophiluria by using the Hansel stain supports a diagnosis of AIN but has limited specificity. In general, AIN should be suspected in a patient who presents with an elevated serum creatinine and urinalysis with leukocytes, leukocyte casts, and possibly eosinophiluria. A definitive diagnosis requires kidney biopsy.

Drug-induced AIN is the most common type of AIN and should be considered in any patient with unexplained AKI who has been exposed to a potentially offending drug. Drug-induced AIN is characterized by a slowly increasing serum creatinine 7 to 10 days after exposure; however, it can occur within 1 day of exposure if the patient has been exposed previously. Drug-induced AIN can also occur months after exposure, as seen with NSAIDs and proton pump inhibitors. The mainstay of treatment is discontinuation of the medication with close follow-up. If no improvement in kidney function occurs within 5 to 7 days, a kidney biopsy should be considered. Although the evidence for glucocorticoids is limited, a trial may be beneficial if given early in the course of the disease and if kidney biopsy results show minimal interstitial fibrosis. If drug-induced AIN is recognized early and the drug stopped immediately, complete renal recovery usually occurs. Irreversible interstitial fibrosis develops between 14 to 21 days after exposure to the offending drug. AIN can also result from connective tissue diseases and infections such as *Legionella*, which should be considered in the appropriate context.

Acute Glomerulonephritis

Acute glomerulonephritis and rapidly progressive glomerulonephritis are kidney diseases characterized by immune-mediated damage to the glomerular basement membrane (GBM), mesangium, and capillary endothelium that presents as AKI. Kidney function progressively declines over days to weeks, and irreversible damage occurs without prompt treatment.

Urine findings of dysmorphic erythrocytes and erythrocyte casts are pathognomonic (see Table 37). Serologic assays for hepatitis B and C, cryoglobulins, serum complement, and antistreptolysin O, anti-DNase B, antinuclear, anti–double-stranded DNA, anti-GBM, and ANCA antibodies can aid in the diagnosis. Complement levels are low in lupus nephritis, endocarditis, acute postinfectious glomerulonephritis, and cryoglobulinemia. Kidney biopsy is often needed for definitive diagnosis. Treatment depends on the underlying cause.

See Glomerular Diseases for more information.

Acute Vascular Syndromes

Large- and small-vessel causes of intrinsic AKI include bilateral renal artery obstruction (thrombosis, emboli, dissection, and vasculitis), bilateral renal vein thrombosis, thrombotic microangiopathy, and atheroembolic disease (see Table 35). Renal artery and renal vein thrombosis commonly present with flank pain, elevated serum LDH, and hematuria due to renal infarction. Treatment usually consists of anticoagulation and supportive care.

Polyarteritis nodosa (PAN) is a systemic vasculitis primarily affecting medium-sized arteries at points of bifurcation. Microaneurysm formation with rupture can result in hemorrhage, thrombosis, and organ ischemia or infarction. The kidneys, skin, peripheral nerves, joints, muscles, and gastrointestinal tract are commonly affected. AKI is caused by ischemic changes in the glomeruli and renal artery vasculitis. In some cases, PAN is associated with active hepatitis B or C infection. See Systemic Vasculitis in MKSAP 17 Rheumatology for more information.

Thrombotic microangiopathy (TMA) is characterized by thrombocytopenia, microangiopathic hemolytic anemia, and AKI occurring from endothelial injury and glomerular capillary thrombosis. Typical examples are thrombotic thrombocytopenic purpura, hemolytic uremic syndrome (HUS), malignant hypertension, the antiphospholipid antibody syndrome, scleroderma renal crisis, preeclampsia-eclampsia, the HELLP (hemolysis, elevated liver enzymes, and low platelets) syndrome, and drug-induced TMA (such as some chemotherapeutic agents and the anti-vascular endothelial growth factor inhibitors, bevacizumab and sunitinib). Free hemoglobin and LDH levels are elevated, whereas haptoglobin levels are low. Urine sediment may be bland or demonstrate hematuria and proteinuria. In patients with Shiga toxin–associated HUS, peripheral blood smear is used to determine whether the anemia is caused by a microangiopathic hemolytic process. Treatment is directed toward the underlying disease. Scleroderma renal crisis is a type of TMA characterized by the

CONT.

acute onset of kidney failure and abrupt onset of moderate to severe hypertension. Urine sediment is usually bland or has mild proteinuria, microscopic hematuria, or rarely erythrocyte casts. Treatment consists of gradual blood pressure control with ACE inhibitors.

Atheroembolic disease can cause irreversible AKI. Patients with atherosclerotic disease may develop atheroembolic AKI several days to weeks after manipulation of the aorta or renal arteries during surgery, angiography, or even spontaneously. Plaque rupture with cholesterol embolization to distal small- and medium-sized arteries causes ischemic end-organ damage through mechanical plugging and inflammation. Atheroemboli can affect the skin, muscle, gastrointestinal tract, liver, and central nervous system in addition to the kidneys. Physical findings include livedo reticularis (**Figure 16**), blue toe syndrome (**Figure 17**), ulcerations, and Hollenhorst plaques on funduscopic examination. Laboratory findings include hypocomplementemia, eosinophilia, and eosinophiluria. Urine may be bland or have minimal proteinuria, occasional microscopic hematuria, or erythrocyte casts. Management is supportive, with secondary prevention of cardiovascular disease (hypertension control, statins, and aspirin).

Intratubular Obstruction

Precipitation of protein or crystals within the tubular lumen can cause AKI. Examples include tubular obstruction from

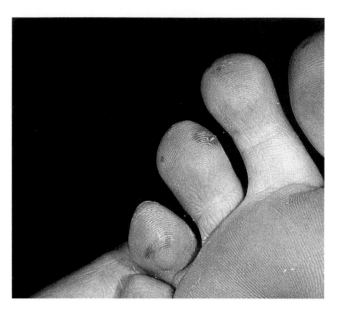

FIGURE 17. Blue toe syndrome presents as a cyanotic toe with necrosis of the skin caused by occlusion of the small vessels from cholesterol emboli as seen in atheroembolic acute kidney injury.

precipitated monoclonal light chains, uric acid from tumor lysis syndrome, calcium oxalate deposition from ethylene glycol, and drugs (see Table 35).

Multiple myeloma can cause several types of kidney disease, with cast nephropathy being the most common form. Cast formation is enhanced by volume depletion, increased urine calcium from hypercalcemia, contrast, NSAIDs, and loop diuretics. The urine is usually bland and the urine dipstick negative or trace positive for protein. The dipstick detects only negatively charged albumin, whereas Bence-Jones proteins are positively charged. The quantification of total protein in the urine leads to the recognition of the discrepancy between the urine dipstick and the actual amount of proteinuria, raising the diagnostic possibility of cast nephropathy. Treatment is directed at treating the myeloma and preventing volume depletion. The role of plasma exchange is controversial. See Kidney Manifestations of Gammopathies for more information.

Ethylene glycol intoxication causes AKI from intratubular precipitation with calcium oxalate crystals, which are often seen on urine microscopy. Ethylene glycol should be suspected in any patient who presents with a high anion gap metabolic acidosis and increased osmolal gap. Treatment includes correction of acidosis, fomepizole, and hemodialysis for severe cases.

Drugs implicated in intratubular obstruction from crystals are listed in Table 35. Hematuria, pyuria, and urine crystals may be present. Predisposing factors include volume depletion, CKD, and changes in urine pH favoring crystal precipitation. AKI is usually reversed after discontinuation of the offending drug. Acute phosphate nephropathy is a potentially irreversible cause of AKI due to oral phosphate–containing bowel preparations. AKI can present weeks to months after

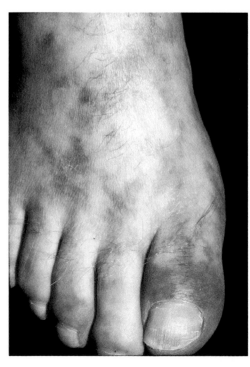

FIGURE 16. Livedo reticularis is a cutaneous reaction pattern that produces a pink, red, or bluish-red, mottled, net-like pattern on the skin. It is caused by slowed blood flow through the superficial cutaneous vasculature and obstruction of capillaries by cholesterol emboli as seen in atheroembolic acute kidney injury. It most commonly affects the lower extremities.

CONT. exposure. Acute phosphate nephropathy causes acute and chronic tubular injury with tubular and interstitial calcium phosphate deposits. Predisposing factors include inadequate hydration, high doses of sodium phosphate, older age, female gender, hypertension, CKD, volume depletion, and use of ACE inhibitors, ARBs, NSAIDs, or diuretics. **H**

KEY POINTS

- Drug-induced acute interstitial nephritis is characterized by a slowly increasing serum creatinine 7 to 10 days after exposure and should be considered in any patient with unexplained acute kidney injury who has been exposed to a potentially offending drug.

- Large- and small-vessel causes of intrinsic acute kidney injury include bilateral renal artery obstruction, bilateral renal vein thrombosis, thrombotic microangiopathy, and atheroembolic disease.

- Intratubular obstruction from precipitated monoclonal light chains, uric acid from tumor lysis syndrome, calcium oxalate deposition from ethylene glycol, and drugs can cause acute kidney injury.

Postrenal Disease

Postrenal AKI results from urinary tract obstruction that is readily reversible if recognized early and corrected promptly (see Table 35). If uncorrected, the elevated tubular pressure can cause CKD and ESKD. Partial or complete obstruction of the urinary tract can occur anywhere from the renal pelvis to the urethral meatus. Obstruction of the upper tract (ureters or renal pelvis) must be bilateral to cause AKI (unless obstruction occurs in a single kidney). Postrenal obstruction should be suspected in patients with a history of benign prostatic hyperplasia, diabetes, nephrolithiasis, abdominal or pelvic surgeries or radiation, pelvic malignancies, or retroperitoneal fibrosis or lymphadenopathy.

The clinical presentation depends upon the site, degree, and rapidity of obstruction. Complete obstruction causes anuria, whereas partial obstruction can present with oliguria, polyuria, unchanged urine output, or fluctuating urine output. Common symptoms of lower tract obstruction include abdominal fullness or pain, urinary frequency, urgency, hesitancy, nocturia, and incomplete voiding. Bladder outlet obstruction (BOO) may reveal a distended bladder on physical examination and should be suspected in patients with prostate enlargement or in the setting of diabetes (neurogenic bladder), pain medications, or anticholinergic medications. Patients with acute ureteral obstruction from nephrolithiasis may present with ureteral colic. In postrenal obstruction, urine sediment is often unremarkable, but microscopic hematuria may be present. Urine chemistries are variable and nondiagnostic (see Table 37).

Evaluation of possible BOO with urinary retention can be diagnosed by a large output of urine volume on bladder catheterization or an elevated postvoid residual bladder volume by ultrasound. Kidney ultrasonography is the modality of choice for diagnosing upper tract obstruction; however, it may not detect early stages of hydronephrosis or obstruction from encasement of the ureter or kidney from retroperitoneal fibrosis or tumor. Noncontrast CT is indicated for suspected nephrolithiasis. Treatment of obstructive uropathy is relief of the obstruction. If the obstruction is relieved within 1 to 2 weeks, recovery of kidney function is excellent. **H**

KEY POINT

- Kidney ultrasonography is the modality of choice for diagnosing upper tract obstruction in patients with postrenal acute kidney injury.

Acute Kidney Injury in Specific Clinical Settings

Contrast-Induced Nephropathy

Contrast-induced nephropathy (CIN) is a common cause of AKI in the hospital setting. Contrast agents are thought to cause ATN through renal vasoconstriction and direct cytotoxicity; however, the mechanisms are not completely understood. Predisposing factors include advanced age, CKD, diabetic nephropathy, conditions of decreased renal perfusion (such as heart failure, hypovolemia, and hemodynamic instability), multiple myeloma, concomitant nephrotoxins, high contrast dose, hyperosmolal contrast agents, and intra-arterial route of administration.

The diagnosis of CIN is based on an increase in the serum creatinine within 24 to 48 hours of contrast exposure. Patients may or may not be oliguric and have coarse granular casts and an FE_{Na} <1%. Patients with CIN typically recover kidney function, with the serum creatinine improving within 3 to 7 days. In high-risk patients, strategies to minimize the development of CIN include intravenous volume expansion with isotonic fluids, use of low- or iso-osmolal contrast media, minimization of contrast volume, and discontinuation of potentially nephrotoxic medications. More recent studies do not support the use of acetylcysteine. Prevention of CIN by dialysis immediately after contrast media administration is not recommended.

Cardiorenal Syndrome

The term *cardiorenal syndrome* (CRS) describes heart and kidney disorders whereby dysfunction in one organ precipitates dysfunction in the other. CRS is characterized by worsening kidney function in the setting of diuretic-resistant heart failure with persistent congestion. CRS is categorized into five types: 1) acute heart failure leading to AKI (CRS1), 2) chronic heart failure leading to CKD, 3) AKI leading to acute heart failure, 4) CKD leading to cardiac dysfunction (heart failure, coronary heart disease, arrhythmias), and 5) systemic conditions leading to simultaneous heart and kidney dysfunction (such as sepsis). Mechanisms of AKI in CRS1 include

CONT.

neurohumoral activation, increased intra-abdominal pressure leading to venous congestion and increased renal venous pressure, reduced renal perfusion, and right ventricular dysfunction.

Management is challenging because treatment of one organ may cause worsening of the other. Treatment is mostly directed toward improving cardiac function with diuretics, ACE inhibitors or ARBs, vasodilators, and inotropes. Many of these medications may worsen kidney function. Ultrafiltration, or the removal of plasma water through an extracorporeal circuit, has been used in patients unresponsive to diuretics; however, current evidence does not support ultrafiltration over intensive diuretic management. Patients presenting with CKD or AKI at presentation of heart failure have an increased mortality.

Hepatorenal Syndrome

Hepatorenal syndrome (HRS) is a reversible form of AKI that occurs in patients with advanced liver cirrhosis or those with fulminant hepatic failure. HRS is characterized by marked reduction in GFR and renal perfusion in the absence of other causes of AKI. AKI in HRS is caused by intense renal vasoconstriction with peripheral arterial vasodilation. Tubular function is preserved with no tubular histologic changes, no proteinuria, normal urine sediment, FE_{Na} <1%, and urine sodium concentration <10 mEq/L (10 mmol/L).

Two subtypes of HRS have been identified based on the rapidity of AKI: type 1 HRS is rapidly progressive AKI defined by the doubling of initial serum creatinine to a level >2.5 mg/dL (221 µmol/L) in <2 weeks, usually with a precipitating event; and type 2 HRS is defined as a more gradual decline in kidney function associated with refractory ascites. Diuretic withdrawal and volume expansion are used to exclude a prerenal cause.

See Hepatorenal Syndrome in MKSAP 17 Gastroenterology and Hepatology for more information.

Tumor Lysis Syndrome

Tumor lysis syndrome (TLS) is characterized by the massive release of uric acid, potassium, and phosphate into the blood from rapid lysis of malignant cells. It is typically seen after initiation of cytotoxic therapy for hematologic malignancies with large tumor burden (such as high-grade lymphomas) or high cell counts (such as acute lymphoblastic leukemia), but TLS can also occur spontaneously. AKI results from intratubular precipitation of uric acid and calcium phosphate crystals. Clinical features include hyperuricemia, hyperkalemia, hyperphosphatemia, and hypocalcemia. General principles for the management of patients at high or intermediate risk for or presenting with TLS are aggressive volume expansion, management of hyperkalemia, and preventive therapy for hyperuricemia. Allopurinol decreases uric acid production, and rasburicase (a recombinant urate oxidase) catalyzes enzymatic oxidation of uric acid into water-soluble allantoin. Rasburicase is usually reserved for those at highest risk; it is contraindicated in patients with glucose-6-phosphate dehydrogenase deficiency because it can induce severe hemolysis and methemoglobinemia. Urine alkalinization in TLS is controversial and can promote calcium phosphate precipitation.

Abdominal Compartment Syndrome

Intra-abdominal hypertension (IAH) is defined as an intra-abdominal pressure (IAP) >12 mm Hg. Abdominal compartment syndrome (ACS) is defined as sustained IAP >20 mm Hg associated with new organ dysfunction. Both IAH and ACS are associated with AKI and increased mortality. ACS occurs in the setting of diminished abdominal wall compliance (abdominal surgery, trauma, prone positioning, respiratory failure, obesity), increased intraluminal contents (gastroparesis, ileus, bowel obstruction), increased intra-abdominal contents (hemoperitoneum, ascites), increased retroperitoneal contents (pancreatitis, retroperitoneal hemorrhage), and capillary leak (secondary to massive fluid resuscitation, coagulopathy, sepsis, burns). Increasing abdominal pressure compresses abdominal viscera and leads to intra-abdominal organ impairment and cardiac, respiratory, and neurologic impairment. Oliguric AKI develops from renal vein and artery compression.

The diagnosis is made by measuring IAP using bladder pressure. Management includes supportive care, management of ascites, correction of positive fluid balance, and abdominal compartment decompression. H

KEY POINTS

- Strategies to minimize the development of contrast-induced nephropathy include intravenous volume expansion with isotonic fluids, use of low- or iso-osmolal contrast media, minimization of contrast volume, and discontinuation of potentially nephrotoxic medications.

- Tumor lysis syndrome is characterized by the massive release of uric acid, potassium, and phosphate into the blood from rapid lysis of malignant cells; management of patients at high or intermediate risk includes aggressive volume expansion, management of hyperkalemia, and preventive therapy for hyperuricemia.

- Abdominal compartment syndrome is defined as sustained intra-abdominal hypertension >20 mm Hg associated with new organ dysfunction; oliguric acute kidney injury develops from renal vein and artery compression in this setting.

Management

General Considerations

Successful management of AKI requires early recognition, correction of the cause, and discontinuation of nephrotoxins. Other supportive measures include optimizing hemodynamics and renal perfusion, preventing further kidney injury, and medically treating complications of AKI. Potassium,

CONT.

magnesium, and phosphate should be restricted. Supplemental bicarbonate can be used to correct metabolic acidosis. Diuretics should be used for volume overload. Nutrition should be managed carefully to ensure adequate caloric and protein intake.

Acute Dialysis

Dialysis is used to control complications of severe AKI. Several specific types of dialysis used in AKI are intermittent hemodialysis (IHD), peritoneal dialysis (PD), continuous renal replacement therapy (CRRT), and hybrid therapies such as prolonged intermittent renal replacement therapy (PIRRT). Absolute indications for dialysis include hyperkalemia, metabolic acidosis, and pulmonary edema refractory to medical therapy; uremic symptoms; uremic pericarditis; and certain drug intoxications.

IHD is delivered 3 to 6 times a week, 3 to 4 hours per session, through a temporary double-lumen hemodialysis catheter inserted into the internal jugular or femoral vein. Advantages of IHD include rapid correction of electrolyte disturbances (such as hyperkalemia) and rapid removal of drug intoxications. The main disadvantage is the risk of hypotension caused by rapid solute and fluid removal.

CRRT is a slow continuous type of dialysis that is delivered 24 hours a day in the ICU for unstable patients. CRRT removes solutes and fluid much more slowly than IHD. As a result, CRRT is used to treat hemodynamically unstable patients who cannot tolerate IHD due to hypotension or in patients in whom IHD cannot adequately control azotemia, acidosis, and volume overload. CRRT often requires anticoagulation.

PIRRT, also known as sustained low-efficiency dialysis (SLED), is slower than IHD and runs for 8 to 12 hours daily. PIRRT combines advantages of both CRRT and IHD: it allows for the improved hemodynamic stability that gradual solute and volume removal provide in CRRT while utilizing the less expensive technology of conventional IHD. PIRRT is an effective alternative to CRRT in hemodynamically unstable patients.

PD is not thought to be as effective as the other RRTs for management of AKI, although direct clinical comparisons are limited. PD may be useful when the other types of dialysis are unavailable or vascular access cannot be obtained. However, PD requires the insertion of a catheter into the peritoneal cavity, which is often complicated by catheter leakage and malfunction. In addition, PD is associated with increased protein losses and is contraindicated in patients with recent abdominal surgery.

Generally, IHD is used for stable patients with AKI, and CRRT or PIRRT for critically ill patients with unstable hemodynamics, multiorgan failure, or high catabolic states. Randomized clinical trials have not shown a benefit of CRRT over IHD or PIRRT for survival or renal recovery. However, CRRT is preferred in patients with acute liver failure and acute brain injury with increased intracranial pressure because rapid fluid and solute shifts in IHD may worsen cerebral edema. **H**

KEY POINT

- In patients with acute kidney injury, absolute indications for dialysis include hyperkalemia, metabolic acidosis, and pulmonary edema refractory to medical therapy; uremic symptoms; uremic pericarditis; and certain drug intoxications.

Kidney Stones
Epidemiology

Kidneys stones are common, with a lifetime incidence between 7% and 13% and a high recurrence rate in the United States. Without treatment, symptomatic nephrolithiasis will recur in 35% to 50% of patients within 5 years and 75% at 20 years. Asymptomatic stones are commonly seen on abdominal imaging and may progress to symptomatic disease in 11% to 32% within 4 years.

Clinical Manifestations

The classic presenting symptom in patients with kidney stones is paroxysmal waxing and waning pain, termed *renal colic*, which usually occurs in the affected flank or back. The pain radiates to the groin, labium, penis, or testicle as the stone travels down the ureter. Kidney stones can produce abdominal pain and symptoms such as nausea, mimicking an acute abdomen.

Diagnosis

On physical examination, patients with kidney stones typically are restless. Although there may be tenderness in the general region of nephrolithiasis, the abdominal examination may be unremarkable.

A complete blood count, complete metabolic profile, and measurement of kidney function are indicated to rule out infection, electrolyte abnormalities, and acute kidney injury. Urinalysis typically reveals hematuria, although the absence of erythrocytes in the urine does not exclude the diagnosis. Urine crystals on microscopy may suggest the chemical composition of the stone, although this finding may not be definitive.

Radiologic imaging is indicated for diagnosis and to guide management based on stone size and location. Plain abdominal radiography has limited utility due to its inability to detect radiolucent uric acid stones and does not provide as much anatomic information as other modalities. However, it may be useful in assessing stone burden in patients with known radiopaque stones. Noncontrast helical CT has traditionally been the most commonly used imaging technique because it detects most stones, provides anatomic information, and visualizes the entire urinary tract; it may also suggest stone composition

CONT.

and potentially provide alternative diagnoses if nephrolithiasis is not detected. However, CT is associated with significant radiation exposure and is contraindicated in pregnant women. Ultrasonography is increasingly being used as an initial diagnostic study. Although less sensitive than CT for nephrolithiasis, particularly for detecting small stones and ureteral stones, ultrasonography does not expose patients to radiation and is usually more readily available and has a lower cost compared with CT; it is also the preferred modality during pregnancy. A positive ultrasound may therefore be adequate for initial diagnosis in patients with a typical presentation for kidney stones, with more complex testing indicated for those with a high clinical suspicion but a nondiagnostic ultrasound or a more complicated clinical presentation. **H**

KEY POINTS

- Noncontrast helical CT is commonly used to evaluate for nephrolithiasis because it detects most stones, provides anatomic information, visualizes the entire urinary tract, may suggest stone composition, and potentially provides alternative diagnoses.

HVC
- Ultrasonography is increasingly being used as an initial diagnostic study for nephrolithiasis due to availability, lack of radiation exposure, and low cost; it is also the preferred modality during pregnancy.

Types of Kidney Stones

Calcium Stones

Approximately 80% of kidney stones contain calcium oxalate, calcium phosphate, or both. Calcium stones are radiopaque on plain radiograph. Hypercalciuria, hyperoxaluria, and hypocitraturia are risk factors for calcium stones.

Hypercalciuria

Hypercalciuria is the most common metabolic risk factor for calcium oxalate stones. In patients with hypercalcemia, increased filtered calcium results in hypercalciuria. However, hypercalciuria is often idiopathic and commonly familial, occurring without associated hypercalcemia.

Hypercalciuria due to hypercalcemia is treated by addressing the cause of increased serum calcium. In patients with other forms of hypercalciuria, thiazide diuretics reduce calcium excretion in the urine by inducing mild hypovolemia, triggering increased proximal sodium reabsorption and passive calcium reabsorption. A low sodium diet enhances the effect thiazides have in promoting calcium reabsorption from the renal tubule. However, restricting dietary calcium intake in patients with hypercalciuria may paradoxically increase the risk of kidney stone formation by causing decreased binding of calcium with oxalate in the gut with increased absorption and excretion of oxalate; therefore, dietary calcium should not be limited unless it is excessive (for example, >2000 mg/d).

Hyperoxaluria

Hyperoxaluria predisposes to calcium oxalate stones and can have several potential causes. Primary hyperoxaluria is a rare inborn error of glyoxylate metabolism resulting in overproduction of oxalate. Excessive dietary oxalate intake (chocolate, spinach, rhubarb, green and black tea) can cause hyperoxaluria. Excessive urinary oxalate may also occur due to significant restriction in dietary calcium intake, which decreases binding of calcium to dietary oxalate in the gut and increases oxalate absorption.

Enteric hyperoxaluria results from malabsorption when excessive free fatty acids in the gastrointestinal lumen bind calcium, increasing free oxalate absorption in the colon. Short bowel syndromes with an intact colon and malabsorptive bariatric procedures (such as Roux-en-Y gastric bypass) are the most common causes of enteric hyperoxaluria.

Avoiding excessive oral intake of oxalate is a primary therapeutic intervention for hyperoxaluria. Specific therapy for enteric hyperoxaluria is oral calcium carbonate or citrate supplementation (up to 4 g/d) to bind intestinal oxalate (the reduction in oxalate absorption counters the potential for increased calcium absorption). Cholestyramine may also be used to decrease oxalate absorption as it binds both oxalate and bile salts in the gut. Patients with primary hyperoxaluria are treated with high-dose pyridoxine.

Hypocitraturia

Urinary citrate inhibits stone formation by binding calcium in the tubular lumen, preventing it from precipitating with oxalate. Hypocitraturia is seen with high animal protein diets and metabolic acidosis from chronic diarrhea, renal tubular acidosis, ureteral diversion, and carbonic anhydrase inhibitors (including seizure medications such as topiramate).

Citrate excretion can be enhanced by alkalinizing the serum with potassium citrate or potassium bicarbonate, which decreases uptake of filtered citrate from the tubular lumen. Increased fruit and vegetable intake also increases citrate excretion, especially in patients who are hypocitraturic.

Struvite Stones

Struvite stones are composed of magnesium ammonium phosphate (struvite) and calcium carbonate-apatite and occur in the presence of urea-splitting bacteria such as *Proteus* or *Klebsiella* in the upper urinary tract. These organisms convert urea to ammonium, which alkalinizes the urine, decreases the solubility of phosphate, and leads to struvite precipitation. Although struvite stones affect less than 10% of patients with kidney stones, they occur more commonly in women and in patients predisposed to chronic or recurrent urinary tract infection, including those with urologic diversions or neurogenic bladder. Struvite stones can rapidly enlarge to fill the entire renal pelvis within weeks to months, taking on a characteristic "staghorn" shape.

Treatment of infections from urea-splitting organisms is the cornerstone of therapy for preventing struvite stone formation. Once struvite stones develop, antibiotic therapy is less effective, particularly for large stones, due to decreased penetration of antimicrobial agents into the stone, allowing for persistent infection and continued stone growth. Surgical stone removal provides definitive therapy.

Uric Acid Stones

Uric acid stones are uncommon (10% of stones), but the incidence increases in hotter, arid climates due to low urine volumes. The main risk factor is low urine pH, which decreases the solubility of uric acid. Hyperuricosuria is not a consistent finding. Comorbid risk factors for uric acid stones include gout, diabetes mellitus, the metabolic syndrome, and chronic diarrhea. Uric acid stones are radiolucent on plain radiograph but are visualized on CT scan or ultrasound.

Preventive measures include maintaining urine output >2 L/24 h and urine alkalinization to a pH of 6.1 to 7.0. Xanthine oxidase inhibitors (such as allopurinol) may be used in patients with hyperuricosuria (>1000 mg/24 h [59 mmol/d]) and patients without hyperuricosuria who have recurrent uric acid stones despite other treatments.

Cystine Stones

Cystine stones occur in cystinuria, a rare autosomal recessive disorder of proximal tubular transport of dibasic amino acids such as cystine. Patients typically present during adolescence, but earlier and later presentations occur. Cystine forms characteristic hexagonal crystals in the urine, and cystine stones can become large and form staghorn calculi. Treatment includes urine alkalinization to increase cystine solubility, dietary sodium and protein restriction to reduce cystine excretion, and thiol-containing agents (penicillamine, tiopronin, captopril) that increase the solubility of cystine.

KEY POINTS

- Hypercalciuria is the most common risk factor for calcium oxalate stones; management includes thiazide diuretics and a low sodium diet.

- Treatment of urea-splitting *Proteus* or *Klebsiella* infections is the cornerstone of therapy for struvite stones, and surgical stone removal provides definitive therapy.

- The main risk factor for uric acid stones is low urine pH; management may involve increased urine volume, urine alkalinization, and xanthine oxidase inhibitors.

Management

Successful management of nephrolithiasis includes risk factor modification, laboratory and radiologic evaluation, dietary changes, and pharmacologic therapy. Referral to nephrology and/or urology may be necessary to treat recurrent or complicated disease.

Acute Management

Acute management of kidney stones includes analgesia, maintenance of adequate hydration, and evaluation for coincident infection. Although most cases may be managed in the ambulatory setting, hospitalization is typically indicated with ureteral obstruction in the presence of urinary tract infection or in a high-risk kidney (solitary or transplanted) or if adequate analgesia cannot be achieved.

Stone collection for chemical analysis is frequently used to guide subsequent therapy. Although there is limited evidence of effectiveness of therapy guided by stone analysis, physiologic and biochemical information suggest that interventions based on stone composition may be helpful in preventing recurrent stone formation. Therefore, it is reasonable to attempt to obtain a stone or its fragments in the acute setting for biochemical analysis.

Stones up to 10 mm can be managed conservatively, although the likelihood of spontaneous passage decreases with increasing size (**Figure 18**). Medical expulsive therapy with α-blocker therapy (such as tamsulosin) or a calcium channel blocker (such as nifedipine) can aid the passage of small stones (≤10 mm in diameter).

Urologic Management

Urgent urologic consultation is indicated for patients with urosepsis, acute kidney injury, anuria, refractory pain, or large stones requiring surgical removal. Complicated cases, including pyelonephritis, bilateral obstruction, and obstruction of a solitary kidney, may require urgent decompression via percutaneous nephrostomy or ureteral stenting depending on the location of the stone and other clinical circumstances. Urologic referral is also indicated for ambulatory patients who do not pass stones with conservative management or who have stones >10 mm in diameter.

Extracorporeal shock wave lithotripsy (ESWL) can be used for stones in the renal pelvis and proximal ureter, but it is less effective for stones located in the mid/distal ureter or the lower pole calyx, larger stones (>15 mm), and hard stones (calcium oxalate monohydrate or cystine). Potential complications of ESWL include incomplete stone fragmentation, kidney injury, and possibly increased blood pressure or new-onset hypertension. Proximal and mid-ureteral stones can also be managed with a percutaneous antegrade approach or retroperitoneal laparoscopy, but these techniques are typically reserved for large, impacted stones.

Ureteroscopy, in which an endoscopic device is introduced in a retrograde fashion into the ureter through the bladder, is most commonly used in the management of mid-ureteral and distal ureteral stones, using a combination of catheter-based stone disintegration methods (such as laser lithotripsy), stone baskets, and ureteral stent placement.

If ESWL and/or ureteroscopy are unsuccessful or if the patient has large complex stones, percutaneous nephrolithotomy may be necessary. Surgical stone removal is the gold standard for staghorn calculi. **H**

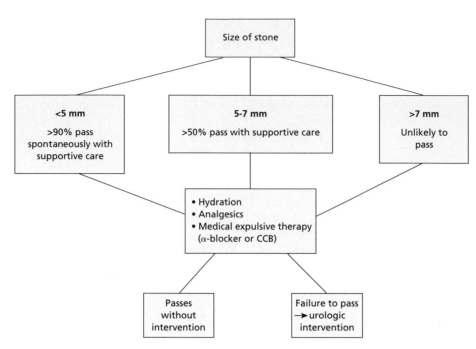

FIGURE 18. Acute management of symptomatic kidney stones. CCB = calcium channel blocker.

TABLE 38.	Prevention Strategies for Nephrolithiasis
Stone Type	**Treatment**
General Stone Advice	
	Fluid intake ≥2 L/d regardless of stone composition; low sodium diet <100 mEq/d (100 mmol/d); age-appropriate calcium intake; consider recommending a low protein diet, 0.8-1 g/kg/d
Calcium[a]	
Idiopathic hypercalciuria	Thiazide diuretics: chlorthalidone, 12.5-25 mg/d, or hydrochlorothiazide, 25 mg twice daily
Hyperoxaluria	All patients: avoid high oxalate foods; reduce soft drink consumption
	Enteric hyperoxaluria: calcium carbonate or citrate, 1-2 g, with meals; cholestyramine, 4 g, with meals
	Primary hyperoxaluria: pyridoxine, 5-20 mg/kg/d
Hypocitraturia	Potassium citrate, 20-30 mEq twice daily; reduce dietary animal protein intake; increase fruit and vegetable intake
Uric Acid	
Urine pH <6.0	Potassium citrate or bicarbonate 40-80 mEq/d (40-80 mmol/d): titrate to urine pH 6.1 to 7.0
Hyperuricosuria	Allopurinol, 100-300 mg/d
Struvite	
Urinary tract infections with urea-splitting organisms	Aggressive treatment of infection; complete removal of stone material
Cystine	
Cystinuria	Potassium citrate or bicarbonate 3-4 mEq/kg/d (3-4 mmol/kg/d) to maintain urine pH >7.0; dietary sodium and protein restriction; chelating agents tiopronin, penicillamine (captopril if hypertension)

[a]The 2014 American College of Physicians Clinical Practice Guideline on the Dietary and Pharmacologic Management to Prevent Recurrent Nephrolithiasis in Adults recommends monotherapy with either a thiazide diuretic, citrate, or allopurinol for patients with calcium composite kidney stones and active disease in which increased fluid intake fails to prevent the recurrence of kidney stones. This recommendation does not apply to patients with hyperparathyroidism or rare causes of nephrolithiasis.

Risk Factor Evaluation and Prevention Strategies

There is evidence that maintaining fluid intake spread throughout the day to achieve at least 2 L of urine per day is effective in reducing the risk of recurrent nephrolithiasis. Less evidence is available for the efficacy of a low protein diet or other dietary interventions to prevent recurrent kidney stones, although they are frequently recommended. There also is evidence that monotherapy with a thiazide diuretic, citrate, or allopurinol is effective in preventing recurrent nephrolithiasis with composite calcium stones if increased fluid intake fails to reduce the formation of stones.

Some clinicians perform a more extensive metabolic evaluation to help guide therapy in patients with recurrent kidney stones or those that occur in the context of an extensive family history of stone disease. If pursued, patients should be instructed to consume their typical diet and level of fluid intake, with at least two 24-hour urine collections to account for dietary variation. Urine collections should include urine volume, pH, creatinine (to assess adequacy of collection), sodium, calcium, phosphate, citrate, oxalate, and uric acid. In the absence of stone analysis, the 24-hour urine results may be suggestive of a particular stone composition but are not definitive.

Prevention strategies for nephrolithiasis are discussed in **Table 38** on page 70.

> **KEY POINTS**
>
> **HVC**
> - For patients with kidney stones ≤10 mm in diameter, conservative management, including analgesia, hydration, and expulsive therapy, may be attempted.
> - Larger stones in the renal pelvis and proximal ureter can be treated with extracorporeal shock wave lithotripsy, whereas mid- and distal ureteral stones can be managed with ureteroscopy.

The Kidney in Pregnancy

Normal Physiologic Changes in Pregnancy

Changes in Hemodynamics

During pregnancy, peripheral vasodilation and loss of response to vasoconstrictive hormones such as angiotensin II and antidiuretic hormone lower blood pressure in the first trimester, reaching maximal effect in the second trimester. Renal sodium and water retention increases plasma volume, which causes increased renal plasma flow and glomerular filtration rate (GFR). Kidney size may increase by up to 1.5 cm. Serum creatinine drops from a normal antepartum value of 0.8 mg/dL (70.7 µmol/L) to 0.5 mg/dL (44.2 µmol/L). Relatively normal serum creatinine levels (>1.0 mg/dL [88.4 µmol/L]) may indicate significant kidney dysfunction.

The increased GFR during pregnancy increases the upper normal limit for proteinuria from 150 mg/24 h to 250 mg/24 h.

Patients with preexisting proteinuria may experience worsening proteinuria during pregnancy that can be difficult to differentiate from preeclampsia.

Changes in the Urinary Tract

The urinary system, including the renal pelvis, calices, and ureters, dilates during pregnancy due to the effects of progesterone or mechanical compression of the ureters at the pelvic brim. These normal physiologic changes may be mistaken for obstruction and take several weeks postpartum to resolve. The dilation increases the risk for ascending pyelonephritis; thus, women should have urine culture screening at the first prenatal visit and be treated for asymptomatic bacteriuria (>100,000 colony-forming units/mL).

Changes in Acid-Base Regulation

Progesterone stimulates the respiratory center during pregnancy, causing hyperventilation and respiratory alkalosis, with an average P_{CO_2} of 30 mm Hg (4.0 kPa) and a serum pH of 7.40 to 7.45. The renal response to hypocapnia is increased bicarbonate excretion, resulting in a serum bicarbonate of 18 to 20 mEq/L (18-20 mmol/L).

Changes in Water Homeostasis

While the plasma volume increases during pregnancy, water retention exceeds the concomitant sodium retention, resulting in mild hypo-osmolality and hyponatremia. The plasma osmolality decreases by 8 to 10 mOsm/kg H_2O, and the serum sodium decreases by 4.0 mEq/L (4.0 mmol/L). These hormonally mediated changes in plasma osmolality and serum sodium do not require therapy. Rarely, women develop gestational diabetes insipidus due to increased metabolism of antidiuretic hormone by the placenta, resulting in polyuria, polydipsia, and hypernatremia.

> **KEY POINTS**
>
> - Pregnancy is associated with increased glomerular filtration rate, decreased serum creatinine, decreased blood pressure, and increased proteinuria.
> - Dilatation of the urinary system during pregnancy increases the risk for ascending pyelonephritis; therefore, urine culture screening and treatment for asymptomatic bacteriuria are appropriate at the first prenatal visit.
> - While the plasma volume increases during pregnancy, water retention exceeds the concomitant sodium retention, resulting in mild hypo-osmolality and hyponatremia.

Hypertension in Pregnancy

Chronic Hypertension

Women with chronic hypertension may experience normal or lower blood pressures during pregnancy. Chronic hypertension may be masked during the first trimester due to the physiologic decrease in blood pressure. Hypertension prior to the 20th week of gestation is most consistent with previously undiagnosed chronic hypertension. Chronic hypertension may be primary (formerly known as essential) or secondary.

The 2013 American College of Obstetricians and Gynecologists (ACOG) guidelines on the management of hypertension in pregnancy recommend treating persistent blood pressure >160/105 mm Hg in women with chronic hypertension or >160/110 mm Hg in women with preeclampsia. Blood pressure goals with medications in chronic hypertension during pregnancy were established at 120-160/80-105 mm Hg. The ACOG guidelines did not establish targets in preeclampsia or gestational hypertension. There is controversy over thresholds for initiating therapy and targets for blood pressure with medications. Evidence of end-organ damage from hypertension (for example, kidney dysfunction, intracranial hemorrhage) may necessitate lower thresholds and targets for blood pressure management. Treatment of milder hypertension (<160/105 mm Hg) during pregnancy is controversial, and benefits of treatment have not been established.

All antihypertensive medications cross the placenta. Some antihypertensive medications are absolutely contraindicated during pregnancy, including ACE inhibitors, angiotensin receptor blockers (ARBs), and, likely, renin inhibitors. Women taking ACE inhibitors or ARBs should be counseled about their teratogenicity throughout all trimesters, and these medications should be stopped if pregnancy is anticipated or possible. There is limited clinical experience with nitroprusside, and its use has been associated with fetal cyanide toxicity. Methyldopa and labetalol have been used safely, although monotherapy with methyldopa may not be sufficient. Although less studied, metoprolol and pindolol have also been used, and atenolol and propranolol may have fetal side effects. Calcium channel blockers (such as long-acting nifedipine) can also be used during pregnancy, whereas diuretics may induce oligohydramnios if initiated during pregnancy.

Gestational Hypertension

Hypertension that develops after 20 weeks of pregnancy without preexisting hypertension, proteinuria, or other end-organ damage is defined as gestational hypertension. Seen in 6% of pregnancies, gestational hypertension resolves within 12 weeks of delivery. Hypertension that persists beyond the 12 weeks is considered chronic hypertension.

Of those who develop gestational hypertension, 15% to 25% progress to preeclampsia, and the rate increases to up to 50% in women who develop hypertension before 30 weeks. Gestational hypertension can recur with subsequent pregnancies and is associated with up to approximately a four-fold increased relative risk for the development of chronic hypertension.

Preeclampsia

Preeclampsia is classically defined as new-onset hypertension with proteinuria (≥300 mg/24 h or a urine protein-creatinine ratio ≥300 mg/g) after 20 weeks of pregnancy. Preeclampsia can also be diagnosed in patients without proteinuria if the hypertension is accompanied by other end-organ damage (**Table 39**). Features of severe preeclampsia include any signs of end-organ damage (excluding proteinuria) or a sustained blood pressure >160/110 mm Hg. Preeclampsia risk factors include preeclampsia with a previous pregnancy, family history, nulliparity, multiple gestations, obesity, chronic kidney disease (CKD), chronic hypertension, diabetes mellitus, and thrombophilia (for example, antiphospholipid antibodies). Eclampsia is the presence of generalized tonic-clonic seizures in women with preeclampsia.

Pathophysiology

The pathophysiology of preeclampsia is complex, as suggested by the multiorgan involvement. Early developmental abnormalities in the placental vasculature result in placental hypoperfusion and increased circulating antiangiogenic factors that result in maternal endothelial dysfunction and end-organ damage.

Clinical Manifestations

Fetal injury (such as growth restriction) and maternal end-organ damage may complicate preeclampsia. Symptoms include headache, altered mental status, visual changes, chest and abdominal pain, and nausea. The HELLP (hemolysis, elevated liver enzymes, low platelets) syndrome may complicate preeclampsia in up to 10% to 20% of cases. The cause of HELLP syndrome is unknown, but it may be related to placental factors. However, it likely represents a separate disorder from preeclampsia.

Prevention and Treatment

Only low-dose aspirin initiated at the end of the first trimester has shown efficacy in preventing preeclampsia. Definitive treatment is delivery, including induction of labor in women at or near term. Severe preeclampsia can be considered an indication for delivery regardless of gestational age given the high

TABLE 39.	Diagnostic Criteria for Preeclampsia
Blood pressure	≥140 mm Hg systolic or ≥90 mm Hg diastolic on two occasions at least 4 hours apart after 20 weeks of pregnancy in a woman with a previously normal blood pressure OR ≥160 mm Hg systolic or ≥110 mm Hg diastolic, hypertension can be confirmed within a short interval (minutes) to facilitate timely antihypertensive therapy
AND	
Proteinuria	≥300 mg/24 h (or this amount extrapolated from a timed collection) OR Urine protein-creatinine ratio ≥300 mg/g OR Dipstick reading of 1+ (used only if other quantitative methods are not available)
OR	
In the absence of proteinuria, new-onset hypertension with the new onset of any of the following:	
Thrombocytopenia	Platelet count <100,000/µL (100 × 10⁹/L)
Kidney dysfunction	Serum creatinine concentration >1.1 mg/dL (97.2 µmol/L) or a doubling of the serum creatinine concentration in the absence of other kidney disease
Impaired liver function	Elevated blood concentrations of liver aminotransaminases to twice the normal concentration
Pulmonary edema	—
Cerebral or visual symptoms	—

With permission from American College of Obstetricians and Gynecologists; Task Force on Hypertension in Pregnancy. Hypertension in pregnancy. Report of the American College of Obstetricians and Gynecologists' Task Force on Hypertension in Pregnancy. Obstet Gynecol. 2013;122(5):1122-31. [PMID: 24150027]

CONT.

risk of maternal morbidity. Women with mild disease and remote from term are managed with maternal and fetal monitoring and antihypertensive therapy as needed. There is no consensus regarding initiation of therapy; however, most experts initiate treatment at blood pressures >150-160/100-110 mm Hg. Antihypertensive medications do not prevent preeclampsia but reduce stroke and heart failure. Intrapartum and postpartum magnesium sulfate is used for seizure prophylaxis in severe preeclampsia but does not reduce the risk of other preeclampsia complications. Close postpartum follow-up of hypertension is recommended. Proteinuria can take months to resolve.

Chronic Kidney Disease in Pregnancy

Women with CKD require preconception counseling because of the greater risk of pregnancy complications such as preeclampsia and declining kidney function when the prepregnancy serum creatinine exceeds 1.4 mg/dL (124 µmol/L). Patients with CKD may develop worsening or new hypertension, increases in chronic proteinuria, and worsening GFR with increasing risk as GFR declines. Patients with more advanced CKD are at risk for worsening CKD and/or acute kidney injury (AKI) requiring dialysis. CKD increases maternal and fetal complications such as gestational hypertension, preterm delivery, preeclampsia, intrauterine growth retardation, and stillbirth. Isolated proteinuria without decreased GFR is also a risk factor for pregnancy complications. Patients with moderate CKD should be advised of the risk of AKI or worsening CKD and the potential need for temporary or permanent dialysis.

Pregnancy is uncommon in dialysis patients because of the more advanced age of many dialysis patients, anovulatory cycles, and comorbid conditions. Diagnosis of pregnancy can be difficult because of elevated β-human chorionic gonadotropin levels due to decreased renal clearance; ultrasonography may be necessary to confirm pregnancy and gestational age. Pregnancy outcomes improve with increased uremic solute clearance through intensive dialysis. Pregnant women on hemodialysis typically receive more than 20 hours of therapy per week on a nearly daily schedule (compared with a three times per week, 9-12 hour/week regimen prior to pregnancy) to maintain blood urea nitrogen levels below 45 to 50 mg/dL (16.1-17.9 mmol/L). Peritoneal dialysis can be technically challenging as the fetus enlarges but can provide adequate clearance with intensified regimens. Additional goals include adequate nutrition, normal electrolytes, blood pressure control, and euvolemia.

Fertility increases after kidney transplantation, although fertility rates remain lower and pregnancy complications higher compared with the general population. Transplant recipients are counseled to wait at least 1 to 2 years after transplant before attempting to conceive. Allograft function (creatinine <1.5 mg/dL [132.6 µmol/L]), immunosuppression regimen, proteinuria (<500 mg/24 h), and other comorbid conditions (such as systemic lupus erythematosus) should be stable prior to conception. Mycophenolate mofetil and sirolimus must be stopped prior to conception due to fetal toxicity. Glucocorticoids, cyclosporine, tacrolimus, and azathioprine have been used during pregnancy. Potential complications from glucocorticoids include infection and adrenal insufficiency.

KEY POINTS

- Women with chronic kidney disease require preconception counseling because of the greater risk of pregnancy complications such as preeclampsia and declining kidney function when the prepregnancy serum creatinine exceeds 1.4 mg/dL (124 µmol/L).

- Kidney transplant recipients should wait at least 1 to 2 years after transplantation and be clinically stable before conception.

- Mycophenolate mofetil and sirolimus must be discontinued prior to conception due to fetal toxicity.

Chronic Kidney Disease
Definition and Staging

Chronic kidney disease (CKD) is defined by the presence of abnormalities of kidney structure or function that persist for >3 months (**Table 40**). The Kidney Disease Improving Global Outcomes (KDIGO) group recently established a definition and staging system for CKD based upon the estimated glomerular

TABLE 40.	Criteria for the Diagnosis of Chronic Kidney Disease[a]
Marker of kidney damage	Moderately increased albuminuria or severely increased albuminuria[b]
	Abnormal urine sediment (such as hematuria)
	Electrolyte or other abnormalities caused by tubular dysfunction
	Histologic abnormalities of the kidney
	Structural kidney abnormalities detected by imaging
	Previous kidney transplantation
AND/OR	
Reduced eGFR	<60 mL/min/1.73 m^2

eGFR = estimated glomerular filtration rate.

[a]Must be present for >3 months.

[b]Moderately increased albuminuria (formerly known as microalbuminuria) is defined as a spot urine albumin-creatinine ratio of 30 to 300 mg/g or a 24-hour excretion of 30 to 300 mg/24 h. Severely increased albuminuria (formerly known as macroalbuminuria) is defined as a spot urine albumin-creatinine ratio of >300 mg/g or a 24-hour excretion of >300 mg/24 h.

filtration rate (eGFR) and albuminuria, with stratification of risk based on these parameters (**Figure 19**). This staging system was designed to improve upon the previously published National Kidney Foundation eGFR-based CKD staging system, which did not incorporate albuminuria quantification. Because

				Persistent albuminuria categories Description and range		
				A1	**A2**	**A3**
				Normal to mildly increased	Moderately increased	Severely increased
				<30 mg/g	30-300 mg/g	>300 mg/g
GFR categories (mL/min/1.73 m^2) Description and range	**G1**	Normal or high	≥90			
	G2	Mildly decreased	60-89			
	G3a	Mildly to moderately decreased	45-59			
	G3b	Moderately to severely decreased	30-44			
	G4	Severely decreased	15-29			
	G5	Kidney failure	<15			

Green: low risk (if no other markers of kidney disease, no CKD); Yellow: moderately increased risk; Orange: high risk; Red: very high risk.

FIGURE 19. KDIGO chronic kidney disease staging system. Prognosis of chronic kidney disease by glomerular filtration rate and albuminuria category. CKD = chronic kidney disease; GFR = glomerular filtration rate; KDIGO = Kidney Disease: Improving Global Outcomes.

eGFR and albuminuria are both associated with mortality, cardiovascular disease, and end-stage kidney disease (ESKD), the KDIGO staging system is better able to identify patients at highest risk of adverse outcomes.

Pathophysiology and Epidemiology

Approximately 7% of U.S. adults over the age of 20 years have an eGFR <60 mL/min/1.73 m^2, and prevalence of CKD increases to 12.3% when those with albuminuria are included. Comorbid conditions associated with increased risk of CKD include diabetes mellitus, hypertension, cardiovascular disease, infection with HIV or hepatitis C, and obesity. The demographic factor most strongly associated with increased risk of CKD is age; 35% of Americans over the age of 60 years have CKD. It is unclear if CKD is more prevalent in black persons; however, CKD is more likely to progress to ESKD in black persons.

The most common causes of ESKD in the United States are diabetic nephropathy (45%), hypertension (29%), and glomerulonephritis (5.5%). After steadily increasing for decades, the incidence of ESKD has recently plateaued. Because mortality of patients with ESKD has been declining, the prevalence of ESKD continues to rise.

Screening

Because patients with CKD are often asymptomatic until the eGFR is <30 mL/min/1.73 m^2 and/or when nephrotic-range proteinuria (>3500 mg/g) develops, most cases are not detected unless patients are screened. However, there is controversy regarding which populations should be screened for CKD. The American College of Physicians (ACP) guidelines recommend against screening for CKD in asymptomatic adults without risk factors for CKD. The guidelines also question the value of screening patients with known risk factors because screening asymptomatic adults for CKD has never been demonstrated to improve clinical outcomes. Moreover, the ACP recommends against testing for proteinuria in patients with or without diabetes who are already taking ACE inhibitors or angiotensin receptor blockers (ARBs) because results would not influence therapy. The United States Preventive Services Task Force (USPSTF) concludes that there is insufficient evidence for screening for CKD in asymptomatic adults. The American Society of Nephrology, however, emphasizes the importance of screening all adults for CKD, including, but not limited to, those with a family history of kidney disease and adults with diabetes, hypertension, or cardiovascular disease.

In patients in whom screening is indicated, a serum creatinine measurement to estimate the GFR and a random urine determination of the albumin-creatinine ratio are recommended.

Clinical Manifestations

As CKD progresses, patients often experience fatigue, worsening signs of volume overload and hypertension, and/or pruritus. When eGFR falls below 10 to 15 mL/min/1.73 m^2 (stage G5), most patients develop more overt symptoms of uremia, including fatigue, anorexia, nausea, vomiting, and confusion (which can progress to delirium and obtundation). Uremia can also induce serositis, especially pericarditis and tamponade.

Diagnosis

Current guidelines suggest staging patients with CKD according to the eGFR and albuminuria (see Figure 19). Establishing the cause is important for guiding treatment and estimating prognosis. The cause may also have important implications with regard to outcomes and management after kidney transplantation.

KEY POINTS

- Chronic kidney disease is defined by the presence of abnormalities of kidney structure or function that persist for >3 months.
- The American College of Physicians recommends against screening for chronic kidney disease (CKD) in asymptomatic adults without risk factors for CKD, whereas the American Society of Nephrology emphasizes the importance of screening all adults for CKD.
- Current guidelines suggest staging patients with chronic kidney disease according to the estimated glomerular filtration rate and albuminuria.

Complications and Management
Cardiovascular Disease

Cardiovascular disease is the most common cause of death in patients with CKD. It has also been increasingly recognized that CKD is one of the strongest risk factors for cardiovascular morbidity and mortality, and the risk increases with decreasing eGFR and increasing albuminuria. Cardiac risk factors should be addressed in patients with CKD. However, many of the landmark studies that underpin the approach for preventing and treating cardiovascular disease excluded patients with CKD (and ESKD in particular) and may not be generalizable to patients with CKD.

Hypertension

Optimal management of hypertension is an important component of evaluating and treating patients with CKD. For patients with CKD, the eighth report from the Joint National Committee (JNC 8) recommends a blood pressure target goal of <140/90 mm Hg, which is higher than the JNC 7 recommendation of <130/80 mm Hg. This change was based on several large clinical trials that failed to show a benefit of a lower blood pressure target on clinical end points. However, in some studies there was a lower risk of a composite kidney failure end point in patients with elevated proteinuria; therefore, some experts still recommend a lower blood pressure goal of <130/80 mm Hg in patients with heavy proteinuria.

The JNC 8 recommends ACE inhibitors or ARBs as first-line therapy for hypertension in most patients with CKD. The JNC 8 recommends that initial therapy in black patients with CKD and proteinuria be with an ACE inhibitor or ARB; in black patients without proteinuria, treatment options include a diuretic, calcium channel blocker, ACE inhibitor, or ARB. Evidence for a beneficial effect of ACE inhibitors or ARBs in slowing CKD progression is limited to patients with albuminuria >300 mg/g (stage A3). See Hypertension for more information.

Dyslipidemia

CKD is most commonly associated with elevated serum triglyceride levels and lower HDL cholesterol levels. LDL cholesterol levels may vary depending upon clinical factors, including nutritional status. Although dyslipidemia is associated with an increased risk of CKD, it is unclear whether treating patients with CKD with lipid-lowering medications prevents CKD progression.

Studies have demonstrated that treatment with statins in patients with an eGFR <60 mL/min/1.73 m^2 (stage G3-G5 not on dialysis) or an eGFR ≥60 mL/min/1.73 m^2 (stage G1-G2) and albuminuria reduces adverse cardiovascular outcomes to a similar or greater extent than in patients with normal kidney function. Current KDIGO guidelines therefore recommend treatment with statins for patients over age 50 years with an eGFR <60 mL/min/1.73 m^2 and/or albuminuria. However, the efficacy of statins in preventing adverse cardiovascular outcomes in patients with ESKD is less clear, with major studies of treating patients on hemodialysis failing to demonstrate a benefit on cardiovascular morbidity or mortality in patients with ESKD with or without diabetes despite control of LDL cholesterol.

Coronary Artery Disease

Patients with CKD have a markedly increased prevalence of coronary artery disease (CAD). This is explained in part by the high prevalence of risk factors such as diabetes or hypertension; however, CKD itself is independently associated with CAD, and the association increases with lower levels of eGFR and higher levels of albuminuria. Despite this excess risk, patients with CKD are paradoxically less likely to be treated for the prevention of CAD. Moreover, patients with CKD are less likely to receive coronary revascularization procedures.

Laboratory studies for the evaluation of CAD must be interpreted with caution in patients with CKD. Reduced GFR may cause decreased clearance of troponins (troponin T in particular) and creatine kinase, leading to false elevation; troponin I is the least likely to be abnormally increased due to CKD. Cardiac enzymes must also be interpreted in the context of the clinical presentation; stable elevations may reflect chronic myocardial injury in uremia, and acute elevations may represent ischemia.

KEY POINTS

- The eighth report from the Joint National Committee (JNC 8) recommends a blood pressure target goal of <140/90 mm Hg for patients with chronic kidney disease (CKD) and ACE inhibitors or angiotensin receptor blockers as first-line therapy for hypertension in most patients with CKD.

- In patients with chronic kidney disease who have an estimated glomerular filtration rate <60 mL/min/1.73 m^2, treatment of dyslipidemia with statins is recommended.

Chronic Kidney Disease-Mineral and Bone Disorder

As kidney function declines, the normal homeostasis of calcium and phosphorus levels by the kidney becomes compromised, resulting in alterations in bone mineralization. The term *chronic kidney disease-mineral and bone disorder* (CKD-MBD) encompasses these changes that commonly occur in patients with CKD. The KDIGO guidelines for the evaluation and management of CKD-MBD are available online at www.kdigo.org.

Calcium and Phosphorus Homeostasis

Calcium and phosphorus homeostasis is regulated primarily by three hormones: parathyroid hormone (PTH), vitamin D, and fibroblast growth factor 23 (FGF-23). FGF-23 is a peptide secreted by osteocytes and osteoclasts and is one of the earliest indicators of CKD-MBD. As the eGFR declines to 30-60 mL/min/1.73 m^2 (stage G3), FGF-23 levels rise, which increases renal phosphorus excretion and helps maintain normal phosphorus levels. However, measurement of this hormone is not routinely done in clinical practice.

Increased FGF-23 and decreased nephron mass reduce the conversion of 25-hydroxy vitamin D to 1,25-dihydroxy vitamin D by renal tubular cells. Reduction in 1,25-dihydroxy vitamin D levels results in lower intestinal absorption of calcium and phosphorus and increased PTH production by the parathyroid glands. Suppression of absorption of calcium and phosphorus in the gut helps mitigate phosphorus retention but contributes to hypocalcemia, especially late in CKD. Hypocalcemia is a potent stimulus for further increases in PTH levels.

Increased plasma PTH occurring as a result of CKD is referred to as *secondary hyperparathyroidism*. Increased PTH levels result in reduced calcium excretion and increased phosphorus excretion by the kidneys and activate osteoclasts, resulting in bone resorption. Early in CKD, the PTH-induced increase in renal phosphorus excretion enables normal phosphorus levels despite reduced renal excretory capacity. However, as CKD progresses, the kidney is unable to compensate for the increased release of phosphorus from bone, and phosphorus levels rise.

This results in a vicious cycle as phosphorus stimulates PTH production. Key factors in the regulation of calcium homeostasis are summarized in **Figure 20**.

Laboratory Abnormalities

Serum calcium and phosphorus levels typically remain in the normal range until the eGFR drops below 20-30 mL/min/1.73 m² (stages G4-G5), at which point the ability of elevated FGF-23 and PTH levels to promote phosphorus excretion becomes overwhelmed and hyperphosphatemia develops. Progressive decline in 1,25-dihydroxy vitamin D levels results in reduced intestinal calcium absorption, and hyperphosphatemia promotes precipitation of calcium and phosphorus in extraskeletal tissues, leading to hypocalcemia.

In addition to reduced conversion of 25-hydroxy vitamin D to 1,25-dihydroxy vitamin D, patients with CKD also have a higher prevalence of 25-hydroxy vitamin D deficiency. KDIGO guidelines state that patients with an eGFR of <60 mL/min/1.73 m² (stage G3-G5) should be screened for 25-hydroxy vitamin D deficiency and supplemented as per guidelines for the general population.

PTH levels are often elevated in patients with an eGFR <60 mL/min/1.73 m² (stage G3-G5) and progressively increase with worsening CKD. KDIGO therefore recommends measuring intact PTH levels in these patients to aid in the detection and management of secondary hyperparathyroidism and its complications.

Vascular Calcification

Numerous studies have documented an increased prevalence of arterial calcification, including the coronary arteries, in patients with CKD; the burden of calcification is highest in patients with ESKD. Arterial calcification reduces vascular compliance and likely contributes to the increased prevalence of left ventricular hypertrophy observed in patients with CKD. Arterial calcification is also strongly associated with cardiovascular and all-cause mortality; KDIGO guidelines therefore suggest treating patients with CKD and arterial calcification as is appropriate for patients in the highest category of cardiovascular risk, although treatments specifically targeted at reducing vascular calcification have not been shown to improve clinical outcomes.

Renal Osteodystrophy

The term *renal osteodystrophy* refers to alteration of bone morphology in patients with CKD, which occurs as part of the systemic disorder of CKD-MBD.

Osteitis Fibrosa Cystica

Osteitis fibrosa cystica is due to abnormally high bone turnover that can occur after prolonged exposure of bone to sustained high levels of PTH in secondary hyperparathyroidism. It is associated with an increased number and activity of osteoblasts and osteoclasts and expansion of osteoid surfaces, resulting in an increased risk of fracture. Patients can be asymptomatic, or they may have bone pain. Classic skeletal changes on radiograph may include subperiosteal resorption of bone, most prominently at the phalanges of the hands.

Adynamic Bone Disease

Adynamic bone disease occurs when there is a lack of bone cell activity and a markedly reduced rate of bone turnover. Histopathologic abnormalities include decreased osteoclast activity with an increase in osteoid, resulting in an increased risk of fracture. Patients have suppressed PTH levels (due to chronic illness or aggressive treatment with vitamin D analogues) and may be asymptomatic or have bone pain. It is important to rule out adynamic bone disease prior to bisphosphonate therapy because these drugs can cause and/or worsen this disease by inhibiting osteoclast activity.

Osteomalacia

Osteomalacia is characterized by decreased mineralization of osteoid at sites of bone turnover. The most common symptoms of osteomalacia include bone pain and tenderness and increased risk of fracture. Although patients with CKD are at increased risk of osteomalacia, CKD does not cause osteomalacia per se, and vitamin D deficiency caused by coexisting factors such as intestinal malabsorption due to gastrointestinal disorders or restricted access to sunlight is often present.

Osteoporosis

Compared with persons with normal kidney function, patients with CKD have many causes of reduced bone density. The diagnosis of osteoporosis therefore cannot be based solely upon reduced bone density detected on dual-energy x-ray

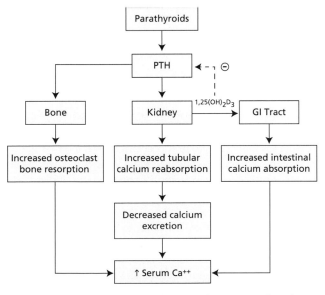

FIGURE 20. Overview of the metabolic systems that maintain calcium homeostasis. PTH stimulates increased 1,25(OH)$_2$D$_3$ synthesis by the kidneys, and 1,25(OH)$_2$D$_3$ causes feedback suppression of PTH production. Ca^{++} = ionized calcium; GI = gastrointestinal; 1,25(OH)$_2$D$_3$ = 1,25-dihydroxy vitamin D$_3$; PTH = parathyroid hormone; ↑ = increased.

absorptiometry (DEXA) scan. Because DEXA has poor predictive value for distinguishing histologic subtypes of bone disease in patients with CKD, KDIGO guidelines do not recommend its routine use in patients with CKD.

Management

In patients with CKD prior to dialysis, the primary goal is to maintain laboratory parameters in the normal range. KDIGO guidelines recommend monitoring calcium, phosphorus, intact PTH, and vitamin D levels in patients with an eGFR <60 mL/min/1.73 m^2 (stages G3-G5).

The approach to managing secondary hyperparathyroidism differs depending upon CKD stage. In patients with an eGFR <60 mL/min/1.73 m^2 not on dialysis, KDIGO guidelines suggest attempting to normalize PTH. The first step in managing secondary hyperparathyroidism is to correct 25-hydroxy vitamin D deficiency and normalize the serum calcium and phosphorus, thus eliminating the stimulus for PTH secretion. If PTH levels remain elevated after correction of 25-hydroxy vitamin D deficiency, calcitriol or calcitriol analogues can be used to further suppress PTH, but monitoring for hyperphosphatemia and/or hypercalcemia due to increased absorption of phosphorus and calcium is necessary. Although KDIGO guidelines suggest attempts to normalize PTH in patients with CKD not on dialysis, it is unclear if this approach improves clinical outcomes. The approach to secondary hyperparathyroidism differs somewhat in patients with ESKD on dialysis. Tertiary hyperparathyroidism is the result of the prolonged PTH stimulation needed to maintain normocalcemia. This prolonged stimulation results in increased calcium levels and severe hyperparathyroid hyperplasia and elevated PTH levels that do not respond to phosphate binders and calcitriol therapy. These patients often require parathyroidectomy for definitive treatment. Further information can be found at www.kdigo.org.

Hyperphosphatemia is an important complication in patients with an eGFR <30 mL/min/1.73 m^2, and the severity is directly associated with mortality. Patients with CKD and hyperphosphatemia should be counseled regarding a low phosphate diet, and most patients require phosphate binders.

KEY POINTS

- The first step in managing secondary hyperparathyroidism is to correct 25-hydroxy vitamin D deficiency and normalize the serum calcium and phosphorus, thus eliminating the stimulus for parathyroid hormone secretion.

- Tertiary hyperparathyroidism is the result of the prolonged parathyroid hormone (PTH) stimulation, resulting in increased calcium levels and severe hyperparathyroid hyperplasia and elevated PTH levels that do not respond to phosphate binders and calcitriol therapy; these patients often require parathyroidectomy.

Anemia

The prevalence of anemia increases as CKD progresses due to several factors, including impaired erythropoietin production, erythropoietin resistance, and reduced erythrocyte life span. Iron deficiency may contribute to erythropoietin resistance. Even if patients do not meet criteria for iron deficiency anemia, it is important to optimize iron stores to maximize the response to endogenous erythropoietin. KDIGO recommendations suggest maintaining transferrin saturation levels of >30% and serum ferritin levels of >500 ng/mL (500 μg/L) using either oral or intravenous iron supplementation.

Initial evaluation for the cause of anemia in patients with CKD includes laboratory studies as would be appropriate for patients without CKD. CKD-related anemia is normocytic. CKD as a cause of a normocytic anemia is a diagnosis of exclusion. There is no specific test to establish the diagnosis. Although erythropoietin levels are often decreased in patients with CKD, there is little evidence to support the utility of measuring erythropoietin levels in patients with CKD.

As the eGFR declines below 30 mL/min/1.73 m^2 (stages G4-G5), anemia can become symptomatic. Erythropoiesis-stimulating agents (ESAs) are highly effective in raising hemoglobin concentrations and alleviating symptoms. Although the use of ESAs can avoid the need for transfusion, the optimal strategy for ESA dosing that balances benefits and risks is unknown. These medications are associated with risks and are expensive. Black box warnings for use of ESAs include the risk of increased mortality and/or tumor progression in patients with active malignancy, increased risk of thromboembolic events for postsurgical patients not on anticoagulant therapy, and increased risk of serious cardiovascular events when ESAs are administered to patients with hemoglobin values >11 g/dL (110 g/L) or history of stroke. It is unknown whether these adverse effects are due to the increased hemoglobin or due to direct effects of high ESA doses. Full KDIGO guidelines for the diagnosis and management of CKD-related anemia can be found at www.kdigo.org.

Metabolic Acidosis

Metabolic acidosis is a common and important complication of CKD that occurs due to progressive loss of the ability of the kidneys to regenerate bicarbonate. Large observational studies have demonstrated a strong association between lower bicarbonate levels and adverse clinical outcomes, including CKD progression and mortality. Recent prospective trials have demonstrated slower progression of CKD in patients treated with alkali to increase serum bicarbonate to at least 23 mEq/L (23 mmol/L). For this reason, KDIGO guidelines now suggest treatment of patients with CKD with alkali to maintain serum bicarbonate in the normal range (23-28 mEq/L [23-28 mmol/L]). However, excessive alkali supplementation above the normal range may also be associated with adverse outcomes with metabolic alkalosis. The most common alkali formulations prescribed are sodium bicarbonate and sodium citrate (citrate is metabolized to bicarbonate). Patients with

CKD who are treated with alkali should be monitored for symptoms of volume overload.

Nephrotoxins

Patients with CKD are at increased risk of acute kidney injury (AKI), and AKI or more indolent kidney injury may promote irreversible CKD progression. The use of potential nephrotoxins should therefore be minimized or avoided in patients with CKD. Patients with CKD should also be counseled to avoid over-the-counter medications such as NSAIDs and to seek medical advice before taking nutritional or herbal preparations because such agents may adversely affect kidney function, can be nephrotoxic, and/or have other harmful effects (Table 41). The use of contrast agents in patients with CKD is discussed in the Imaging section of Special Considerations.

Proteinuria

The severity of proteinuria is strongly associated with adverse clinical outcomes, including progression of CKD to ESKD, cardiovascular morbidity, and mortality. Several large prospective randomized controlled studies have demonstrated that ACE inhibitors or ARBs decrease proteinuria and slow the progression of proteinuric kidney diseases. However, there is substantial evidence that using ACE inhibitors, ARBs, or renin inhibitors in combination to treat patients with CKD and proteinuria does not improve clinical outcomes and is associated with increased risk of hypotension and hyperkalemia.

Protein Restriction

Protein-restricted diets have been shown to slow the progression of kidney disease in animal models. The mechanism is thought to be due at least in part to reduced glomerular filtration pressure, preventing progressive injury and fibrosis. In the Modification of Diet in Renal Disease study, no definitive benefit was seen in renal outcomes in patients randomly assigned to the low protein (0.6 g/kg/d) group.

Although there is insufficient evidence to recommend routine use of low protein diets to slow progression of CKD, high protein diets may precipitate or exacerbate symptoms of uremia. Small studies suggest that low protein diets might delay the onset of symptomatic uremia and the need for renal replacement therapy in selected patients.

KEY POINTS

- Chronic kidney disease as a cause of a normocytic anemia is a diagnosis of exclusion; erythropoietin levels are not diagnostic.
- Erythropoiesis-stimulating agents are associated with an increased risk of serious cardiovascular events when administered to patients with hemoglobin values ≥11 g/dL (110 g/L) or a history of stroke.
- Metabolic acidosis in patients with chronic kidney disease should be treated with alkali to maintain serum bicarbonate in the normal range.
- ACE inhibitors or angiotensin receptor blockers slow progression of chronic kidney disease in patients with proteinuria.

Special Considerations

Imaging

Important risk factors for AKI due to contrast, known as contrast-induced nephropathy (CIN), include severity of CKD, reduced renal perfusion (due to poor cardiac function or

TABLE 41.	Over-the-Counter Medications to Avoid or Use With Great Caution in Chronic Kidney Disease	
Class	**Medication/Supplement**	**Adverse Effect(s)**
Analgesics	NSAIDs (including COX-2 inhibitors)	AKI; hyperkalemia; increased blood pressure
Vasoconstricting decongestants	Pseudoephedrine; ephedrine; phenylephrine; oxymetazoline	Increased blood pressure
Laxatives	Magnesium hydroxide	Hypermagnesemia
	Sodium phosphate (oral or enema)	Hyperphosphatemia
Antacids	Aluminum hydroxide	Aluminum toxicity; osteomalacia
	Magnesium hydroxide	Hypermagnesemia
	Sucralfate	Aluminum toxicity
Nutritional supplements	Creatine	Fluid overload; factitious increase in creatinine; AKI (rarely)
	Germanium	AKI
	Salt substitutes	Hyperkalemia
Herbal remedies	Aristolochia/aristolochic acid	AKI; chronic tubulointerstitial fibrosis
	Ephedra (ma huang)	Increased blood pressure; myocardial infarction; stroke; AKI

AKI = acute kidney injury; COX = cyclooxygenase.

CONT.

volume depletion), higher dose of contrast, use of early generation high osmolar ionic contrast, repeated doses of contrast, and concomitant use of NSAIDs. The most effective ways to prevent CIN are to avoid contrast by using alternative studies and to correct all modifiable risk factors. Patients with CKD should receive intravenous hydration with isotonic saline or bicarbonate-containing solutions before and after receiving contrast. Although the risk of CIN is clearly increased in patients with CKD, risks and benefits should be judged on a case-by-case basis. See Acute Kidney Injury for more information on CIN.

Gadolinium-containing MRI contrast agents are associated with the risk of nephrogenic systemic fibrosis (NSF) in patients with CKD. NSF is characterized by hardened and thickened skin on the trunk and the extremities, along with widening and fibrosis of the dermis and infiltration with CD34 fibrocytes on skin biopsy. Although most cases have occurred in patients with ESKD, isolated cases have been reported in patients with AKI, cirrhosis, or CKD not on dialysis. Therefore, gadolinium contrast must be avoided in patients with an eGFR <30 mL/min/1.73 m^2 unless there is a compelling clinical indication with informed patient consent. If gadolinium is used, prior nephrology consult should be obtained to assess risks of gadolinium administration and guide the use of dialysis in advanced CKD and ESKD. See MKSAP 17 Dermatology for more information on NSF. H

Vaccination

Patients with CKD are at increased risk of infections that can be prevented by vaccination; however, these patients also have impaired immune responses to vaccines. Patients with CKD should receive vaccinations according to guidelines with a few exceptions. Current Centers for Disease Control (CDC) guidelines state that vaccinations in patients with CKD may be more effective when performed before the need for chronic dialysis or kidney transplantation. All susceptible patients with CKD should be vaccinated against hepatitis B virus. Patients with CKD should also receive the 23- and 13-valent pneumococcal vaccines, with revaccination with the 23-valent vaccine after a minimum of 5 years. The influenza vaccine should be administered annually to patients with CKD; importantly, these patients should only receive the inactivated influenza vaccine due to the risks associated with the live vaccine in immunocompromised patients. More information on vaccinations is available at http://itunes.apple.com/us/app/acp-immunization-advisor/id503636536.

Vascular Access

Patients with progressive or severe CKD may ultimately require renal replacement therapy with hemodialysis; vascular access is therefore a major clinical consideration in these patients. Patients who receive hemodialysis via an arteriovenous fistula (AVF) have superior clinical outcomes and fewer vascular complications or episodes of infection compared with arteriovenous grafts (AVGs) or catheters. Therefore, great care should be taken to protect peripheral veins in patients with CKD from venipuncture-induced trauma. Specific measures to protect peripheral veins include restricting phlebotomy, limiting intravenous (IV) catheter sites to hands, and protecting the nondominant arm for possible AVF placement. Because AVF placement can be technically challenging and may require several months for full maturation, referral to an experienced surgeon many months before dialysis is critical.

It is important to avoid peripherally inserted central venous catheters and subclavian catheters on either side due to the risk of sclerosis of peripheral veins and subclavian stenosis in patients at risk of developing ESKD.

In patients with ESKD on dialysis, it is critical to protect the arm with an existing AVF or AVG against trauma from blood pressure measurements, venipuncture, or other procedures. Other veins in the arms should also be protected in case they are needed for future vascular access.

Older Patients

CKD is highly prevalent in the older population, and the incidence of dialysis initiation is increasing most rapidly among patients over the age of 75 years. Management of CKD can be complicated by the high burden of comorbidities; interdisciplinary coordination of care is therefore essential. Particular care needs to be taken when evaluating older patients with impending ESKD. Decisions regarding initiation of renal replacement therapy and/or referral for evaluation for kidney transplantation in an older patient with impending ESKD must take into account comorbid medical conditions, functional status, expected outcomes, and patient preferences regarding goals of care. H

KEY POINTS

- Gadolinium-containing MRI contrast agents are associated with the risk of nephrogenic systemic fibrosis and should be avoided in patients with an estimated glomerular filtration rate <30 mL/min/1.73 m^2.
- The incidence of dialysis initiation is increasing most rapidly among patients over the age of 75 years; decisions regarding initiation of renal replacement therapy in an older patient with impending end-stage kidney disease must take into account comorbid medical conditions, functional status, expected outcomes, and patient preferences regarding goals of care.

HVC

End-Stage Kidney Disease

Although declining in recent years, mortality for U.S. patients initiating dialysis is approximately 10 times higher than for age-matched controls. The most common causes of death in patients with ESKD are cardiovascular disease and infection. Efforts to decrease mortality in this vulnerable population are therefore primarily focused upon preventing cardiovascular and infectious complications.

Planning for ESKD treatment should begin many months, and ideally more than 1 year, prior to the need for renal replacement because the rate of CKD progression can be unpredictable. Several recent studies have demonstrated no benefit in starting dialysis in asymptomatic patients early based upon an arbitrary eGFR cutoff compared with waiting until patients develop very low eGFR (<8-10 mL/min/1.73 m²) or clinical indications for dialysis are present.

Patients with an eGFR <30 mL/min/1.73 m² should receive education regarding treatment options, including peritoneal dialysis and hemodialysis, transplantation, and non-dialytic management of ESKD. Patients who opt for hemodialysis should be referred for arteriovenous fistula (AVF) placement before their eGFR drops below 15 mL/min/1.73 m² (stage G5) to allow sufficient time for AVF maturation. Placement of arteriovenous graft (AVG) or peritoneal dialysis catheters can occur a few weeks prior to therapy but should be planned months ahead.

Suitable candidates for kidney transplantation should be referred for evaluation once their eGFR is <20 mL/min/1.73 m². The reasons for timely referral for transplant are twofold. First, the best clinical outcomes occur with "preemptive transplants," in which patients receive the transplant prior to dialysis. Second, because the waiting list for kidneys can be extremely long (>7 years in some parts of the United States), it is important that patients start accruing time on the transplant list as early as possible to maximize the chances that they will receive a transplant while they are still healthy enough to tolerate the procedure and benefit from it. ▪

KEY POINTS

- Suitable candidates for kidney transplantation should be referred for evaluation once their estimated glomerular filtration rate is <20 mL/min/1.73 m².

- Preemptive kidney transplants are associated with better clinical outcomes compared with transplantation after dialysis.

 ## Dialysis
Hemodialysis

Most U.S. patients with ESKD receive hemodialysis three times a week during 3.5- to 4-hour in-center sessions. Recent data suggest that more frequent and/or longer dialysis sessions provided in-center or at home may provide some health benefits, including better control of volume and electrolytes (particularly phosphorus). Patients receiving more frequent and/or longer dialysis are also usually able to liberalize their diet with regard to potassium, phosphorus, and fluid intake. Because longer and/or more frequent hemodialysis has not yet been demonstrated to decrease mortality in a randomized controlled trial, the choice of hemodialysis modality and site of dialysis must incorporate patient preference and other factors, including availability of adequate home resources and support.

See Vascular Access for information on vascular access in patients undergoing hemodialysis.

Peritoneal Dialysis

In patients receiving peritoneal dialysis (PD), a dialysate solution is intermittently instilled into the peritoneal cavity via an indwelling catheter, and excess water and solutes are removed by osmosis and diffusion across the peritoneal membrane into the dialysis solution. Clinical outcomes, including mortality, are equivalent for patients on PD compared with hemodialysis, although there is a trend toward superior outcomes for PD in patients with new-onset ESKD who have significant residual kidney function. This may be explained in part by the fact that residual kidney function is preserved longer in patients on PD than in those on hemodialysis. Peritonitis is one of the most important complications of PD and can damage the peritoneum, reducing the efficacy of dialysis. PD-associated peritonitis is uncommon, with one episode of peritonitis every 2 to 3 years, usually caused by bacteria from skin introduced by poor sterile technique and often easily treated with antibiotics.

PD provides patients with more autonomy than in-center hemodialysis but requires that patients or their caregiver be capable of learning to connect/disconnect dialysis bags with a sterile technique and to have access to clean space and sufficient storage for supplies. Absolute contraindications to PD include documented loss of peritoneal function and uncorrectable mechanical defects of the peritoneum or abdominal wall that prevent effective dialysis or increase the risk of infection.

Non-dialytic Therapy

Some patients with ESKD may elect not to initiate dialysis, and others who are already undergoing chronic dialysis may decide to withdraw from treatment. Non-dialytic therapy for patients with ESKD is a viable treatment option that entails active management of symptoms with a primary focus on maximizing quality of life. The life expectancy of some patients with ESKD with advanced age and severe comorbidities can be extremely short and may not be improved by dialysis. Palliative medicine and hospice services can be used to manage symptoms in patients who choose non-dialytic ESKD therapy. In patients with minimal residual kidney function who withdraw from dialysis, most die within 2 weeks. ▪

KEY POINTS

- Clinical outcomes are equivalent for patients on peritoneal dialysis (PD) compared with hemodialysis, although there is a trend toward superior outcomes for PD in patients with new-onset end-stage kidney disease who have significant residual kidney function.

- Non-dialytic therapy for patients with end-stage kidney disease is a viable treatment option that entails active management of symptoms with a primary focus on maximizing quality of life.

Kidney Transplantation

Patients who receive kidney transplants for treatment of ESKD have markedly improved life expectancy and quality of life, and transplantation is the preferred therapy for eligible candidates. However, there is a severe shortage of available donor organs in the United States. The waiting list for transplants varies markedly by region within the United States. Because the best outcomes occur in patients who receive a preemptive transplant from a living donor, early referral for transplant evaluation to identify suitable living donors is important. If no living donor is available, early transplant listing is essential to minimize waiting time for a transplant.

Patients and donors are carefully screened for potential issues that may affect the safety and/or outcome of the transplant, including the presence of active malignancy, coronary ischemia, or active infection, and to ensure that there are adequate social supports and financial resources available.

Patients are usually managed by transplant nephrologists for at least the first 3 to 6 months posttransplant and subsequently co-managed with general nephrologists and/or internists, especially for comorbidities. The KDIGO Clinical Practice Guideline for the Care of Kidney Transplant Patients can be found at www.kdigo.org.

Immunosuppressive Therapy

Patients with kidney transplants must receive immunosuppressive medications to prevent their immune system from rejecting the kidney allograft. Doses are typically highest immediately after transplant and are tapered gradually over several months to minimize toxicities associated with these medications while maintaining adequate immunosuppression.

The most commonly used immunosuppressants in the immediate posttransplant period for immunosuppression induction are anti–T cell and interleukin-2 receptor blocking antibodies. The most commonly prescribed medications for chronic maintenance immunosuppression include calcineurin inhibitors (tacrolimus or cyclosporine), antimetabolites (mycophenolate mofetil or azathioprine), and glucocorticoids. Although these medications are usually well tolerated, they can have significant side effects (**Table 42**).

Risks of Transplantation

Immediately after kidney transplantation, patients must be monitored closely for acute rejection and postsurgical complications. In the ensuing months, the focus shifts toward minimizing the risks of infection and side effects of medications while maintaining adequate immunosuppression to maintain optimal graft function.

Infection

Patients with kidney transplants are at increased risk for several infections, and the type of organism varies depending upon the time after transplant. In the first month, the most common infectious complications are wound infections and urinary tract infections.

TABLE 42. Common Side Effects of Medications Used for Chronic Maintenance Immunosuppression After Kidney Transplantation

Class	Medication	Common Side Effects
Calcineurin inhibitor	Cyclosporine	Hypertension; decreased GFR; dyslipidemia; hirsutism
	Tacrolimus	New-onset diabetes mellitus; decreased GFR; hypertension; gastrointestinal symptoms
Antimetabolite, blocker of de novo purine synthesis	Mycophenolate mofetil	Diarrhea; nausea/vomiting; leukopenia; anemia
	Azathioprine	Leukopenia
mTOR inhibitor	Sirolimus; everolimus	Proteinuria; dyslipidemia; new-onset diabetes mellitus; anemia; leukopenia
Glucocorticoid receptor agonist	Prednisone	Osteopenia; hypertension; edema; new-onset diabetes mellitus

GFR = glomerular filtration rate; mTOR = mammalian target of rapamycin.

After the first month, opportunistic infections become more important. Cytomegalovirus (CMV) is an important pathogen in kidney transplant patients, and the risk of CMV infection depends upon the serologic status of the kidney donor and recipient at the time of transplant. The highest risk occurs when a seronegative recipient (one who has never had a CMV infection) receives a kidney from a seropositive donor. Signs and symptoms of CMV infection include fever, hepatitis, pneumonitis, and gastrointestinal ulceration. Due to the relatively high incidence of CMV infection posttransplantation, most guidelines suggest that kidney transplant recipients receive prophylactic valganciclovir. Similar to other patients receiving strongly immunosuppressive medications, kidney transplant recipients should also receive prophylaxis against *Pneumocystis jirovecii* pneumonia.

Polyoma BK virus is an opportunistic infection that induces kidney injury in approximately 5% of kidney transplant recipients. The most common clinical manifestation of BK virus infection is an acute or indolent rise in serum creatinine due to BK-induced renal tubular cell injury and tubulointerstitial nephritis or, less commonly, due to ureteral stenosis. Because more intense immunosuppression is associated with higher risk of BK nephropathy, reduction of immunosuppression is the mainstay of prevention and must be balanced with risk of rejection.

Cancer

Immunosuppression of kidney transplant recipients increases the incidence and progression of several types of malignancies.

CONT.

The most common malignancies arising in transplant recipients are non-melanoma skin cancers, predominantly squamous cell carcinomas. Therefore, transplant recipients should be carefully screened for skin cancer and educated on the importance of protection from ultraviolet radiation.

Kaposi sarcoma (KS) is much more common in kidney transplant recipients than in the general population. The risk is highest in men of Jewish, Mediterranean, Arabic, Caribbean, or African ancestry, which parallels the regions where human herpesvirus-8, the causative factor in KS, is endemic. The most commonly used approaches to managing KS are reducing the intensity of immunosuppression and switching to sirolimus-based immunosuppression for its antiproliferative effects.

Posttransplant lymphoproliferative disease (PTLD) is caused by unrestricted proliferation of B lymphocytes, which is usually associated with Epstein-Barr virus (EBV) infection and impaired surveillance by T lymphocytes induced by immunosuppression. The most important risk factors for PTLD are the degree of immunosuppression and negative recipient EBV serostatus pretransplant. The most common treatments for PTLD are reduction of immunosuppression and administration of the anti-B-cell antibody rituximab in patients with CD20+ tumors.

Because several other types of cancer are also more prevalent and/or have worse outcomes in kidney transplant recipients, it is important to screen potential kidney recipients and donors for the presence of active malignancy prior to transplant.

Special Considerations in Transplant Recipients

Acute Kidney Injury

Kidney transplant recipients have an increased risk of AKI, which can occur immediately posttransplant or years later. Although acute rejection is an important cause of AKI, it occurs relatively early posttransplant and is less likely to occur after the first few months in patients who are adherent with their immunosuppressant medications. Other common reversible causes of AKI in transplant recipients with a previously functioning graft include volume depletion/prerenal causes, calcineurin inhibitor toxicity, acute interstitial nephritis, acute tubular necrosis, BK nephropathy, and ureteral or bladder outlet obstruction.

Disease Recurrence

Many forms of primary kidney disease can recur in the transplant allograft, including many glomerular diseases. In patients with ESKD due to autoimmune glomerulonephritis, including lupus or ANCA-associated glomerulonephritis, it is important that the disease be quiescent for several months prior to transplant. Some common causes of ESKD such as diabetic nephropathy and IgA nephropathy can recur in the allograft, although they are unlikely to cause allograft failure. However, recurrence of some primary kidney diseases, including focal segmental glomerulosclerosis and thrombotic microangiopathy, can worsen allograft outcomes and may warrant aggressive treatment.

Cardiovascular Disease

Because cardiovascular disease is the most common cause of death in kidney transplant recipients, aggressive management of cardiac risk factors is warranted (See Complications and Management, Cardiovascular Disease). Immunosuppressive medications, including calcineurin inhibitors, sirolimus, and glucocorticoids, contribute to dyslipidemia. Although clinical studies on the efficacy of statins in preventing cardiovascular mortality have yielded conflicting results, a large proportion of kidney transplant recipients receive these medications. KDIGO guidelines state that fluvastatin, atorvastatin, rosuvastatin, pravastatin, or simvastatin may be used in transplant recipients. Cyclosporine increases serum levels of statins; therefore, clinicians should consider reducing the dose of statins in patients taking cyclosporine.

Bone Disease

Kidney transplant recipients are at increased risk of bone disease due to several factors, including secondary or tertiary hyperparathyroidism, side effects of immunosuppressive medications, and high prevalence of vitamin D deficiency. Glucocorticoids can cause osteopenia and/or osteonecrosis, and tacrolimus can induce phosphate wasting. Secondary hyperparathyroidism usually improves after kidney transplantation but may not fully resolve and should be managed as described in the Chronic Kidney Disease-Mineral and Bone Disorder section.

Vaccination

Patients with CKD should receive all appropriate vaccinations prior to transplantation as outlined in the Vaccination section of Special Considerations. Most transplant centers avoid immunizations in the first 3 to 6 months after transplant when patients are more immunosuppressed and less likely to have an adequate response to immunization, with the exception of the influenza vaccine, which can be given within 1 month of transplantation in unvaccinated patients in the setting of an influenza outbreak. Vaccination using live attenuated viruses is generally contraindicated in kidney transplant recipients.

Nonadherence

Successful transplant outcomes depend heavily upon the ability of patients to adhere to medications, scheduled appointments, dietary advice, and abstinence from smoking or illicit drug use. It is therefore critical that patients be evaluated prior to transplant for adherence to medical therapy and adequacy of social support. Lack of medical insurance and financial resources is also an important factor that can prevent patients from being able to afford immunosuppressive medications. A multidisciplinary team approach that includes psychiatric services, nursing, and social work is therefore essential to promote patient adherence.

Risks of Kidney Donation

Persons who wish to be considered for living kidney donation must undergo extensive testing to ensure that they have normal kidney function and excellent health with low risk of future kidney or cardiac disease. In the United States, potential donors must be assigned an Independent Living Donor Advocate who is not directly affiliated with the transplant center or team and who advocates solely for the interests of the donor. Although long-term donor outcomes are generally excellent and similar to healthy non-donor controls, potential donors must be fully educated regarding short-term surgical risks and potential long-term risks, especially if they have a family history of kidney disease or are from racial or ethnic groups with increased susceptibility to kidney disease.

KEY POINTS

- Wound and urinary tract infections are most common in the first month following kidney transplantation; after the first month, opportunistic infections with cytomegalovirus, *Pneumocystis jirovecii*, and polyoma BK virus are most common.

- Immunosuppression of kidney transplant recipients increases the incidence and progression of several types of malignancies, including non-melanoma skin cancers, Kaposi sarcoma, and posttransplant lymphoproliferative disease.

- The dose of statins should be reduced in kidney transplant recipients taking cyclosporine.

Complications of End-Stage Kidney Disease

Cardiovascular Disease

The most common cause of death in patients with ESKD is arrhythmia/sudden cardiac death. The reasons for this propensity are unclear, but important factors include abnormalities in serum electrolyte concentrations that may rapidly change during hemodialysis, chronic fluid overload that likely contributes to high prevalence of left ventricular hypertrophy and cardiac fibrosis, and uremic toxins. Arterial calcification may also promote cardiac disease due to reduced vascular compliance and other factors. It is therefore important to attenuate electrolyte disturbances, especially hyperkalemia, to avoid rapid changes in extracellular potassium during dialysis, which may precipitate arrhythmias. Also, promoting adherence to dietary fluid restriction may prevent intradialytic hypotension caused by rapid fluid removal during dialysis, which can cause cardiovascular and central nervous system injury.

Infection

Infection is the second-leading cause of death in patients with ESKD. Catheter-associated bacteremia and sepsis contribute to morbidity and mortality. Patients with suspected bacteremia due to infection of a tunneled cuffed catheter should have blood cultures drawn and receive empiric antibiotics while awaiting culture results. Indications for immediate catheter removal are listed in **Table 43**. Afebrile patients who have received at least 48 hours of appropriate antibiotics and who do

TABLE 43. Indications for Immediate Removal of Cuffed Tunnel Hemodialysis Catheters in Patients With Known or Suspected Catheter-Related Bacteremia

Severe sepsis
Hemodynamic instability
Evidence of metastatic infection
Infection of catheter exit site or tunnel
Persistent fever and/or bacteremia >48-72 h despite adequate antibiotic coverage and no other suspected source
Infection due to high risk and difficult-to-cure organisms, including *Staphylococcus aureus*, *Pseudomonas*, or fungi

not have an indication for immediate catheter removal can safely have their catheter exchanged over a guidewire to minimize venous trauma associated with de novo catheter placement. Attempting to salvage a hemodialysis catheter in a patient with bacteremia is rarely advisable due to poor rates of success, except in patients in whom the risks outweigh benefits.

Acquired Cystic Kidney Disease

Acquired kidney cysts often develop in patients with severe CKD and are frequently detected during routine kidney ultrasound or incidentally noted on abdominal CT or MRI scan. Acquired cystic kidney disease becomes more common and progresses during the course of ESKD, and some studies suggest that it may affect >50% of patients who have had ESKD for >3 years. The epithelial cells lining these cysts may undergo malignant transformation by poorly understood mechanisms. Patients with ESKD have a markedly increased risk for renal cell carcinoma. Although current guidelines do not support routine screening for renal cell carcinoma in all patients with CKD, a high level of suspicion is warranted in patients with symptoms such as new-onset gross hematuria or unexplained flank pain.

KEY POINT

- Complications of end-stage kidney disease include cardiovascular disease, infection, and acquired cystic kidney disease.

Bibliography

Clinical Evaluation of Kidney Function

Corapi KM, Chen JL, Balk EM, Gordon CE. Bleeding complications of native kidney biopsy: a systematic review and meta-analysis. Am J Kidney Dis. 2012 Jul;60(1):62-73. [PMID: 22537423]

Davis R, Jones JS, Barocas DA, et al; American Urological Association. Diagnosis, evaluation and follow-up of asymptomatic microhematuria (AMH) in adults: AUA guideline. J Urol. 2012 Dec;188(6 suppl):2473-81. [PMID: 23098784]

Inker LA, Eckfeldt J, Levey AS, et al. Expressing the CKD-EPI (Chronic Kidney Disease Epidemiology Collaboration) cystatin C equations for estimating GFR with standardized serum cystatin C values. Am J Kidney Dis. 2011 Oct;58(4):682-4. [PMID: 21855190]

Levey AS, Fan L, Eckfeldt JH, Inker LA. Cystatin C for glomerular filtration rate estimation: coming of age. Clin Chem. 2014 Jul;60(7):916-9. [PMID: 24871681]

Margulis V, Sagalowsky AI. Assessment of hematuria. Med Clin North Am. 2011 Jan;95(1):153-9. [PMID: 21095418]

Moyer VA; U.S. Preventive Services Task Force. Screening for bladder cancer: U.S. Preventive Services Task Force recommendation statement. Ann Intern Med. 2011 Aug 16;155(4):246–51. [PMID: 21844550]

Perazella MA, Coca SG, Hall IE, Iyanam U, Koraishy M, Parikh CR. Urine microscopy is associated with severity and worsening of acute kidney injury in hospitalized patients. Clin J Am Soc Nephrol. 2010 Mar;5(3):402–8. [PMID: 20089493]

Perazella MA, Coca SG, Kanbay M, Brewster UC, Parikh CR. Diagnostic value of urine microscopy for differential diagnosis of acute kidney injury in hospitalized patients. Clin J Am Soc Nephrol. 2008 Nov;3(6):1615–9. [PMID: 18784207]

Piccoli GB, Daidola G, Attini R, et al. Kidney biopsy in pregnancy: evidence for counselling? A systematic narrative review. BJOG. 2013 Mar;120(4):412–27. [PMID: 23320849]

Stacul F, van der Molen AJ, Reimer P, et al; Contrast Media Safety Committee of European Society of Urogenital Radiology (ESUR). Contrast induced nephropathy: updated ESUR Contrast Media Safety Committee guidelines. Eur Radiol. 2011 Dec;21(12):2527–41. [PMID: 21866433]

Stevens LA, Coresh J, Greene T, Levey AS. Assessing kidney function–measured and estimated glomerular filtration rate. N Engl J Med. 2006 Jun 8;354(23): 2473–83. [PMID: 16760447]

Thomsen HS, Morcos SK, Almén T, et al; ESUR Contrast Medium Safety Committee. Nephrogenic systemic fibrosis and gadolinium–based contrast media: updated ESUR Contrast Medium Safety Committee guidelines. Eur Radiol. 2013 Feb;23(2):307–18. [PMID: 22865271]

Zoungas S, Ninomiya T, Huxley R, et al. Systematic review: sodium bicarbonate treatment regimens for the prevention of contrast-induced nephropathy. Ann Intern Med. 2009 Nov 8;151(9):631–8. [PMID: 19884624]

Fluids and Electrolytes

Adrogue HJ, Madias NE. Hypernatremia. N Engl J Med. 2000 May 18;342(20):1493–9. [PMID: 10816188]

Bedford JJ, Weggery S, Ellis G, et al. Lithium–induced nephrogenic diabetes insipidus: renal effects of amiloride. Clin J Am Soc Nephrol. 2008 Sep;3(5):1324–31. [PMID: 18596116]

Berl T. Impact of solute intake on urine flow and water excretion. J Am Soc Nephrol. 2008;19(6):1076–8. [PMID: 18337482]

Berl T, Quittnat-Pelletier F, et al; Investigators SALTWATER. Oral tolvaptan is safe and effective in chronic hyponatremia. J Am Soc Nephrol. 2010 Jun;21(4):705–12. [PMID: 20185637]

Berl T, Rastegar A. A patient with severe hyponatremia and hypokalemia: osmotic demyelination following potassium repletion. Am J Kidney Dis. 2010 Apr;55(4):742–8. [PMID: 20338465]

Christensen BM, Zuber AM, Loffing J, et al. alphaENaC–mediated lithium absorption promotes nephrogenic diabetes insipidus. J Am Soc Nephrol. 2011 Feb;22:253–61. [PMID: 21051735]

Feldman BJ, Rosenthal SM, Vargas GA, et al. Nephrogenic syndrome of inappropriate antidiuresis. N Engl J Med. 2005 May 5;352(18):1884–90. [PMID: 15872203]

Felsenfeld AJ, Levine BS. Approach to treatment of hypophosphatemia. Am J Kidney Dis. 2012 Oct;60(4):655–61. [PMID: 22863286]

Mohmand HK, Issa D, Ahmad Z, Cappuccio JD, Kouides RW, Sterns RH. Hypertonic saline for hyponatremia: risk of inadvertent overcorrection. Clin J Am Soc Nephrol. 2007 Nov;2(6):1110–7. [PMID: 17913972]

Perianayagam A, Sterns RH, Silver SM, et al. DDAVP is effective in preventing and reversing inadvertent overcorrection of hyponatremia. Clin J Am Soc Nephrol. 2008 Mar;3(2):331–6. [PMID: 18235152]

Roscioni SS, de Zeeuw D, Bakker SJ, Lambers Heerspink HJ. Management of hyperkalaemia consequent to mineralocorticoid–receptor antagonist therapy. Nat Rev Nephrol. 2012 Dec;8(12):691–9. [PMID: 23070570]

Sterns RH, Nigwekar SU, Hix JK: The treatment of hyponatremia. Semin Nephrol. 2009 May;29(3):282–99. [PMID: 19523575]

Unwin RJ, Luft FC, Shirley DG. Pathophysiology and management of hypokalemia: a clinical perspective. Nat Rev Nephrol. 2011 Feb;7(2):75–84. [PMID: 21278718]

Acid-Base Disorders

Gennari FJ. Pathophysiology of metabolic alkalosis: a new classification based on the centrality of stimulated collecting duct ion transport. Am J Kidney Dis. 2011;58(4):626–36. [PMID: 21849227]

Izzedine H, Launay-Vacher V, Isnard-Bagnis C, Deray G. Drug-induced Fanconi's syndrome. Am J Kidney Dis. 2003;41(2):292–309. [PMID: 12552490]

Karet FE. Inherited distal renal tubular acidosis. J Am Soc Nephrol. 2002;13(8): 2178–84. [PMID: 12138152]

Kraut JA, Kurtz I. Toxic alcohol ingestions: clinical features, diagnosis, and management. Clin J Am Soc Nephrol. 2008;3(1):208–25. [PMID: 18045860]

Kraut JA, Nagami GT. The serum anion gap in the evaluation of acid-base disorders: what are its limitations and can its effectiveness be improved? Clin J Am Soc Nephrol. 2013;8(11):2018–24. [PMID: 23833313]

Madias NE. Renal acidification responses to respiratory acid-base disorders. J Nephrol. 2010;23(suppl 16):S85–S91. [PMID: 21170892]

Melcescu E, Phillips J, Moll G, Subauste JS, Koch CA. 11Beta-hydroxylase deficiency and other syndromes of mineralocorticoid excess as a rare cause of endocrine hypertension. Horm Metab Res. 2012;44(12):867–78. [PMID: 22932914]

Nakhoul F, Nakhoul N, Dorman E, et al. Gitelman's syndrome: a pathophysiological and clinical update. Endocrine. 2012;41(1):53–7. [PMID: 22169961]

Raimondi GA, Gonzalez S, Zaltsman J, Menga G, Adrogué HJ. Acid-base patterns in acute severe asthma. J Asthma. 2013;50(10):1062–1068. [PMID: 23947392]

Rastegar A. Use of the DeltaAG/DeltaHCO3-ratio in the diagnosis of mixed acid-base disorders. J Am Soc Nephrol 2007;18(9):2429–31. [PMID: 17656477]

Rodriguez Soriano J. Renal tubular acidosis: the clinical entity. J Am Soc Nephrol. 2002;13(6):2160–70. [PMID: 12138150]

Treger R, Pirouz S, Kamangar N, Corry D. Agreement between central venous and arterial blood gas measurements in the intensive care unit. Clin J Am Soc Nephrol. 2010;5(3):390–4. [PMID: 20019117]

Hypertension

ACCORD Study Group, Cushman WC, Evans GW, Byington RP, et al. Effects of intensive blood-pressure control in type 2 diabetes mellitus. N Engl J Med. 2010 Apr 29;362(17):1575–85. [PMID: 20228401]

Calhoun DA, Jones D, Textor S, et al; American Heart Association Professional Education Committee. 2008 Resistant hypertension: diagnosis, evaluation, and treatment: a scientific statement from the American Heart Association Professional Education Committee of the Council for High Blood Pressure Research. Circulation. 2008 Jun 24;117(25):e510–26. [PMID: 18574054]

Chobanian AV, Bakris GL, Black HR, et al; Joint National Committee on Prevention, Detection, Evaluation, and Treatment of High Blood Pressure. National Heart, Lung, and Blood Institute; National High Blood Pressure Education Program Coordinating Committee. 2003 Seventh Report of the Joint National Committee on Prevention, Detection, Evaluation, and Treatment of High Blood Pressure. Hypertension. 2003 Dec;42(6):1206–52. [PMID: 14656957]

Cornelissen VA, Smart NA. Exercise training for blood pressure: a systematic review and meta-analysis. J Am Heart Assoc. 2013 Feb 1;2(1):e004473. [PMID: 23525435]

Eckel RH, Jakicic JM, Ard JD, et al; American College of Cardiology/American Heart Association Task Force on Practice Guidelines. 2013 AHA/ACC guideline on lifestyle management to reduce cardiovascular risk: a report of the American College of Cardiology/American Heart Association Task Force on Practice Guidelines. J Am Coll Cardiol. 2014 Jul 1;63(25 Pt B):2960–84. [PMID: 24239922]

Fried LF, Emanuele N, Zhang JH, et al; VA NEPHRON-D Investigators. Combined angiotensin inhibition for the treatment of diabetic nephropathy. N Engl J Med. 2013;369(20):1892–903. [PMID: 24206457]

Furberg CD, Wright JT, Davis BR, et al. Major outcomes in high-risk hypertensive patients randomized to angiotensin-converting enzyme inhibitor or calcium channel blocker vs diuretic: The Antihypertensive and Lipid-Lowering Treatment to Prevent Heart Attack Trial (ALLHAT). JAMA. 2002 Dec 18;288(23):2981–97. [PMID: 12479763]

Hermida RC, Ayala DE, Mojón A, Fernández JR. Bedtime dosing of antihypertensive medications reduces cardiovascular risk in CKD. J Am Soc Nephrol. 2011 Dec;22(12):2313–21. [PMID: 22025630]

James PA, Oparil S, Carter BL, et al. 2014 evidence-based guideline for the management of high blood pressure in adults: report from the panel members appointed to the Eighth Joint National Committee (JNC 8). JAMA. 2014 Feb 5;311(5):507–20. [PMID: 24352797]

Kidney Disease: Improving Global Outcomes (KDIGO) Blood Pressure Work Group. KDIGO Clinical Practice Guideline for the Management of Blood Pressure in Chronic Kidney Disease. Kidney Inter. Suppl. 2012; 2:337–414. Available at www.kdigo.org/clinical_practice_guidelines/pdf/CKD/KDIGO_2012_CKD_GL.pdf. Accessed December 12, 2014.

Pierdomenico SD, Cuccurullo F. Prognostic value of white-coat and masked hypertension diagnosed by ambulatory monitoring in initially untreated subjects: an updated meta-analysis. Am J Hypertens. 2011 Jan;24(1):52–8. [PMID: 20847724]

Bibliography

Stergiou GS, Asayama K, Thijs L, et al; International Database on HOme blood pressure in relation to Cardiovascular Outcome (IDHOCO) Investigators. Prognosis of white-coat and masked hypertension: international database of home blood pressure in relation to cardiovascular outcome. Hypertension. 2014 Apr;63(4):675-82. [PMID: 24420553]

Zennaro MC, Rickard AJ, Boulkroun S. Genetics of mineralocorticoid excess: an update for clinicians. Eur J Endocrinol. 2013;169(1):R15-25. [PMID: 23610123]

Chronic Tubulointerstitial Diseases

Bleyer AJ, Hart PS, Kmoch S. Hereditary interstitial kidney disease. Semin Nephrol. 2010;30(4):366-73. [PMID: 20807609]

Bollée G, Dahan K, Flamant M, et al. Phenotype and outcome in hereditary tubulointerstitial nephritis secondary to UMOD mutations. Clin J Am Soc Nephrol. 2011;6(10):2429-38. [PMID: 21868615]

Gökmen MR, Cosyns JP, Arlt VM, et al. The epidemiology, diagnosis, and management of aristolochic acid nephropathy: a narrative review. Ann Intern Med. 2013;158(6):469-77. [PMID: 23552405]

Stone JH, Zen Y, Deshpande V. IgG4-related disease. N Engl J Med. 2012;366(6):539-51. [PMID: 22316447]

Glomerular Diseases

American Diabetes Association: Standards of medical care in diabetes-2014. Diabetes Care. 2014 Jan;37(suppl 1):S14-80. [PMID: 24357209]

Appel GB, Contreras G, Dooley MA, et al. Mycophenolate mofetil versus cyclophosphamide for induction treatment of lupus nephritis. J Am Soc Nephrol. 2009 May;20(5):1103-12. [PMID: 19369404]

D'Agati VD, Fogo AB, Bruijn JA, Jennette JC. Pathologic classification of focal segmental glomerulosclerosis: a working proposal. Am J Kidney Dis. 2004 Feb;43(2):368-82. [PMID: 14750104]

D'Agati VD, Kaskel FJ, Falk RJ. Focal segmental glomerulosclerosis. N Engl J Med. 2011 Dec 22;365(25):2398-2411. [PMID: 22187987]

Hogan J, Radhakrishnan J. The treatment of minimal change disease in adults. J Am Soc Nephrol. 2013 Apr;24(5):702-11. [PMID: 23431071]

Jennette JC, Falk RJ, Bacon PA, et al. 2012 Revised International Chapel Hill Consensus Conference Nomenclature of Vasculitides. Arth Rheum. 2013 Jan;65(1):1-11. [PMID: 23045170]

Nasr SH, Radhakrishnan J, D'Agati VD. Bacterial infection-related glomerulonephritis in adults. Kidney Int. 2013 May;83(5):792-803. [PMID: 23302723]

Pusey CD. Anti-glomerular basement membrane disease. Kidney Int. 2003 Oct;64(4):1535-50. [PMID: 12969182]

Qin W, Beck LH Jr, Zeng C, et al. Anti-phospholipase A2 receptor antibody in membranous nephropathy. J Am Soc Nephrol. 2011 Jun;22(6):1137-43. [PMID: 21566055]

Sethi S, Fervenza FC. Membranoproliferative glomerulonephritis-a new look at an old entity. N Eng J Med. 2012 Mar 22;366(12):1119-31. [PMID: 22435371]

Siddall EC, Radhakrishnan J. The pathophysiology of edema formation in the nephrotic syndrome. Kidney Int. 2012 Sep;82(6):635-42. [PMID: 22718186]

Specks U, Merkel PA, Seo P, et al. Efficacy of remission-induction regimens for ANCA-associated vasculitis. N Eng J Med. 2013 Aug 1;369(5):417-27. [PMID: 23902481]

Waldman M, Austin HA 3rd. Treatment of idiopathic membranous nephropathy. J Am Soc Nephrol. 2012 Oct;23(10):1617-30. [PMID: 22859855]

Waldman M, Crew RJ, Valeri A, et al. Adult minimal-change disease: clinical characteristics, treatment, and outcomes. Clin J Am Soc Nephrol. 2007 May;2(3):445-53. [PMID: 17699450]

Weening JJ, D'Agati VD, Schwartz MM, et al; International Society of Nephrology Working Group on the Classification of Lupus Nephritis; Renal Pathology Society Working Group on the Classification of Lupus Nephritis. The classification of glomerulonephritis in systemic lupus erythematosus revisited. Kidney Int 2004 Feb;65(2):521-30. [PMID: 14717922]

Working Group of the International IgA Nephropathy Network and the Renal Pathology Society, Roberts IS, Cook HT, et al. The Oxford classification of IgA nephropathy: pathology definitions, correlations, and reproducibility. Kidney Int. 2009 Sep;76(5):546-56. [PMID: 19571790]

Wyatt RJ, Julian BA. IgA nephropathy. N Eng J Med. 2013 Jun 20;368(25):2402-14. [PMID: 23782179]

Kidney Manifestations of Gammopathies

Leung N, Bridoux F, Hutchison CA, et al. Monoclonal gammopathy of renal significance: when MGUS is no longer undetermined or insignificant. Blood. 2012 Nov 22;120(22):4292-95. [PMID: 23047823]

Rosenstock JL, Markowitz GS, Valeri AM, Sacchi G, Appel GB, D'Agati VD. Fibrillary and immunotactoid glomerulonephritis: distinct entities with different clinical and pathologic features. Kidney Int. 2003 Apr;63:1450-61. [PMID: 12631361]

Genetic Disorders and Kidney Disease

Brown EJ, Pollak MR, Barua M. Genetic testing for nephrotic syndrome and FSGS in the era of next-generation sequencing. Kidney Int. 2014 May;85(5):1030-8. [PMID: 24599252]

Chaki M, Hoefele J, Allen SJ, et al. Genotype-phenotype correlation in 440 patients with NPHP-related ciliopathies. Kidney Int. 2011 Dec;80(11):1239-45. [PMID: 21866095]

Feriozzi S, Torras J, Cybulla M, et al; Investigators FOS: The effectiveness of long-term agalsidase alfa therapy in the treatment of Fabry nephropathy. Clin J Am Soc Nephrol. 2012 Jan;7(1):60-9. [PMID: 22246281]

Pollak MR, Genovese G, Friedman DJ. APOL1 and kidney disease. Curr Opin Nephrol Hypertens. 2012 Mar 21(2):179-82. [PMID: 22257798]

Schrier RW. Renal volume, renin-angiotensin-aldosterone system, hypertension, and left ventricular hypertrophy in patients with autosomal dominant polycystic kidney disease. J Am Soc Nephrol. 2009 Sept;20(9):1888-93. [PMID: 19696226]

Torres VE, Chapman AB, Devuyst O, et al; Investigators TT. Tolvaptan in patients with autosomal dominant polycystic kidney disease. N Engl J Med. 2012 Dec 20;367(25):2407-18. [PMID: 23121377]

Trudu M, Janas S, Lanzani C, et al; Swiss Kidney Project on Genes in Hypertension. Common noncoding UMOD gene variants induce salt-sensitive hypertension and kidney damage by increasing uromodulin expression. Nat Med. 2013 Dec;19(12):1655-60. [PMID: 24185693]

Acute Kidney Injury

Bart BA, Goldsmith SR, Lee KL, et al; Heart Failure Clinical Research Network. Ultrafiltration in decompensated heart failure with cardiorenal syndrome. N Engl J Med. 2012 Dec 13;367(24):2296-2304. [PMID: 23131078]

Cruz DN, Goh CY, Marenzi G, et al. Renal replacement therapies for prevention of radiocontrast-induced nephropathy: a systematic review. Am J Med. 2012 Jan;125(1):66-78. [PMID: 22195531]

Kidney Disease: Improving Global Outcomes (KDIGO) Acute Kidney Injury Work Group. KDIGO Clinical Practice Guideline for Acute Kidney Injury. Kidney Inter, Suppl. 2012;2:1-138. Available at: www.kdigo.org/clinical_practice_guidelines/pdf/KDIGO%20AKI%20Guideline.pdf. Accessed 8/21/14.

Lopez-Olivo MA, Pratt G, Palla SL, Salahudeen A. Rasburicase in tumor lysis syndrome of the adult: a systematic review and meta-analysis. Am J Kidney Dis. 2013 Sep;62(3):481-92. [PMID: 23684124]

Mohmand H, Goldfarb S. Renal dysfunction associated with intra-abdominal hypertension and the abdominal compartment syndrome. J Am Soc Nephrol. 2011 Apr;22(4):615-21. [PMID: 21310818]

Mutter TC, Ruth CA, Dart AB. Hydroxyethyl starch (HES) versus other fluid therapies: effects on kidney function. Cochrane Database Syst Rev. 2013 Jul 23;7:CD007594. [PMID: 23881659]

Nadim MK, Kellum JA, Davenport A, et al; ADQI Workgroup Hepatorenal syndrome: the 8th International Consensus Conference of the Acute Dialysis Quality Initiative (ADQI) Group. Crit Care. 2012 Feb 9;16(1):R23. [PMID: 22322077]

van Hal SJ, Paterson DL, Lodise TP. Systematic review and meta-analysis of vancomycin-induced nephrotoxicity associated with dosing schedules that maintain troughs between 15 and 20 milligrams per liter. Antimicrob Agents Chemother. 2013 Feb;57(2):734-44. [PMID: 23165462]

Wilson FP, Berns JS. Onco-nephrology: tumor lysis syndrome. Clin J Am Soc Nephrol. 2012 Oct;7(10):1730-9. [PMID: 22879434]

Zimmerman JL, Shen MC. Rhabdomyolysis. Chest. 2013 Sep;144(3):1058-65. [PMID: 24008958]

Kidney Stones

Eisner BH, Goldfarb DS, Pareek G. Pharmacologic treatment of kidney stone disease. Urol Clin North Am. 2013 Feb;40(1):21-30. [PMID: 23177632]

Fink HA, Wilt TJ, Eidman KE, et al. Medical management to prevent recurrent nephrolithiasis in adults: a systematic review for an American College of Physicians Clinical Guideline. Ann Intern Med. 2013 Apr;158(7):535-43. [PMID: 23546565]

Goldfarb DS, Arowojolu O. Metabolic evaluation of first-time and recurrent stone formers. Urol Clin North Am. 2013 Feb;40(1):13-20. [PMID: 23177631]

Heilberg IP, Goldfarb DS. Optimum nutrition for kidney stone disease. Adv Chronic Kidney Dis. 2013 Mar;20(2):165-74. [PMID: 23439376]

Pearle MS. Shock-wave lithotripsy for renal calculi. N Engl J Med. 2012 Jul 5;367(1):50-7. [PMID: 22762318]

Pearle MS, Goldfarb DS, Assimos DG, et al; American Urological Association. Medical management of kidney stones: AUA guideline. J Urol. 2014 Aug;192:316-24. [PMID: 24857648]

Qaseem A, Dallas P, Forciea MA, Starkey M, Denberg TD, Clinical Guidelines Committee of the American College of Physicians. Dietary and pharmacologic management to prevent recurrent nephrolithiasis in adults: a clinical practice guideline from the American College of Physicians. Ann Intern Med. 2014 Nov 4;161(9):659-67. [PMID: 25364887]

Sakhaee K, Maalouf NM, Sinnott B. Clinical review. Kidney stones 2012: pathogenesis, diagnosis, and management. J Clin Endocrinol Metab. 2012 Jun;97(6):1847-60. [PMID: 22466339]

Viprakasit DP, Sawyer MD, Herrell SD, Miller NL. Changing composition of staghorn calculi. J Urol. 2011 Dec;186(6):2285-90. [PMID: 22014820]

The Kidney in Pregnancy

Abalos E, Duley L, Steyn DW. Antihypertensive drug therapy for mild to moderate hypertension during pregnancy. Cochrane Database Syst Rev. 2014 Feb 6;2:CD002252. [PMID: 24504933]

American College of Obstetricians and Gynecologists; Task Force on Hypertension in Pregnancy. Hypertension in pregnancy. Report of the American College of Obstetricians and Gynecologists' Task Force on Hypertension in Pregnancy. Obstet Gynecol. 2013 Nov;122(5):1122-31. [PMID: 24150027]

Cheung KL, Lafayette RA. Renal physiology of pregnancy. Adv Chronic Kidney Dis. 2013 May;20(3):209-14. [PMID: 23928384]

Kattah AG, Garovic VD. The management of hypertension in pregnancy. Adv Chronic Kidney Dis. 2013 May;20(3):229-39. [PMID: 23928387]

Nadeau-Fredette AC, Hladunewich M, Hui D, Keunen J, Chan CT. End-stage renal disease and pregnancy. Adv Chronic Kidney Dis. 2013 May;20(3):246-52. [PMID: 23928389]

Vellanki K. Pregnancy in chronic kidney disease. Adv Chronic Kidney Dis. 2013 May;20(3):223-8. [PMID: 23928386]

Chronic Kidney Disease

Baigent C, Landray MJ, Reith C, et al; SHARP Investigators. The effects of lowering LDL cholesterol with simvastatin plus ezetimibe in patients with chronic kidney disease (Study of Heart and Renal Protection): a randomised placebo-controlled trial. Lancet. 2011 Jun 25;377(9784):2181-92. [PMID: 21663949]

Chandna SM, Da Silva-Gane M, Marshall C, Warwicker P, Greenwood RN, Farrington K. Survival of elderly patients with stage 5 CKD: comparison of conservative management and renal replacement therapy. Nephrol Dial Transplant. 2011 May;26(5):1608-14. [PMID: 21098012]

Cooper BA, Branley P, Bulfone L, et al. A randomized, controlled trial of early versus late initiation of dialysis. N Engl J Med. 2010 Aug 12;363(7):609-19. [PMID: 20581422]

de Brito-Ashurst I, Varagunam M, Raftery MJ, Yaqoob MM. Bicarbonate supplementation slows progression of CKD and improves nutritional status. J Am Soc Nephrol. 2009 Sep;20(9):2075-84. [PMID: 19608703]

Fellstrom BC, Jardine AG, Schmieder RE, et al; AURORA Study Group. Rosuvastatin and cardiovascular events in patients undergoing hemodialysis. N Engl J Med. 2009 Apr 2;360(14):1395-407. [PMID: 19332456]

FHN Trial Group, Chertow GM, Levin NW, et al. In-center hemodialysis six times per week versus three times per week. N Engl J Med. 2010 Dec 9;363(24):2287-300. [PMID: 21091062]

Fried LF, Emanuele N, Zhang JH, et al; VA NEPHRON-D Investigators. Combined angiotensin inhibition for the treatment of diabetic nephropathy. N Engl J Med. 2013 Nov 14;369(20):1892-903. [PMID: 24206457]

Ibrahim HN, Foley R, Tan L, et al. Long-term consequences of kidney donation. N Engl J Med. 2009 Jan 29;360(5):459-69. [PMID: 19179315]

Kidney Disease: Improving Global Outcomes (KDIGO) Anemia Work Group. KDIGO Clinical Practice Guideline for Anemia in Chronic Kidney Disease. Kidney Int Suppl. 2012;2:279-335.

Kidney Disease: Improving Global Outcomes (KDIGO) CKD Work Group. KDIGO 2012 Clinical Practice Guideline for the Evaluation and Management of Chronic Kidney Disease. Kidney Int Suppl. 2013;3:1-150.

Kidney Disease: Improving Global Outcomes (KDIGO) CKD-MBD Work Group. KDIGO clinical practice guideline for the diagnosis, evaluation, prevention, and treatment of chronic kidney disease–mineral and bone disorder (CKD–MBD). Kidney Int Suppl. 2009 Aug;(113):S1-130. [PMID: 19644521]

Kidney Disease: Improving Global Outcomes (KDIGO) Transplant Work Group. KDIGO clinical practice guideline for the care of kidney transplant recipients. Am J Transplant. 2009 Nov;9 Suppl 3:S1-155. [PMID: 19845597]

Kurella Tamura M, Covinsky KE, Chertow GM, Yaffe K, Landefeld CS, McCulloch CE. Functional status of elderly adults before and after initiation of dialysis. N Engl J Med. 2009 Oct 15;361(16):1539-47. [PMID: 19828531]

Mann JF, Schmieder RE, McQueen M, et al; ONTARGET investigators. Renal outcomes with telmisartan, ramipril, or both, in people at high vascular risk (the ONTARGET study): a multicentre, randomised, double-blind, controlled trial. Lancet. 2008 Aug 16;372(9638):547-53. [PMID: 18707986]

Palmer SC, Hayen A, Macaskill P, et al. Serum levels of phosphorus, parathyroid hormone, and calcium and risks of death and cardiovascular disease in individuals with chronic kidney disease: a systematic review and meta-analysis. JAMA. 2011 Mar 16;305(11):1119-27. [PMID: 21406649]

Ravani P, Palmer SC, Oliver MJ, et al. Associations between hemodialysis access type and clinical outcomes: a systematic review. J Am Soc Nephrol. 2013 Feb;24(3):465-73. [PMID: 23431075]

Solomon SD, Uno H, Lewis EF, et al; Trial to Reduce Cardiovascular Events with Aranesp Therapy (TREAT) Investigators. Erythropoietic response and outcomes in kidney disease and type 2 diabetes. N Engl J Med. 2010 Sep 16;363(12):1146-55. [PMID: 20843249]

Tamaru MK, Covinsky KE, Chertow JM, Yaffe K, Landefeld CS, McCulloch CE. Functional status of elderly adults before and after initiation of dialysis. N Engl J Med. 2009 Oct 15;361(16):1539-47. [PMID: 19828531]

U.S. Food and Drug Administration. FDA Drug Safety Communication: erythropoiesis-stimulating agents (ESAs): Procrit, Epogen and Aranesp. www.fda.gov/Drugs/DrugSafety/PostmarketDrugSafetyInformationfor PatientsandProviders/ucm200297.htm. Accessed March 21, 2014.

Wanner C, Krane V, Marz W, et al; German Diabetes and Dialysis Study Investigators. Atorvastatin in patients with type 2 diabetes mellitus undergoing hemodialysis. N Engl J Med. 2005 Jul 21;353(3):238-48. [PMID: 16034009]

Weinhandl ED, Foley RN, Gilbertson DT, Arneson TJ, Snyder JJ, Collins AJ. Propensity-matched mortality comparison of incident hemodialysis and peritoneal dialysis patients. J Am Soc Nephrol. 2010 Mar;21(3):499-506. [PMID: 20133483]

Nephrology Self-Assessment Test

This self-assessment test contains one-best-answer multiple-choice questions. Please read these directions carefully before answering the questions. Answers, critiques, and bibliographies immediately follow these multiple-choice questions. The American College of Physicians is accredited by the Accreditation Council for Continuing Medical Education (ACCME) to provide continuing medical education for physicians.

The American College of Physicians designates MKSAP 17 **Nephrology** for a maximum of **19** *AMA PRA Category 1 Credits*™. Physicians should claim only the credit commensurate with the extent of their participation in the activity.

Earn "Instantaneous" CME Credits Online

Print subscribers can enter their answers online to earn CME credits instantaneously. You can submit your answers using online answer sheets that are provided at mksap.acponline.org, where a record of your MKSAP 17 credits will be available. To earn CME credits, you need to answer all of the questions in a test and earn a score of at least 50% correct (number of correct answers divided by the total number of questions). Take any of the following approaches:

➤ Use the printed answer sheet at the back of this book to record your answers. Go to mksap.acponline.org, access the appropriate online answer sheet, transcribe your answers, and submit your test for instantaneous CME credits. There is no additional fee for this service.

➤ Go to mksap.acponline.org, access the appropriate online answer sheet, directly enter your answers, and submit your test for instantaneous CME credits. There is no additional fee for this service.

➤ Pay a $15 processing fee per answer sheet and submit the printed answer sheet at the back of this book by mail or fax, as instructed on the answer sheet. Make sure you calculate your score and fax the answer sheet to 215-351-2799 or mail the answer sheet to Member and Customer Service, American College of Physicians, 190 N. Independence Mall West, Philadelphia, PA 19106-1572, using the courtesy envelope provided in your MKSAP 17 slipcase. You will need your 10-digit order number and 8-digit ACP ID number, which are printed on your packing slip. Please allow 4 to 6 weeks for your score report to be emailed back to you. Be sure to include your email address for a response.

If you do not have a 10-digit order number and 8-digit ACP ID number or if you need help creating a username and password to access the MKSAP 17 online answer sheets, go to mksap.acponline.org or email custserv@acponline.org.

CME credit is available from the publication date of December 31, 2015, until December 31, 2018. You may submit your answer sheets at any time during this period.

*Each of the numbered items is followed by lettered answers. Select the **ONE** lettered answer that is **BEST** in each case.*

Self-Assessment Test

Item 1

A 43-year-old man is evaluated during a routine physical examination. He has no current symptoms and no prior medical history. Family history is notable for diabetes mellitus and hypertension in two first-degree relatives. He takes no medications.

On physical examination, initial blood pressure measurement is 144/86 mm Hg; repeat measurement after 5 minutes of rest are 136/86 mm Hg and 134/88 mm Hg. BMI is 32. The remainder of the examination is normal.

Laboratory studies show normal serum creatinine and plasma glucose levels.

In addition to lifestyle modifications, which of the following is the most appropriate next step in the management of this patient's blood pressure?

(A) Initiate a low-dose ACE inhibitor
(B) Initiate low-dose chlorthalidone
(C) Order ambulatory blood pressure monitoring
(D) Recheck blood pressure in 1 year

Item 2

A 74-year-old woman is evaluated for a 1-week history of intermittent painless gross hematuria. She has a 3-year history of stage G4/A3 chronic kidney disease due to diabetic nephropathy, a 12-year history of type 2 diabetes mellitus, diabetic retinopathy, and hypertension. Medications are lisinopril, furosemide, insulin glargine, and insulin lispro.

On physical examination, temperature is 37.0 °C (98.6 °F), blood pressure is 128/85 mm Hg, pulse rate is 76/min, and respiration rate is 15/min. BMI is 28. The lungs are clear. There are no abdominal masses or costovertebral angle tenderness. There is no edema.

Laboratory studies:

Creatinine	2.6 mg/dL (230 µmol/L)
Estimated glomerular filtration rate	23 mL/min/1.73 m²
Urinalysis	2+ protein; 25-50 erythrocytes/hpf; 0 leukocytes/hpf; no erythrocyte casts

Which of the following is the most appropriate diagnostic test to perform in this patient?

(A) Contrast-enhanced CT of the abdomen and pelvis
(B) Gadolinium-enhanced MRI of the abdomen and pelvis
(C) Radiography of the abdomen and pelvis
(D) Ultrasonography of the abdomen and pelvis

Item 3

A 45-year-old man is evaluated during a new patient visit. He immigrated to the United States from Serbia 4 years ago and was diagnosed with Balkan endemic nephropathy at that time. His kidney function has remained stable, and his only symptoms are mild nocturia and urinary frequency. Medical history is otherwise unremarkable. He takes no medications.

On physical examination, temperature is 37.1 °C (98.7 °F), blood pressure is 138/82 mm Hg, pulse rate is 76/min, and respiration rate is 12/min. BMI is 26. The remainder of the examination is normal.

Laboratory studies:

Hemoglobin	9.6 g/dL (96 g/L)
Electrolytes	Normal
Creatinine	1.7 mg/dL (150.1 µmol/L)
Glucose	Normal
Estimated glomerular filtration rate	35 mL/min/1.73 m²
Urinalysis	Specific gravity 1.005; 2+ glucose; 10-20 erythrocytes/hpf

An increased risk of which of the following is most likely in this patient?

(A) Diabetes mellitus
(B) Intracranial cerebral aneurysm
(C) Renal cell carcinoma
(D) Transitional cell carcinoma

Item 4

A 64-year-old man is evaluated for a 6-week history of intermittent red-colored urine. He notes fatigue but otherwise feels well. Medical history includes hypertension, mechanical mitral valve replacement due to myxomatous degeneration, and calcium oxalate nephrolithiasis. He is a current smoker with a 60-pack-year history. Medications are amlodipine, warfarin, and aspirin.

On physical examination, temperature is 37.6 °C (99.7 °F), blood pressure is 112/72 mm Hg, and pulse rate is 98/min. BMI is 30. Examination of the heart reveals a metallic click with a grade 2/6 cardiac systolic murmur that radiates to the axilla. The lungs are clear. There is no costovertebral angle tenderness. The remainder of the examination is unremarkable.

Urinalysis is dipstick positive for 3+ blood, 1+ protein, and no leukocyte esterase or nitrites; on microscopic examination, there are no cells or casts, although calcium oxalate crystals are seen.

Which of the following is the most likely cause of this patient's clinical findings?

(A) Bladder cancer
(B) Glomerulonephritis
(C) Hemoglobinuria
(D) Nephrolithiasis

Item 5

A 62-year-old man is evaluated during a follow-up visit for hypertension. His clinic blood pressure readings during the past year have been persistently above 140/90 mm Hg, and home blood pressure readings have been in the range of 150-170/90-96 mm Hg. He reports no symptoms. Medical history is otherwise unremarkable. Medications are maximal doses of lisinopril, nifedipine, and atenolol.

On physical examination, temperature is 36.8 °C (98.2 °F), blood pressure is 168/100 mm Hg in both arms with no orthostasis, pulse rate is 60/min, and respiration rate is 16/min. BMI is 29. Retinal examination shows copper wiring of the arteries. An S_4 is heard on cardiac auscultation. There are no bruits heard over the carotids or abdomen. Neurologic and peripheral vascular examinations are normal. There is no edema.

Laboratory studies:

Creatinine	1.5 mg/dL (132.6 µmol/L)
Potassium	4.1 mEq/L (4.1 mmol/L)
Estimated glomerular filtration rate	45 mL/min/1.73 m²
Urinalysis	No protein, blood, or cells

Electrocardiogram shows left ventricular hypertrophy with repolarization abnormalities. Kidney ultrasound is normal.

Which of the following is the most appropriate next step in management?

(A) Add chlorthalidone
(B) Add clonidine transdermal patch
(C) Add minoxidil
(D) Switch nifedipine to amlodipine

Item 6

A 68-year-old man is evaluated for a 6-month history of progressive dyspnea on exertion, dizziness on standing, lower extremity edema, and burning pain with numbness in his extremities. He also notes intermittent loose stools up to 6 times daily. Medical history is otherwise unremarkable, and he takes no medications. He is current with scheduled health maintenance screening interventions, and laboratory studies obtained 3 years ago for an insurance physical examination were normal.

On physical examination, temperature is normal, pulse rate is 90/min, and respiration rate is 20/min. Blood pressure is 140/70 mm Hg sitting; upon standing, blood pressure drops to 90/60 mm Hg with dizziness. BMI is 27. Estimated central venous pressure is 7 cm H_2O. Decreased breath sounds are heard at the lung bases bilaterally. Heart examination does not reveal a rub or gallop. Abdominal examination reveals mild hepatosplenomegaly. On neurologic examination, there is impaired touch and vibration sense in a glove and stocking distribution. Bilateral lower extremity edema is noted to the level of the ankles.

Laboratory studies:

Albumin	2.8 g/dL (28 g/L)
Creatinine	1.6 mg/dL (141.4 µmol/L)
Electrolytes	Normal
Fasting plasma glucose	98 mg/dL (5.4 mmol/L)
Urinalysis	3+ protein; no blood or cells
Urine protein-creatinine ratio	4800 mg/g

Which of the following is the most likely diagnosis on kidney biopsy?

(A) AL amyloidosis
(B) Diabetic nephropathy
(C) Myeloma nephropathy
(D) Primary focal segmental glomerulosclerosis

Item 7

A 55-year-old woman is evaluated for persistent hyperkalemia. She is asymptomatic. Medical history is significant for type 2 diabetes mellitus complicated by nephropathy and peripheral neuropathy; she also has hypertension. Medications are insulin, rosuvastatin, amlodipine, amitriptyline, and aspirin.

On physical examination, temperature is 36.3 °C (97.4 °F), blood pressure is 130/72 mm Hg, pulse rate is 64/min, and respiration rate is 18/min. BMI is 32. Estimated central venous pressure is 6.0 cm H_2O. There is hyperesthesia of the feet bilaterally but no edema. The remainder of the examination is unremarkable.

Laboratory studies:

Creatinine	1.9 mg/dL (168 µmol/L)
Electrolytes:	
Sodium	138 mEq/L (138 mmol/L)
Potassium	5.1 mEq/L (5.1 mmol/L)
Chloride	112 mEq/L (112 mmol/L)
Bicarbonate	18 mEq/L (18 mmol/L)
Glucose	142 mg/dL (7.9 mmol/L)
Phosphorus	4.5 mg/dL (1.5 mmol/L)
Estimated glomerular filtration rate	27 mL/min/1.73 m²
Urinalysis	pH 5.0

Which of the following is the most likely cause of this patient's metabolic findings?

(A) Kidney failure
(B) Type 1 (hypokalemic distal) renal tubular acidosis
(C) Type 2 (proximal) renal tubular acidosis
(D) Type 4 (hyperkalemic distal) renal tubular acidosis

Item 8

A 37-year-old woman is evaluated for an episode of blood in her urine. She notes the passage of red-colored urine that resolved spontaneously and was not associated with her menstrual cycle. She reports having had several similar episodes in the past. She has no other symptoms such as abdominal pain or dysuria. Medical history is otherwise unremarkable, and she takes no medications.

On physical examination, the patient is afebrile. Blood pressure is 128/78 mm Hg, pulse rate is 82/min, and respiration rate is 13/min. Cardiopulmonary and abdominal examinations are normal. There is no flank tenderness to palpation. The remainder of the examination is unremarkable.

Laboratory studies show a normal complete blood count and metabolic profile and a serum creatinine level of 0.9 mg/dL (79.6 µmol/L). Dipstick urinalysis is positive for blood and protein but is negative for leukocyte esterase and nitrites.

Microscopy of the urine sediment is shown.

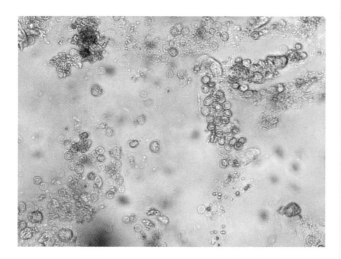

Which of the following is the most appropriate next step in the evaluation of this patient?

(A) Cystoscopy

(B) Evaluation for glomerular disease

(C) Noncontrast helical abdominal CT

(D) Serum creatine kinase measurement

Item 9

A 22-year-old woman is evaluated for persistent hematuria initially discovered following treatment of a urinary tract infection. She is asymptomatic. Family history is significant for persistent hematuria in her father and brother without kidney failure. Medical history is unremarkable, and she takes no medications.

On physical examination, temperature is 37.0 °C (98.6 °F), blood pressure is 110/74 mm Hg, pulse rate is 74/min, and respiration rate is 16/min. BMI is 22. Hearing is normal, and examination of the eyes is unremarkable. Cardiopulmonary examination is normal. Skin examination shows no lesions. Neurologic examination is unremarkable.

Laboratory studies:

Blood urea nitrogen	18 mg/dL (6.4 mmol/L)
Creatinine	0.9 mg/dL (79.6 µmol/L)
Urinalysis	pH 5.0; 2+ blood; no protein; 10-20 erythrocytes/hpf

Kidney ultrasound shows normal-sized kidneys without evidence of obstruction or cysts.

Which of the following is the most likely diagnosis?

(A) Fabry disease

(B) Hereditary nephritis

(C) Thin glomerular basement membrane disease

(D) Tuberous sclerosis complex

Item 10

A 51-year-old man is evaluated during a follow-up visit for management of newly diagnosed hypertension and diabetes mellitus. He has started a program of lifestyle modification for his diabetes but has not yet started antihypertensive therapy. He is currently taking no medications.

On physical examination, blood pressure is 148/92 mm Hg, and pulse rate is 76/min. BMI is 33. The remainder of the examination is unremarkable.

Laboratory studies show a serum creatinine level of 1.5 mg/dL (132.6 µmol/L) (estimated glomerular filtration rate of 52 mL/min/1.73 m^2) and a serum potassium level of 4.2 mEq/L (4.2 mmol/L); a urine dipstick demonstrates no hematuria or proteinuria, and a spot urine protein-creatinine ratio is 50 mg/g.

Which of the following is the most appropriate antihypertensive treatment for this patient?

(A) Hydrochlorothiazide

(B) Lisinopril

(C) Lisinopril and amlodipine

(D) Lisinopril and hydrochlorothiazide

(E) Lisinopril and losartan

Item 11

A 73-year-old man is evaluated during a routine examination. He feels well but notes a gradual weight gain of 9.1 kg (20 lb) over the past 5 years. He reports his blood pressure to be around 155/85 mm Hg on several determinations at his local pharmacy. Medical history is significant for mild benign prostatic hyperplasia, gout, and hyperlipidemia. Medications are atorvastatin and as-needed colchicine.

On physical examination, blood pressure is 158/87 mm Hg, pulse rate is 85/min, and respiration rate is 12/min. BMI is 29. Cardiac examination is normal, and the remainder of the physical examination is unremarkable.

Laboratory studies show a normal chemistry panel; a urine dipstick demonstrates no blood or protein.

An electrocardiogram shows no evidence of left ventricular hypertrophy.

Which of the following is the most appropriate next step in management?

(A) Doxazosin

(B) Hydrochlorothiazide

(C) Metoprolol

(D) Lifestyle modifications

(E) Repeat blood pressure determination in 6 months

Item 12

A 24-year-old man is evaluated in the hospital for progressively worsening kidney function. He was admitted 5 days ago with fevers and was diagnosed with endocarditis with methicillin-resistant *Staphylococcus aureus*. Intravenous vancomycin was started and adjusted daily to target levels of 15 to 20 µg/mL (10.4-13.8 µmol/L). Since admission, his fevers have resolved, but his serum creatinine level has gradually increased. Medical history includes two previous admissions for staphylococcal endocarditis treated with prolonged courses of antibiotics. He has occasionally used injection drugs, including heroin, during the past 4 years. His only medication is vancomycin.

On physical examination, temperature is 37.3 °C (99.2 °F), blood pressure is 110/70 mm Hg, pulse rate is 92/min, and respiration rate is 18/min. BMI is 22. Cardiac examination is notable for a soft diastolic murmur along the left sternal border. There is trace lower extremity edema. There is no skin rash or arthritis.

Laboratory studies:

C3	Low
C4	Normal
Creatinine	2.8 mg/dL (247.5 µmol/L) (1.5 mg/dL [132.6 µmol/L] on admission)
Cryoglobulins	Negative
Urinalysis	3+ blood; 2+ protein; 30-40 erythrocytes/hpf; 10-15 leukocytes/hpf; erythrocyte casts

Transthoracic ultrasound shows moderate aortic regurgitation without vegetations (confirmed on transesophageal ultrasound). Kidney ultrasound shows normal-sized, mildly echogenic kidneys. Doppler study of the renal arteries and veins is normal.

Which of the following is the most appropriate management?

(A) Initiate glucocorticoids

(B) Schedule a kidney biopsy

(C) Switch vancomycin to daptomycin

(D) Continue current therapy

Item 13

A 58-year-old man is evaluated during a follow-up visit for a 15-year history of hypertension. Medical history is significant for hypertensive nephropathy. He states that he feels well and is without current complaints. Medications are lisinopril and hydrochlorothiazide.

On physical examination, the patient is afebrile, blood pressure is 138/82 mm Hg, pulse rate is 83/min, and respiration rate is 12/min. BMI is 29. Cardiovascular examination is unremarkable. The lungs are clear. There is no peripheral edema.

Laboratory studies are significant for a serum creatinine level of 1.7 mg/dL (150.3 µmol/L) and a urine albumin-creatinine ratio of 200 mg/g.

Which of the following is the most appropriate management?

(A) Add losartan

(B) Increase lisinopril dose

(C) Replace lisinopril with amlodipine

(D) Continue current medications

Item 14

A 20-year-old woman is evaluated during a new-patient visit for persistent dipstick-positive hematuria initially discovered 2 years ago when she was evaluated for a possible urinary tract infection. Two subsequent urinalyses have shown dipstick-positive hematuria and 10-15 erythrocytes/hpf on microscopic examination without other abnormalities. She has not noted any episodes of gross hematuria or

other urinary tract symptoms. She reports no fever, rash, or arthritis. Family history is notable for her mother and maternal aunt who have hematuria; there is no family history of kidney disease. Medical history is otherwise negative, and the patient takes no medications.

On physical examination, the patient is afebrile, blood pressure is 118/78 mm Hg, pulse rate is 64/min, and respiration rate is 14/min. BMI is 22. The remainder of the physical examination is normal.

Laboratory studies:

Complements (C3 and C4)	Normal
Creatinine	0.6 mg/dL (53 µmol/L)
Hepatitis B and C serologies	Negative
Antinuclear antibodies	Negative
ANCA	Negative
Urinalysis	2+ blood; no protein; 10-15 erythrocytes/hpf; no casts
Urine protein-creatinine ratio	110 mg/g

Kidney ultrasound is normal.

Which of the following is the most appropriate management?

(A) Abdominal CT with contrast

(B) Cystoscopy

(C) Kidney biopsy

(D) Serial kidney function and urine protein determinations

(E) Urine cytology

Item 15

A 48-year-old woman is evaluated during a follow-up visit for hypertension. Blood pressure measurements taken at the past three visits have been in the range of 135 to 146 mm Hg systolic and 86 to 92 mm Hg diastolic. Twenty-four hour ambulatory blood pressure monitoring shows an overall mean blood pressure of 136/84 mm Hg; daytime readings average 138/85 mm Hg, and nighttime readings average 130/82 mm Hg. She has no other pertinent personal or family history. She takes no medications.

On physical examination, blood pressure is 146/92 mm Hg, and pulse rate is 76/min. BMI is 29. The remainder of the examination is unremarkable.

Laboratory studies show a normal chemistry panel; a urine dipstick demonstrates no protein.

Which of the following is the most appropriate next step in management?

(A) Begin lisinopril

(B) Begin melatonin

(C) Recheck blood pressure in the office in 6 months

(D) Recheck blood pressure in the office in 1 year

(E) Repeat 24-hour ambulatory blood pressure monitoring in 1 year

Item 16

A 36-year-old man is evaluated following his second episode of nephrolithiasis. His initial kidney stone occurred

6 months ago and passed spontaneously. The stone was recovered and on analysis was found to be a pure uric acid stone. He was advised to increase his urine output to at least 2 L/d and has been adherent to this recommendation. His second episode occurred last week. He again passed the stone spontaneously, which was submitted for analysis and shown to be a pure uric acid stone. Medical history is significant for type 2 diabetes mellitus, but he has never had evidence of gout. Medications are metformin and rosuvastatin.

On physical examination, temperature is 36.9 °C (98.5 °F), blood pressure is 135/87 mm Hg, pulse rate is 78/min, and respiration rate is 12/min. BMI is 31. There is no costovertebral angle tenderness. No joint abnormalities or gouty tophi are noted.

Laboratory studies:

Electrolytes	Normal
Kidney function studies	Normal
Urate	7.6 mg/dL (0.45 mmol/L)
Urinalysis	pH 5.8; no blood; no cells or crystals
24-Hour uric acid excretion	850 mg/24 h (5 mmol/24 h)

In addition to continuing oral hydration, which of the following is the most appropriate next step in therapy?

(A) Allopurinol
(B) Cholestyramine
(C) Hydrochlorothiazide
(D) Urine alkalinization

Item 17

A 45-year-old man is evaluated during a routine follow-up visit. Medical history is significant for difficult-to-control hypertension, type 2 diabetes mellitus complicated by proliferative retinopathy and sensory and autonomic neuropathy, and chronic kidney disease. He has no new symptoms. Medications are lisinopril, amlodipine, hydrochlorothiazide, and insulin.

On physical examination, temperature is 36.9 °C (98.4 °F), blood pressure is 180/100 mm Hg in both arms, pulse rate is 66/min, and respiration rate is 14/min. BMI is 34. There is bilateral lower extremity edema to the mid calf.

Laboratory studies are significant for a serum creatinine level of 2.2 mg/dL (194.5 µmol/L), a serum potassium level of 4.2 mEq/L (4.2 mmol/L), and a urine protein-creatinine ratio of 4000 mg/g.

Which of the following is the most appropriate treatment?

(A) Add aliskiren
(B) Add clonidine
(C) Add minoxidil
(D) Switch hydrochlorothiazide to furosemide

Item 18

An 85-year-old man arrives with his daughter to discuss options for end-stage kidney disease (ESKD) management. He has stage G5/A3 chronic kidney disease due to diabetic nephropathy and hypertension. History is also significant for a 3-year history of Alzheimer disease and heart failure with a left ventricular ejection fraction of 35%. Medications are aspirin, losartan, furosemide, carvedilol, and calcium acetate. The patient is a resident of a nursing facility.

On physical examination, the patient appears comfortable but is not oriented to place or time. Temperature is 37.0 °C (98.6 °F), blood pressure is 142/70 mm Hg, pulse rate is 82/min, and respiration rate is 18/min. BMI is 21. The lungs are clear. There is trace bipedal edema. The remainder of the examination is unremarkable.

Laboratory studies are notable for a blood urea nitrogen level of 82 mg/dL (29.3 mmol/L), a serum creatinine level of 5.1 mg/dL (450.8 µmol/L), and an estimated glomerular filtration rate of 9 mL/min/1.73 m^2.

Which of the following is the most appropriate recommendation for management of this patient's ESKD?

(A) Hemodialysis in a dialysis unit
(B) Hemodialysis at the nursing facility
(C) Nocturnal peritoneal dialysis
(D) Non-dialytic therapy

Item 19

A 48-year-old woman is evaluated during a follow-up visit for newly diagnosed hypertension, confirmed by multiple measurements at home and in the office. Medical history is notable for hyperlipidemia, for which she takes atorvastatin. Lifestyle modifications have been recommended.

On physical examination, blood pressure is 160/92 mm Hg, and pulse rate is 64/min. BMI is 32. The remainder of the examination is unremarkable.

Laboratory studies show a serum creatinine level of 1.1 mg/dL (97.2 µmol/L), a fasting plasma glucose level of 114 mg/dL (6.3 mmol/L), and a serum potassium level of 4.0 mEq/L (4.0 mmol/L); a urine dipstick demonstrates no blood or protein.

Which of the following is most likely to be effective in controlling this patient's hypertension?

(A) Amlodipine
(B) Lisinopril
(C) Losartan
(D) Lisinopril and amlodipine
(E) Losartan and lisinopril

Item 20

A 55-year-old woman is evaluated during a follow-up visit for elevated blood pressure noted on several previous clinic visits. She checks her blood pressure at home with a device checked in the clinic for accuracy and reports measurements typically in the "120s over 80s." She is asymptomatic except for occasional palpitations associated with episodes of anxiety. Medical history is notable for depression, for which she takes citalopram.

On physical examination, blood pressure is 152/88 mm Hg, and pulse rate is 88/min. BMI is 24. The remainder of the examination is unremarkable.

Laboratory studies show a normal chemistry panel; a urine dipstick demonstrates no blood or protein.

A resting electrocardiogram is normal.

Which of the following is the most appropriate diagnostic test to perform next?

(A) 24-Hour ambulatory blood pressure monitoring

(B) 24-Hour urine testing for fractionated metanephrines

(C) Ambulatory electrocardiography

(D) Echocardiography

(E) Plasma aldosterone-plasma renin ratio

Item 21

A 65-year-old man is hospitalized for an ischemic, nonhealing right lower extremity ulcer with associated biopsy-proven osteomyelitis. On hospital day 1, he was started on cefazolin and underwent angiography and stenting of the iliac artery using a low osmolar contrast agent. On day 2, he became febrile and was switched to vancomycin and gentamicin based on culture sensitivity data. On day 3, his fever resolved and his serum creatinine was at baseline (1.5 mg/dL [132.6 µmol/L]). On day 10, his serum creatinine increased to 3.0 mg/dL (265.2 µmol/L) with a urine output of 0.5 mL/kg/h. Medical history is notable for type 2 diabetes mellitus, hypertension, dyslipidemia, coronary artery disease, and chronic kidney disease. Medications are rosuvastatin, amlodipine, carvedilol, aspirin, insulin, vancomycin, and gentamicin.

On physical examination, blood pressure is 150/78 mm Hg, and pulse rate is 72/min. There is no rash. The lower extremities have decreased peripheral pulses. The right foot has a 1-cm clean-appearing ulcer on the tip of the second toe. The remainder of the physical examination is normal.

Laboratory studies on day 10:

Hemoglobin	11.2 g/dL (112 g/L)
Leukocyte count	8500/µL (8.5 × 10⁹/L) with 58% polymorphonuclear leukocytes, 20% lymphocytes, 3% eosinophils
Creatinine	3.0 mg/dL (265.2 µmol/L) (baseline, 1.5 mg/dL [132.6 µmol/L])
Urine sodium	40 mEq/L (40 mmol/L)
Fractional excretion of sodium	2.1%
Urinalysis	Specific gravity 1.012; pH 5.5; trace blood; trace protein; 1-3 normal-appearing erythrocytes/hpf; granular casts; tubular epithelial cells

Kidney ultrasound is normal.

Which of the following is the most likely cause of this patient's acute kidney injury?

(A) Cefazolin

(B) Cholesterol emboli

(C) Contrast

(D) Gentamicin

Item 22

A 59-year-old man is evaluated during a follow-up visit for a 6-year history of end-stage kidney disease and a 20-year history of hypertension. He had a kidney transplant 3 months ago with an unremarkable postoperative course. Current medications are tacrolimus, mycophenolate mofetil, nifedipine, losartan, valganciclovir, and prednisone, 5 mg/d.

On physical examination, temperature is 37.0 °C (98.6 °F), blood pressure is 165/95 mm Hg, pulse rate is 86/min, and respiration rate is 14/min. BMI is 28. There are no oral lesions. There is no jugular venous distention. Heart sounds are normal. The lungs are clear. The abdomen is nontender with no bruits. There is a well-healed scar in the right lower abdomen over the kidney allograft. There is 1+ peripheral edema.

Laboratory studies are notable for a serum creatinine level of 1.0 mg/dL (88.4 µmol/L).

Monitoring for which of the following complications is indicated in this patient?

(A) Hyperphosphatemia

(B) Hyperthyroidism

(C) Hypoparathyroidism

(D) New-onset diabetes mellitus and dyslipidemia

Item 23

A 36-year-old man is evaluated in the emergency department for right flank pain of 2 days' duration and an episode of gross hematuria. He reports no fever, nausea, or gastrointestinal symptoms. He has no other pertinent medical history, and he takes no medications. Family history is notable for a father with kidney stones.

On physical examination, the patient is in moderately painful discomfort. Temperature is 37.1 °C (98.7 °F), blood pressure is 123/76 mm Hg, pulse rate is 78/min, and respiration rate is 12/min. BMI is 21. There is no costovertebral angle tenderness. The abdomen is normal without rebound or guarding. The remainder of the examination is unremarkable.

Laboratory studies show a normal complete blood count, electrolyte panel, and kidney function. Urinalysis is significant for large blood on dipstick and >50,000 erythrocytes/hpf.

Noncontrast abdominal CT scan reveals a 12-mm stone in the right renal pelvis.

Which of the following is the most appropriate management?

(A) Mechanical stone removal

(B) Nifedipine

(C) Oral glucocorticoids

(D) Tamsulosin

Item 24

A 54-year-old woman is evaluated for fatigue, anorexia, polyuria, and nocturia of several weeks' duration. She had otherwise felt well until the onset of her current symptoms. Medical history is significant for autoimmune pancreatitis diagnosed 1 year ago, treated with a prednisone taper that was completed 8 months ago with resolution of her symptoms. She takes no medications.

On physical examination, temperature is 36.2 °C (97.2 °F), blood pressure is 110/58 mm Hg, pulse rate is 72/min, and respiration rate is 16/min. BMI is 25. Estimated central venous pressure is 7 cm H$_2$O. The lungs are clear. There are no murmurs or extra heart sounds. Abdominal examination is unremarkable. There is no edema.

Laboratory studies:

Blood urea nitrogen	56 mg/dL (20 mmol/L)
Creatinine	5.2 mg/dL (459.7 µmol/L)
Serum free light chain ratio	Normal
Urinalysis	pH 5.0; 1+ protein; 3-5 erythrocytes/hpf; 5-10 leukocytes/hpf; occasional leukocyte casts

Chest radiograph is normal. Kidney ultrasound shows slightly enlarged kidneys without evidence of obstruction.

Which of the following is the most likely diagnosis?

(A) ANCA-associated vasculitis

(B) Anti–glomerular basement membrane antibody disease

(C) IgG4-related interstitial nephritis

(D) Lupus nephritis

Item 25

A 46-year-old woman is evaluated in the emergency department for fatigue and weakness of 5 days' duration. The patient also reports recurrent lower extremity swelling. She is vague when asked about medication or drug use.

On physical examination, blood pressure is 108/62 mm Hg, pulse rate is 98/min, and respiration rate is 16/min. Upon standing, systolic blood pressure decreases by 15 mm Hg, and pulse rate increases by 10/min. BMI is 26. The remainder of the examination is unremarkable, with no evidence of lower extremity edema.

Laboratory studies:

Serum bicarbonate	29 mEq/L (29 mmol/L)
Serum creatinine	1.2 mg/dL (106.1 µmol/L)
Serum potassium	3.1 mEq/L (3.1 mmol/L)
Urine chloride	53 mEq/L (53 mmol/L)
Urine potassium	25 mEq/L (25 mmol/L)
Urine sodium	42 mEq/L (42 mmol/L)

Which of the following is the most appropriate diagnostic test to perform next?

(A) 24-Hour urine free cortisol excretion

(B) Plasma aldosterone-plasma renin ratio

(C) Serum thyroid-stimulating hormone level

(D) Urine diuretic screening

Item 26

A 77-year-old woman is evaluated 4 months following a left middle cerebral artery ischemic stroke. The severity of her stroke required prolonged initial hospitalization and a 3-month stay in a rehabilitation center before returning home. Residual deficits include dense right-sided hemiparesis and dysphagia requiring oral feeding with thickened

liquids. Medical history is otherwise significant for hypertension and diabetes mellitus. Current medications are aspirin, chlorthalidone, lisinopril, tolterodine, and insulin.

On physical examination, temperature is 37.2 °C (99.0 °F), blood pressure is 136/86 mm Hg, and pulse rate is 86/min. BMI is 18. The general medical examination is unremarkable. Neurologic examination reveals dysarthria, left-sided facial droop, 1/5 strength in the right arm and leg, and bilateral distal sensory neuropathy.

Laboratory studies:

Hemoglobin A$_{1c}$	7.2%
Albumin	2.4 g/dL (24 g/L)
Blood urea nitrogen	12 mg/dL (4.3 mmol/L) (4 months ago: 28 mg/dL [10 mmol/L])
Creatinine	0.8 mg/dL (70.7 µmol/L) (4 months ago: 1.4 mg/dL [123.8 µmol/L])
Urinalysis	Normal

Which of the following is the most likely cause of this patient's decreased serum creatinine level?

(A) Decrease in muscle mass

(B) Improvement in diabetic kidney disease

(C) Initiation of chlorthalidone

(D) Initiation of lisinopril

Item 27

A 60-year-old man is evaluated during a routine visit. He has stage G4/A3 chronic kidney disease due to membranous glomerulopathy. He received treatment with cyclosporine and prednisone and received rituximab 2 years ago. Current medications are lisinopril, atorvastatin, furosemide, and calcium carbonate/vitamin D. He received the complete hepatitis B immunization series, pneumococcal polysaccharide, tetanus and diphtheria combined with acellular pertussis, and influenza immunizations 6 months ago.

On physical examination, vital signs are normal. BMI is 27. The remainder of the examination is noncontributory.

Which of the following is an appropriate approach to pneumococcal vaccination in this patient?

(A) Administer the pneumococcal conjugate vaccine now

(B) Administer the pneumococcal conjugate vaccine in 6 months

(C) Administer the pneumococcal polysaccharide and pneumococcal conjugate vaccines in 6 months

(D) Repeat the pneumococcal polysaccharide vaccine now

Item 28

A 26-year-old woman is evaluated for muscle weakness developing over the past several months. She has no focal symptoms and states that she otherwise feels well. Medical history is unremarkable, and there is no pertinent family history. She takes no medications.

On physical examination, blood pressure is 98/62 mm Hg, pulse rate is 98/min, and respiration rate is 16/min. BMI is 19. There is no lower extremity edema. The remainder of the examination is unremarkable.

Laboratory studies:

Serum electrolytes:
Sodium	142 mEq/L (142 mmol/L)
Potassium	3.1 mEq/L (3.1 mmol/L)
Chloride	120 mEq/L (120 mmol/L)
Bicarbonate	15 mEq/L (15 mmol/L)
Serum creatinine	1.2 mg/dL (106.1 μmol/L)

Urine electrolytes:
Sodium	18 mEq/L (18 mmol/L)
Potassium	8.0 mEq/L (8.0 mmol/L)
Chloride	32 mEq/L (32 mmol/L)
Urine pH	5.0
Urine dipstick	No blood or protein

Which of the following is the most likely cause of this patient's acid-base and electrolyte abnormalities?

(A) Bulimia nervosa

(B) Gitelman syndrome

(C) Laxative abuse

(D) Surreptitious diuretic use

(E) Type 1 (hypokalemic distal) renal tubular acidosis

Item 29

A 65-year-old man is evaluated during a follow-up visit for a preemptive living donor kidney transplant 6 months ago, with a postoperative course complicated by an episode of acute cellular rejection requiring antithymocyte antibody induction. He has done well since then. He has a 10-year history of chronic kidney disease due to diabetic nephropathy and a 35-year history of type 1 diabetes mellitus. Basal cell carcinoma was removed from his nose 2 years ago. Current medications are tacrolimus, mycophenolate mofetil, valganciclovir, and prednisone, 5 mg/d.

On physical examination, temperature is 37.0 °C (98.6 °F), blood pressure is 135/78 mm Hg, pulse rate is 80/min, and respiration rate is 14/min. BMI is 22. There is no lymphadenopathy. Actinic keratoses are present on the forehead. The lungs are clear. The abdomen is nontender without organomegaly. The kidney allograft in the left pelvis is nontender with a well-healed scar. There is no peripheral edema.

Laboratory studies show a serum creatinine level of 1.2 mg/dL (106.1 μmol/L).

In addition to age- and sex-appropriate screening, which of the following should this patient be evaluated for?

(A) Colon cancer

(B) Lung cancer

(C) Prostate cancer

(D) Skin cancer

(E) No additional screening

Item 30

A 68-year-old woman is hospitalized for coronary artery bypass surgery for multi-vessel coronary artery disease. Medical history includes atherosclerotic cardiovascular disease, hypertension, type 2 diabetes mellitus, hyperlipidemia, and chronic kidney disease. Home medications are simvastatin, lisinopril, furosemide, amlodipine, aspirin, and glimepiride.

On physical examination, blood pressure is 150/82 mm Hg, and pulse rate is 76/min. BMI is 25. The remainder of the physical examination is unremarkable.

Laboratory studies are significant for a baseline serum creatinine level of 2.3 mg/dL (203.3 μmol/L), with an estimated glomerular filtration rate (eGFR) of 25 mL/min/1.73 m².

Which of the following is considered the strongest predictor of the development of acute kidney injury in the perioperative period for this patient?

(A) Baseline eGFR

(B) BMI

(C) Hypertension

(D) Perioperative lisinopril use

(E) Perioperative statin use

Item 31

A 72-year-old woman is evaluated for a 3-year history of progressively worsening low back pain involving the lumbar spine, sacroiliac joints, and hips. She reports progressive difficulty with rising from a squat and climbing stairs. She also has had several spontaneous fractures over the past year. At the time of presentation, she cannot walk without support. Medical history is also notable for type 2 diabetes mellitus, hypertension, and hyperlipidemia. Medications are glipizide, quinapril, rosiglitazone, atorvastatin, and hydrocodone/acetaminophen.

On physical examination, blood pressure is 147/84 mm Hg, and pulse rate is 82/min. There is a small swelling over the proximal phalanx of the left index finger. There is tenderness upon palpation of the ribs. Examination of the joints and spine is normal. Decreased strength in the proximal muscles of the lower limbs is noted.

Laboratory studies:
Albumin	3.9 g/dL (39 g/L)
Alkaline phosphatase	436 U/L
Calcium	9.0 mg/dL (2.3 mmol/L)
Creatinine	0.9 mg/dL (79.6 μmol/L)
Phosphorus	1.7 mg/dL (0.55 mmol/L)
Intact parathyroid hormone	22 pg/mL (22 ng/L)
1,25-Dihydroxy vitamin D	5.0 pg/mL (12 pmol/L)
25-Hydroxy vitamin D	40 ng/mL (99.8 nmol/L)
24-Hour urine phosphate	1.4 g/24 h (45 mmol/24 h) (normal range, 0.4-1.3 g/24 h [12.9-42 mmol/24 h])

Which of the following is the most likely cause of this patient's hypophosphatemia?

(A) Nutritional vitamin D deficiency

(B) Oncogenic osteomalacia

(C) Primary hyperparathyroidism

(D) X-linked hypophosphatemic rickets

Item 32

A 47-year-old man is admitted to the medical ICU with severe sepsis, multi-lobar pneumonia, and acute respiratory distress syndrome. He developed oliguric acute kidney injury on hospital day 3; he has produced only 240 mL of urine over the past 24 hours despite adequate intravenous hydration. He is mechanically ventilated and requires 80% FIO_2. Medical history is unremarkable, and current medications are piperacillin/tazobactam, vancomycin, norepinephrine, vasopressin and propofol infusions, and a proton pump inhibitor.

On physical examination the patient is intubated and sedated. Temperature is 38.5 °C (101.3 °F), blood pressure is 95/60 mm Hg, and pulse rate is 130/min. Estimated central venous pressure is 14 cm H_2O. There is no rash. Generalized anasarca is noted. Examination of the chest reveals coarse breath sounds and inspiratory crackles throughout both lungs.

Laboratory studies:

Blood urea nitrogen	103 mg/dL (36.8 mmol/L)
Creatinine	4.3 mg/dL (380.1 µmol/L)
Electrolytes	
Sodium	137 mEq/L (137 mmol/L)
Potassium	6.0 mEq/L (6.0 mmol/L)
Chloride	97 mEq/L (97 mmol/L))
Bicarbonate	16 mEq/L (16 mmol/L)
Phosphorus	7.2 mg/dL (2.33 mmol/L)
Serum pH	7.2
Urinalysis	3+ blood; 0-2 erythrocytes/hpf; multiple granular casts and tubular epithelial cells

Which of the following is the most appropriate treatment for this patient's kidney failure?

(A) Initiate continuous renal replacement therapy
(B) Initiate intermittent hemodialysis
(C) Initiate slow continuous ultrafiltration
(D) Start a furosemide infusion

Item 33

A 50-year-old man is hospitalized with acute onset of shortness of breath and fatigue. In the emergency department, he coughed up a large quantity of blood followed by hypoxic respiratory failure, for which he was intubated.

On physical examination, the patient is well developed. He is afebrile; blood pressure is 140/90 mm Hg, and heart rate is 98/min. There is no jugular venous distension. Coarse crackles are heard in the lung fields. There is trace lower extremity edema. The remainder of the physical examination is normal.

Laboratory studies:

Hemoglobin	9.0 g/dL (90 g/L)
Blood urea nitrogen	38 mg/dL (13.6 mmol/L)
Creatinine	3.2 mg/dL (282.9 µmol/L)
Liver chemistry tests	Normal
Urinalysis	3+ blood; 2+ protein; 20-30 erythrocytes/hpf; 5-10 leukocytes/hpf
Urine protein-creatinine ratio	2200 mg/g

A chest radiograph shows bilateral pulmonary infiltrates.

A kidney biopsy is performed, which shows necrotizing, crescentic glomerulonephritis with linear staining of IgG along the glomerular basement membrane.

Which of the following is the most likely diagnosis?

(A) Anti–glomerular basement membrane antibody disease
(B) Cardiorenal syndrome
(C) Membranous nephropathy
(D) Microscopic polyangiitis

Item 34

A 54-year-old woman is evaluated during a follow-up visit for chronic osteomyelitis. She has type 2 diabetes mellitus complicated by nephropathy and peripheral neuropathy and was recently diagnosed with osteomyelitis of the left foot associated with a chronic neuropathic ulcer. Bone biopsy and culture demonstrated methicillin-sensitive *Staphylococcus aureus*, and 1 week ago she was started on oral high-dose trimethoprim-sulfamethoxazole and rifampin based on sensitivity data for a planned 6-week course of therapy. Medical history is also significant for hypertension. Medications are trimethoprim-sulfamethoxazole, rifampin, glipizide, and atorvastatin.

On physical examination today, temperature is 37.2 °C (99.0 °F), blood pressure is 126/66 mm Hg, and pulse rate is 78/min. Chest, heart, and abdominal examinations are unremarkable. There is loss of sensation to light touch on the feet bilaterally to the ankles. The ulcer overlying the first metatarsal head on the plantar aspect of the left foot is clean and dry.

Current laboratory studies:

Blood urea nitrogen	28 mg/dL (10 mmol/L) (pretreatment baseline: 26 mg/dL [9.3 mmol/L])
Creatinine	1.8 mg/dL (159.1 µmol/L) (pretreatment baseline: 1.4 mg/dL [123.8 µmol/L])
Potassium	4.7 mEq/L (4.7 mmol/L)

Which of the following is the most appropriate management?

(A) Discontinue rifampin
(B) Discontinue trimethoprim-sulfamethoxazole
(C) Order a urine eosinophil test
(D) Continue current therapy

Item 35

A 57-year-old man is evaluated in the emergency department for a 3-day history of left inguinal pain and gross hematuria. He reports no history of kidney stones or kidney disease. Medical history is notable for hypertension and dyslipidemia. Medications are amlodipine and atorvastatin.

On physical examination, temperature is 37.2 °C (98.9 °F), blood pressure is 129/78 mm Hg, pulse rate is 96/min, and respiration rate is 12/min. BMI is 24. There is no left costovertebral angle tenderness.

Laboratory studies show normal complete blood count, serum electrolytes, blood urea nitrogen, and serum creatinine. Dipstick urinalysis reveals 3+ blood, trace protein, and negative leukocyte esterase and nitrites. Urine microscopy shows 1-2 leukocytes/hpf, too numerous to count erythrocytes, and no casts.

A kidney ultrasound shows normal-appearing kidneys, no hydronephrosis, and no nephrolithiasis.

Which of the following is the most appropriate diagnostic test to perform next?

(A) Doppler ultrasonography of the renal veins

(B) Kidney biopsy

(C) Noncontrast helical abdominal CT

(D) Urine culture

Item 36

A 72-year-old man is admitted to the ICU with a 3-day history of worsening shortness of breath and edema. He is found to have pulmonary edema with severe hypoxia requiring intubation and mechanical ventilation. Medical history is significant for ischemic cardiomyopathy, coronary artery disease, myocardial infarction, hypertension, hyperlipidemia, and benign prostatic hyperplasia. Medications on admission are aspirin, lisinopril, carvedilol, atorvastatin, and as-needed furosemide.

On physical examination, the patient is afebrile, blood pressure is 92/60 mm Hg, and pulse rate is 112/min. Estimated central venous pressure is 14 cm H_2O. Diffuse crackles are heard throughout both lung fields. Cardiovascular examination reveals an S_3 gallop. There is lower extremity edema to the knees.

A dobutamine infusion is started. A urinary catheter is inserted, and he is given intravenous furosemide with a urine output of 230 mL over the next 4 hours.

Laboratory studies:

Blood urea nitrogen	76 mg/dL (27.1 mmol/L)
Serum creatinine	3.0 mg/dL (265.2 µmol/L) (baseline: 1.9 mg/dL [168 mmol/L])
Serum electrolytes	Normal
Urine sodium	64 mEq/L (64 mmol/L)
Fractional excretion of sodium	1.9%
Fractional excretion of urea	8.8%
Urinalysis	Specific gravity 1.018; pH 5.5; 1+ protein; 1-2 erythrocytes/hpf; 2-4 leukocytes/hpf; moderate hyaline and fine granular casts

Which of the following is the most likely diagnosis?

(A) Acute interstitial nephritis

(B) Acute tubular necrosis

(C) Obstructive uropathy

(D) Prerenal acute kidney injury

Item 37

A 24-year-old woman is evaluated for fever, lower extremity edema, and worsening malar rash. She was diagnosed

with systemic lupus erythematosus 2 years ago. Her initial evaluation showed normal kidney function, trace proteinuria, and an otherwise normal urinalysis; periodic monitoring of her kidney function and urinalysis has been unchanged. She has been treated with hydroxychloroquine and prednisone, 5 mg/d, since the time of her diagnosis with good control of her symptoms. Medical history is otherwise unremarkable, and she takes no additional medications.

On physical examination, blood pressure is 140/92 mm Hg. A malar rash is present. Mild erythema and effusion in the left knee and bilateral wrist joints are noted. The remainder of the examination is unremarkable.

Laboratory studies:

Hemoglobin	9.2 g/dL (92 g/L)
C3	Low
C4	Low
Creatinine	1.0 mg/dL (88.4 µmol/L)
Liver chemistry tests	Normal
Anti–double stranded DNA antibodies	Elevated
Urinalysis	3+ blood; 2+ protein; 20-30 erythrocytes/hpf; 5-10 leukocytes/hpf
Urine protein-creatinine ratio	2200 mg/g

A kidney biopsy shows a diffuse proliferative glomerulonephritis with immunofluorescence microscopy showing granular deposits in the subendothelial, mesangial, and subepithelial areas (IgG, IgM, IgA, C3, and C1q), which are confirmed by electron microscopy, and is classified as class IV lupus nephritis.

Which of the following is the most appropriate treatment?

(A) Increase prednisone

(B) Increase prednisone and add mycophenolate mofetil

(C) Increase prednisone and perform plasmapheresis

(D) Continue current therapy and rebiopsy in 3 months

Item 38

A 70-year-old woman is evaluated during a new-patient visit. She is asymptomatic. Medical history is significant for osteoporosis and borderline blood pressure elevations; she was advised by her previous physician to periodically check her blood pressures at home. She reports that over the past year these readings have been consistently between 140 and 150 mm Hg systolic and 82 and 86 mm Hg diastolic. She follows a low salt diet and exercises regularly three times a week. Family history is notable for both parents who were diagnosed with hypertension after the age of 65 years. Medications are alendronate and calcium with vitamin D.

On physical examination, temperature is 36.9 °C (98.4 °F), pulse rate is 68/min, and respiration rate is 14/min. Blood pressure is 146/86 mm Hg, with a repeat measurement of 148/86 mm Hg; there are no orthostatic changes.

Laboratory studies show a serum creatinine level of 0.7 mg/dL (61.9 µmol/L) and a serum potassium level of 4.0 mEq/L (4.0 mmol/L); urinalysis is normal.

Electrocardiogram is normal.

Which of the following is the most appropriate next step in management?

(A) Begin hydrochlorothiazide
(B) Begin lisinopril
(C) Obtain echocardiography
(D) Continue clinical observation

Item 39

A 25-year-old man is evaluated for dark-colored urine for 2 days, swelling of the face and hands for 1 day, and severe headaches this morning. He reports having an upper respiratory tract infection 1 week ago with fever, sore throat, and swollen glands, but had otherwise felt well. Medical history is otherwise unremarkable, and he takes no medications.

On physical examination, temperature is 37.2 °C (99.0 °F), blood pressure is 180/90 mm Hg, pulse rate is 88/min, and respiration rate is 14/min. Cardiopulmonary and abdominal examinations are normal. No skin rash or arthritis is present. There is bilateral lower extremity edema to the mid shins.

Laboratory studies:

Albumin	3.3 g/dL (33 g/L)
C3	Low
C4	Normal
Creatinine	1.4 mg/dL (124 µmol/L)
Antistreptolysin O antibodies	Elevated
Urinalysis	3+ blood; 2+ protein; too numerous to count erythrocytes/hpf; 10-15 leukocytes/hpf; numerous erythrocyte casts
Urine protein-creatinine ratio	1900 mg/g
Rapid streptococcal antigen test	Positive

Which of the following is the most likely diagnosis?

(A) IgA nephropathy
(B) Infection-related glomerulonephritis
(C) Lupus nephritis
(D) Small-vessel vasculitis

Item 40

A 54-year-old woman is hospitalized for management of acute kidney injury. Medical history is significant for obesity but is otherwise unremarkable. She reports that she was seen in a weight loss clinic 1 month ago and was prescribed an unknown weight reduction drug, which she has been taking since that time. She takes no other medications.

On physical examination, blood pressure is 140/70 mm Hg, and pulse rate is 72/min. BMI is 40. Estimated central venous pressure is 10 cm H_2O. There are crackles at the lung bases. Heart examination is unremarkable. There is lower extremity edema to the mid-calf bilaterally. The remainder of the examination is unremarkable.

Laboratory studies show a serum creatinine level of 5.1 mg/dL (450.8 µmol/L). Urinalysis is dipstick positive for trace protein, and urine sediment is notable for 0-2 erythrocytes/hpf, 0-5 leukocytes/hpf, and numerous calcium oxalate crystals.

Kidney ultrasound demonstrates normal-sized kidneys with slightly increased echogenicity and no hydronephrosis. Kidney biopsy demonstrates deposition of calcium oxalate crystals within the tubules and the interstitium.

Which of the following is the most likely cause of this patient's acute kidney injury?

(A) Aristolochic acid
(B) Ephedrine
(C) Orlistat
(D) Phentermine

Item 41

A 35-year-old man is evaluated in the emergency department for dyspnea of 24 hours' duration. He also reports progressive lower extremity edema for 1 month. He has no other pertinent personal or family medical history, and he takes no medications.

On physical examination, the patient is afebrile, blood pressure is 120/78 mm Hg, pulse rate is 100/min, and respiration rate is 22/min. Oxygen saturation on ambient air is 88%. BMI is 25. The chest is clear. Examination of the heart is unremarkable. There is bilateral lower extremity pitting edema to the knees. The remainder of the examination is normal.

Laboratory studies:

Albumin	1.8 g/dL (18 g/L)
Creatinine	1.1 mg/dL (97.2 µmol/L)
Urinalysis	Negative for blood; 3+ protein; no cells
Urine protein-creatinine ratio	5500 mg/g

Chest radiograph is normal. CT angiogram of the chest shows a right pulmonary artery embolism.

The patient is started on supplemental oxygen and heparin.

Which of the following is the most likely underlying diagnosis?

(A) Acute interstitial nephritis
(B) Membranous glomerulopathy
(C) Poststreptococcal glomerulonephritis
(D) Thrombotic microangiopathy

Item 42

A 32-year-old man is evaluated during a follow-up visit for high blood pressure. During a recent insurance examination, his blood pressure was 180/80 mm Hg. He rechecked his blood pressure in a pharmacy, and it was 138/80 mm Hg. Medical history is unremarkable. Family history is notable for both parents who have hypertension; his father experienced a stroke at age 60 years. The patient takes no medications. He has a 10-pack-year history of smoking but stopped smoking 5 years ago. He is asymptomatic, exercises regularly, and follows a heart-healthy, low salt diet.

On physical examination, temperature is 36.8 °C (98.3 °F), blood pressure is 190/90 mm Hg, pulse rate is 90/min, and respiration rate is 14/min. BMI is 28. Blood pressure taken 5 minutes later is 160/80 mm Hg. The blood pressure readings are symmetric in all four limbs, with no postural drop. Retinal examination is normal. Cardiovascular examination is normal.

Laboratory studies show normal serum creatinine and electrolyte levels, and a urinalysis is unremarkable.

Electrocardiogram is normal.

Ambulatory blood pressure monitoring results:

Average blood pressure	121/81 mm Hg
Systolic blood pressure readings >140 mm Hg	15%
Diastolic blood pressure readings >90 mm Hg	20%
Awake/sleep blood pressure decrease	16%/12%

Which of the following is the most appropriate next step in management?

(A) Order echocardiography

(B) Order a plasma aldosterone-plasma renin ratio

(C) Start amlodipine

(D) Continue clinical follow-up

Item 43

A 72-year-old man was diagnosed with colon cancer 12 months ago, and surgical resection was performed. He presented with metastatic lesions to the liver 2 months ago, for which he was started on a chemotherapy regimen that includes oxaliplatin with 5-fluorouracil and leucovorin with bevacizumab. He has been experiencing progressive headaches and lower extremity swelling over the past 3 weeks. He reports no diarrhea, mental status changes, or shortness of breath.

On physical examination, temperature is 36.8 °C (98.2 °F), blood pressure is 180/120 mm Hg, pulse rate is 80/min, and respiration rate is 16/min. BMI is 32. There is 2+ pedal edema.

Laboratory studies show a hemoglobin level of 7.5 g/dL (75 g/L), a platelet count of 90,000/µL (90 × 10^9/L), and a serum creatinine level of 2.2 mg/dL (194 µmol/L); a peripheral blood smear shows numerous schistocytes.

Which of the following is the most likely cause of this patient's clinical picture?

(A) 5-Fluorouracil

(B) Bevacizumab

(C) Leucovorin

(D) Oxaliplatin

Item 44

A 54-year-old woman is evaluated during a follow-up visit for stage G4/A3 chronic kidney disease due to diabetic nephropathy. She is asymptomatic except for mild fatigue and peripheral edema and reports a good appetite. Medications are ramipril, furosemide, and calcium acetate.

On physical examination, temperature is 37.0 °C (98.6 °F), blood pressure is 128/73 mm Hg, pulse rate is 80/min, and respiration rate is 14/min. BMI is 29. Pallor and pale mucous membranes are noted. There is no jugular venous distention. There is no pericardial friction rub. The lungs are clear. There is no asterixis. Neurologic examination is normal.

Laboratory studies are significant for a serum creatinine level of 2.6 mg/dL (229.8 µmol/L) and an estimated glomerular filtration rate of 19 mL/min/1.73 m^2 (1 year ago: 30 mL/min/1.73 m^2).

After discussing the goals of care, the patient wishes to explore renal replacement options and kidney transplantation.

Which of the following is the most appropriate management?

(A) Nephrologist referral now

(B) Nephrologist referral in 6 months

(C) Repeat creatinine measurement in 2 weeks

(D) Continue current management

Item 45

A 54-year-old woman is evaluated during a follow-up examination. She has a 22-year history of type 2 diabetes mellitus complicated by sensory neuropathy and proliferative retinopathy, for which she has received laser photocoagulation. She also has hypertension and hyperlipidemia. Medications are metformin, glipizide, atorvastatin, and lisinopril, 20 mg/d.

On physical examination, temperature is normal, blood pressure is 132/78 mm Hg, pulse rate is 72/min, and respiration rate is 12/min. BMI is 29. Cardiopulmonary and abdominal examinations are normal. There is no lower extremity edema. There is decreased sensation to monofilament testing in the feet.

Laboratory studies:

Hemoglobin A$_{1c}$	6.8%
Creatinine	1.2 mg/dL (106.1 µmol/L) (2 years ago: 0.8 mg/dL [70.7 µmol/L])
Electrolytes	Normal
Urine albumin-creatinine ratio	460 mg/g (5 years ago: <30 mg/g)

Which of the following is the most appropriate management of this patient's hypertension?

(A) Add amlodipine

(B) Add losartan

(C) Reduce lisinopril dose

(D) Continue current therapy

Item 46

A 54-year-old man is hospitalized for necrotizing pancreatitis. His course has been complicated by acute respiratory distress syndrome requiring ventilator support. He is hemodynamically unstable and requires an intravenous norepinephrine infusion to maintain a mean arterial blood pressure of 65 mm Hg. On the third hospital day, he develops increasing norepinephrine and oxygen requirements and increasing ventilator airway pressures, and he becomes oliguric. Medications are propofol and fentanyl.

On physical examination, blood pressure is 80/60 mm Hg, pulse rate is 92/min, and respiration rate is 12/min. Estimated central venous pressure is 12 cm H_2O. Heart sounds are normal. There are diffuse pulmonary crackles. The abdomen is modestly distended and tense. Bilateral lower extremity and flank edema are present.

Laboratory studies:

Hemoglobin	9.0 g/dL (90 g/L)
INR	2.0
Creatinine	2.1 mg/dL (185.6 µmol/L) (on admission, 0.9 mg/dL [79.6 µmol/L])
Urine sodium	<10 mEq/L (10 mmol/L)
Urinalysis	Specific gravity 1.022; pH 6.0; 0-1 erythrocytes/hpf; 0-2 leukocytes/hpf; occasional hyaline casts

Kidney ultrasound reveals normal sized kidneys and no hydronephrosis.

Which of the following is the most appropriate next step in management?

(A) Bladder pressure measurement
(B) Erythrocyte transfusion to a target hemoglobin of 11 g/dL (110 g/L)
(C) Isotonic saline bolus, 500 mL
(D) Pulmonary artery catheter placement

Item 47

A 68-year-old woman is evaluated for myalgia and generalized weakness. Medical history is significant for hypertension, hyperlipidemia, hypothyroidism, and chronic kidney disease. One week ago, she was hospitalized with symptoms of a transient ischemic attack. Carotid ultrasound revealed 50% stenosis of her left internal carotid. Her serum creatinine level during hospitalization was 1.5 mg/dL (132.6 µmol/L), and her thyroid-stimulating hormone level was 18 µU/mL (18 mU/L). She states that she had not been regularly adherent with her medications prior to admission, but that since discharge she has been taking her medications as prescribed. Current medications are aspirin, high-dose atorvastatin, lisinopril, hydrochlorothiazide, and levothyroxine.

On physical examination, blood pressure is 152/78 mm Hg, and pulse rate is 82/min. She is not orthostatic. Skin turgor is normal. The lung fields are clear. Cardiovascular examination reveals a left carotid bruit and a fourth heart sound. There is diffuse tenderness to palpation of the major muscle groups. Trace lower extremity edema is present.

Laboratory studies:

Complete blood count	Normal
Creatinine	3.0 mg/dL (265.2 µmol/L)
Electrolytes:	
Sodium	132 mEq/L (132 mmol/L)
Potassium	5.6 mEq/L (5.6 mmol/L)
Chloride	100 mEq/L (100 mmol/L)
Bicarbonate	22 mEq/L (22 mmol/L)
Phosphorus	6.0 mg/dL (1.9 mmol/L)
Urinalysis	4+ blood; 0-1 erythrocytes/hpf; 0-2 leukocytes/hpf; numerous granular casts

Which of the following medications is the most likely cause of this patient's acute kidney injury?

(A) Atorvastatin
(B) Hydrochlorothiazide
(C) Levothyroxine
(D) Lisinopril

Item 48

A 42-year-old man is evaluated during a follow-up visit for chronic kidney disease due to vesicoureteral reflux that progressed to end-stage kidney disease 10 years ago; he has been receiving hemodialysis for 5 years. He is anuric but feels well and reports no other symptoms. Medical history is otherwise unremarkable.

On physical examination, temperature is 37.0 °C (98.6 °F), blood pressure is 145/95 mm Hg, pulse rate is 85/min, and respiration rate is 14/min. BMI is 26. The lungs are clear. The abdominal examination is normal, and there is no costovertebral angle tenderness. The remainder of the examination is normal.

An abdominal ultrasound was recently performed to evaluate a complaint of abdominal discomfort, which has since resolved. This study was remarkable for bilateral small echogenic kidneys with innumerable cysts and a 4-cm mass in the right renal parenchyma.

Which of the following is the most likely diagnosis?

(A) Hemorrhagic kidney cyst
(B) Renal angiomyolipoma
(C) Renal cell carcinoma
(D) Transitional cell carcinoma

Item 49

A 45-year-old man is evaluated during an annual routine health maintenance visit. History is notable for type 2 diabetes mellitus (diet controlled) diagnosed 3 months ago. Family history is significant for his father who developed end-stage kidney disease due to diabetes at age 68 years. He reports no symptoms and takes no medications.

On physical examination, temperature is 37.0 °C (98.6 °F), blood pressure is 135/78 mm Hg, pulse rate is 70/min, and respiration rate is 12/min. BMI is 31. Cardiac examination reveals no murmur or gallop. The lungs are clear. There is 1+ peripheral edema.

Laboratory studies show a serum creatinine level of 1.0 mg/dL (88.4 µmol/L).

Which of the following is the most appropriate next step in management?

(A) Measure urine albumin excretion

(B) Order kidney ultrasonography

(C) Perform dipstick urinalysis

(D) Start an angiotensin receptor blocker

Item 50

A 65-year-old man is evaluated for a slowly rising serum creatinine level from 0.8 mg/dL (70.7 µmol/L) to 1.4 mg/dL (124 µmol/L) noted on laboratory testing over the past 8 months. Medical history is significant for benign prostatic hyperplasia and gastroesophageal reflux disease. He feels well and has no current symptoms. Medications are tamsulosin and omeprazole.

On physical examination, temperature is 37.1 °C (98.7 °F), blood pressure is 134/84 mm Hg, pulse rate is 76/min, and respiration rate is 12/min. BMI is 26. There is no rash. The remainder of the examination is unremarkable.

Laboratory studies:

Complete blood count with differential	Normal
Blood urea nitrogen	38 mg/dL (13.6 mmol/L)
Creatinine	1.4 mg/dL (124 µmol/L)
Electrolytes	Normal
Urinalysis	Positive for protein; no blood, glucose, leukocyte esterase, or nitrites; <3 erythrocytes/hpf; 3-5 leukocytes/hpf; no casts or crystals
Urine protein-creatinine ratio	470 mg/g

Kidney ultrasound shows normal-sized kidneys without hydronephrosis or calculi.

Which of the following is the most appropriate next step in management?

(A) Discontinue omeprazole

(B) Discontinue tamsulosin

(C) Order a 24-hour urine collection for creatinine clearance and proteinuria

(D) Perform duplex ultrasonography

Item 51

A 56-year-old woman is hospitalized for acute decompensated heart failure. Medical history is significant for ischemic cardiomyopathy, coronary artery disease, hypertension, and hyperlipidemia. Medications on admission are aspirin, lisinopril, carvedilol, spironolactone, rosuvastatin, and as-needed furosemide.

Baseline medications are continued, and intravenous diuretics are started resulting in a 2.0-kg negative fluid balance over the initial 36 hours with improvement of her symptoms. However, her serum creatinine level increased to 1.5 mg/dL (132.6 µmol/L) from her baseline of 1.2 mg/dL (106.1 µmol/L).

On physical examination, the patient is afebrile, blood pressure is 112/82 mm Hg, pulse rate is 68/min, and respiration rate is 16/min. Oxygen saturation is 92% on 2 L oxygen by nasal cannula. Estimated central venous pressure is 12 cm H_2O. Examination of the lungs reveals bibasilar crackles, improved from admission. Cardiac examination reveals an S_3 gallop. There is lower extremity edema to the mid-calf.

In addition to continuing her baseline medications, which of the following is the most appropriate next step in management?

(A) Add nesiritide and continue intravenous diuretics

(B) Continue intravenous diuretics

(C) Discontinue intravenous diuretics and begin ultrafiltration

(D) Hold intravenous diuretics for 24 hours

Item 52

A 32-year-old woman is evaluated during a follow-up visit. She is at 12 weeks' gestation of her first pregnancy. Her pregnancy has been uncomplicated except for persistently elevated blood pressures measured at her obstetric visits. She otherwise feels well. She has no urinary symptoms such as dysuria, hematuria, or foamy urine. She did not receive routine medical care prior to her pregnancy. Family history is notable for hypertension in her parents and one older sibling. Her only medication is a prenatal vitamin.

On physical examination, temperature is 37.1 °C (98.8 °F), blood pressure is 154/93 mm Hg, pulse rate is 87/min, and respiration rate is 16/min. BMI is 24. Funduscopic and neurologic examinations are normal. Chest and cardiac examinations are normal. Abdominal examination is unremarkable. There is trace lower extremity edema.

Laboratory studies show normal liver chemistries and kidney function. A complete blood count is normal except for a hemoglobin level of 10.9 g/dL (109 g/L). Urinalysis is normal.

Which of the following is the most likely diagnosis?

(A) Chronic hypertension

(B) Gestational hypertension

(C) Normal pregnancy

(D) Preeclampsia

Item 53

A 65-year-old man is evaluated in the emergency department for polyuria, polydipsia, and nocturia. Medical history is notable for diabetes mellitus, for which he takes metformin. He has a 45-pack-year history of smoking and does not drink alcohol.

On physical examination, the patient is alert and oriented. Blood pressure is 110/70 mm Hg supine and 100/65 mm Hg standing, pulse rate is 88/min supine and 95/min standing, and respiration rate is 20/min. BMI

CONT.

is 20. Occasional expiratory wheezing is noted in the right posterior lung field.

Laboratory studies:

Blood urea nitrogen	30 mg/dL (10.7 mmol/L)
Total cholesterol	250 mg/dL (6.48 mmol/L)
Electrolytes:	
Sodium	130 mEq/L (130 mmol/L)
Potassium	4.5 mEq/L (4.5 mmol/L)
Chloride	92 mEq/L (92 mmol/L)
Bicarbonate	24 mEq/L (24 mmol/L)
Glucose	800 mg/dL (44.4 mmol/L)
Plasma osmolality	319 mOsm/kg H_2O

Chest radiograph shows a 2-cm cavitary mass in the right upper lobe.

Which of the following conditions is the most likely cause of this patient's hyponatremia?

(A) Adrenal insufficiency
(B) Hyperglycemia
(C) Hyperlipidemia
(D) Reset osmostat
(E) Syndrome of inappropriate antidiuretic hormone secretion

 Item 54

A 76-year-old woman is evaluated in the emergency department for altered sensorium. Medical records indicate a history of osteoarthritis. Listed medications are acetaminophen, naproxen, aspirin, and tramadol.

On physical examination, the patient is not communicative. Temperature is 36.5 °C (97.7 °F), blood pressure is 108/62 mm Hg, pulse rate is 104/min, and respiration rate is 12/min. BMI is 24. Lung examination reveals no crackles or wheezing. Neurologic examination is remarkable for somnolence but with appropriate responsiveness to noxious stimuli.

Laboratory studies:

Creatinine	1.2 mg/dL (106.1 µmol/L)
Electrolytes:	
Sodium	139 mEq/L (139 mmol/L)
Potassium	3.9 mEq/L (3.9 mmol/L)
Chloride	102 mEq/L (102 (mmol/L)
Bicarbonate	26 mEq/L (26 mmol/L)
Arterial blood gas studies:	
pH	7.30
P_{CO_2}	55 mm Hg (7.3 kPa)
P_{O_2}	65 mm Hg (8.6 kPa)

Overdose of which of the following is the most likely cause of this patient's findings?

(A) Acetaminophen
(B) Aspirin
(C) Naproxen
(D) Tramadol

 Item 55

A 65-year-old woman is hospitalized for pneumonia and sepsis. She has no pertinent personal or family medical history and takes no medications.

On physical examination, the patient is intubated and mechanically ventilated. Temperature is 39.0 °C (102.2 °F), blood pressure is 90/60 mm Hg, pulse rate is 100/min, and respiration rate is 24/min. Estimated central venous pressure is 6 cm H_2O. Central venous oxygen saturation is 60%.

Intravenous fluid resuscitation is to be initiated.

Which of the following resuscitation therapies is contraindicated in this patient?

(A) Albumin
(B) Hydroxyethyl starch
(C) Isotonic crystalloids
(D) Lactated Ringer solution

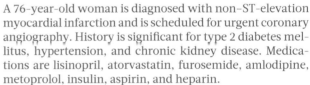 **Item 56**

A 76-year-old woman is diagnosed with non–ST-elevation myocardial infarction and is scheduled for urgent coronary angiography. History is significant for type 2 diabetes mellitus, hypertension, and chronic kidney disease. Medications are lisinopril, atorvastatin, furosemide, amlodipine, metoprolol, insulin, aspirin, and heparin.

On physical examination, blood pressure is 152/84 mm Hg, pulse rate is 82/min, and respiration rate is 14/min. There is no jugular venous distention. Cardiac examination reveals regular rhythm with an S_4 but no murmurs. The lungs are clear. There is mild lower extremity edema at the ankles.

Laboratory studies are significant for a serum creatinine level of 2.0 mg/dL (176.8 µmol/L) and an estimated glomerular filtration rate of 30 mL/min/1.73 m²; urinalysis reveals 2+ protein.

In addition to discontinuing diuretic therapy, which of the following is the most appropriate periprocedural management of this patient?

(A) Begin intravenous isotonic saline
(B) Begin oral N-acetylcysteine
(C) Begin prophylactic hemodialysis within 2 hours after procedure
(D) Discontinue lisinopril for at least 24 hours before procedure

Item 57

A 57-year-old man is evaluated for a diagnosis of acute kidney injury. He was diagnosed with gastroesophageal reflux disease 3 weeks ago and was prescribed omeprazole. Several days ago he noticed lower extremity swelling and decreased frequency of urination. Laboratory evaluation showed a serum creatinine level of 2.2 mg/dL (194.5 µmol/L). Medical history is otherwise unremarkable, and he takes no other medications. He reports no allergies.

On physical examination, the patient is afebrile, blood pressure is 135/77 mm Hg, pulse rate is 88/min, and respiration rate is 12/min. There is no rash. Cardiac examination and estimated central venous pressure are normal. The lungs are clear. Lower extremity edema to the ankles is present bilaterally.

Dipstick urinalysis reveals blood and trace protein, and urine sediment is notable for 5-10 erythrocytes/hpf, 10-20 leukocytes/hpf, and 1 leukocyte cast.

In addition to discontinuing omeprazole, which of the following is the most appropriate next step in management?

(A) Kidney biopsy

(B) Oral glucocorticoids

(C) Repeat kidney function testing in 5 to 7 days

(D) Urine eosinophil testing

Item 58

A 53-year-old woman is evaluated during a follow-up visit for recurrent urinary tract infections. She has been treated for three episodes of urinary tract infection with *Klebsiella* over the past 4 months. Despite an initial response to antibiotics, her urinary tract symptoms return once the antibiotics are stopped. She has no systemic symptoms, including fever or chills. Medical history is otherwise unremarkable. She currently takes no medications.

On physical examination, temperature is 37.1 °C (98.8 °F), blood pressure is 124/74 mm Hg, pulse rate is 72/min, and respiration rate is 12/min. BMI is 22. There is no costovertebral angle tenderness to palpation. The remainder of the examination is unremarkable.

Urine dipstick reveals a pH of 9.0 and is positive for leukocyte esterase and nitrites; urine microscopy shows 8-10 leukocytes/hpf and many coffin-lid–shaped crystals consistent with struvite.

Kidney ultrasound shows a 1.2-cm irregularly shaped stone in the left renal pelvis.

Which of the following is the most appropriate next step in management?

(A) Chronic antibiotic therapy

(B) Low phosphate diet

(C) Stone removal

(D) Urine acidification

Item 59

A 28-year-old man is evaluated for a 2-month history of progressive lower extremity edema, weight loss, and fatigue. Medical history is significant for recreational use of inhaled cocaine; he denies injection drug use. He has no other known medical issues and takes no medications.

On physical examination, temperature is 37.2 °C (99.0 °F), blood pressure is 130/90 mm Hg, pulse rate is 90/min, and respiration rate is 20/min. BMI is 28. Temporal wasting is present. The lungs are clear. Cardiac examination is normal, and no pericardial rub is detected. There is no hepatosplenomegaly or evidence of ascites on abdominal examination. The lower extremities show edema to the knees bilaterally. Skin and joint examinations are normal. Mild asterixis is noted.

Laboratory studies:

Albumin	2.5 g/dL (25 g/L)
Liver chemistry studies	Normal
Blood urea nitrogen	98 mg/dL (35 mmol/L)
Creatinine	6.8 mg/dL (601.1 μmol/L)
Urinalysis	1+ blood; 3+ protein; 5 erythrocytes/hpf; 0-2 leukocytes/hpf
Urine protein-creatinine ratio	3700 mg/g

Kidney ultrasound shows mildly enlarged and echogenic kidneys without obstruction.

Kidney biopsy results are indicative of the collapsing variant of focal segmental glomerulosclerosis (FSGS).

Which of the following tests is most likely to establish the cause of this patient's FSGS?

(A) Hepatitis B and C serologies

(B) HIV antibody test

(C) Serum and urine electrophoresis

(D) Treponemal antibody test

Item 60

A 60-year-old woman is evaluated for a 3-week history of fever, fatigue, and arthralgia. She also notes intermittent low back pain and weight loss of 4.5 kg (10 lb) during the past 2 months. She reports no dysuria or night sweats. Medical history is significant for urinary tract infections once every 1 to 2 years and osteoarthritis. She has a 25-pack-year smoking history but stopped 15 years ago. Her only medication is as-needed ibuprofen.

On physical examination, temperature is 38.2 °C (100.8 °F), blood pressure is 152/94 mm Hg, pulse rate is 92/min, and respiration rate is 16/min. BMI is 26. Lung, heart, and abdominal examinations are normal. There is no costovertebral angle tenderness. Skin examination reveals nonblanching erythematous palpable papules and macules on the lower legs.

Laboratory studies:

Creatinine	1.8 mg/dL (159.1 μmol/L) (baseline: 0.9 mg/dL [79.6 μmol/L])
Urinalysis	2+ blood; 2+ protein; positive for leukocyte esterase; 20-30 erythrocytes/hpf; 5-10 leukocytes/hpf; no crystals

Urine microscopy results are shown.

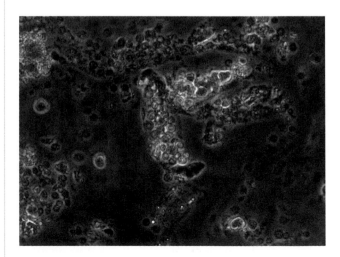

Which of the following is the most appropriate next step in management?

(A) Antibiotics

(B) Cystoscopy

(C) Kidney biopsy

(D) Kidney ultrasonography

CONT.

Item 61

A 52-year-old woman is evaluated in the hospital following admission for gastroenteritis and hyponatremia. She reports a 5-day history of diarrhea, nausea, and vomiting, and had been drinking water to maintain hydration. On evaluation in the emergency department earlier today, she was noted to be mildly volume contracted with an initial serum sodium level of 114 mEq/L (114 mmol/L) with normal plasma glucose and minimally elevated blood urea nitrogen levels. Her mental status was normal. She was given 2 liters of normal saline and admitted to the hospital. Medical history is unremarkable, and she takes no medications.

On physical examination, the patient feels better. Temperature is normal, blood pressure is 120/70 mm Hg, pulse rate is 84/min, and respiration rate is 16/min. BMI is 22. Estimated central venous pressure is 6 cm H_2O. Cardiopulmonary examination is unremarkable, and the abdomen is mildly tender to palpation diffusely. The neurologic examination is normal.

Current laboratory studies:

Blood urea nitrogen	14 mg/dL (5 mmol/L)
Creatinine	1.0 mg/dL (88.4 µmol/L)
Electrolytes:	
Sodium	128 mEq/L (128 mmol/L)
Potassium	4.0 mEq/L (4.0 mmol/L)
Chloride	94 mEq/L (94 mmol/L)
Bicarbonate	24 mEq/L (24 mmol/L)
Glucose	90 mg/dL (5 mmol/L)

Which of the following is the most appropriate management of this patient's hyponatremia?

(A) Desmopressin intravenously

(B) Desmopressin intravenously with 5% dextrose

(C) Fluid restriction of 800 mL/d

(D) Fluid restriction of 800 mL/d and salt tablets

(E) No additional intervention

Item 62

A 40-year-old woman is evaluated during a follow-up visit for a diagnosis of autosomal dominant polycystic kidney disease (ADPKD). She is asymptomatic but is questioning whether she should be screened for a brain aneurysm. Medical history is otherwise significant for hypertension treated with enalapril. Family history is notable for her father who has ADPKD and is on hemodialysis and her paternal grandmother who died of chronic kidney disease, although she does not know the type. She is not aware of any family history of stroke or other neurologic abnormalities. She works as an administrator in an office.

On physical examination, temperature is 37.0 °C (98.6 °F), blood pressure is 140/90 mm Hg, pulse rate is 80/min, and respiration rate is 15/min. BMI is 22. Cardiovascular, pulmonary, and neurologic examinations are

normal. On abdominal examination, nontender masses are palpable bilaterally.

Which of the following is the most appropriate screening regimen for this patient?

(A) One-time MR angiography now

(B) One-time MR angiography at age 50 years

(C) MR angiography now and every 5 years

(D) No screening

Item 63

A 65-year-old woman is evaluated in the emergency department for dysuria, urgency, and polyuria occurring for 4 days. She has no neurologic symptoms. Medical history is significant for depression. Her only medication is fluoxetine, which was started 8 weeks ago.

On physical examination, temperature is 38.0 °C (100.4 °F), blood pressure is 140/90 mm Hg, pulse rate is 85/min, and respiration rate is 15/min. BMI is 30. Cardiovascular, pulmonary, and neurologic examinations are normal. Mild tenderness to palpation of the mid lower abdomen is noted. There is no costovertebral angle tenderness.

Laboratory studies:

Blood urea nitrogen	10 mg/dL (3.6 mmol/L)
Creatinine	1.0 mg/dL (88.4 µmol/L)
Electrolytes:	
Sodium	123 mEq/L (123 mmol/L)
Potassium	4.0 mEq/L (4.0 mmol/L)
Chloride	91 mEq/L (91 mmol/L)
Bicarbonate	24 mEq/L (24 mmol/L)
Glucose	120 mg/dL (6.7 mmol/L)
Plasma osmolality	260 mOsm/kg/H_2O
Urine sodium	40 mEq/L (40 mmol/L)
Urine osmolality	600 mOsm/kg/H_2O
Urinalysis	Too numerous to count leukocytes/hpf

Antibiotics for a urinary tract infection are started.

In addition to discontinuing fluoxetine, which of the following is the most appropriate management of this patient's hyponatremia?

(A) Fluid restriction

(B) Hypertonic saline infusion

(C) Isotonic saline infusion

(D) Oral demeclocycline

(E) Tolvaptan

Item 64

A 76-year-old woman is evaluated during a follow-up visit for hypertension. She notes fluctuating home blood pressure measurements, with systolic blood pressure measurements in the range of 140 to 150 mm Hg. History is notable for osteoporosis, hip fracture and subsequent hip replacement, and vertebral fracture. Medications are amlodipine, alendronate, calcium, and vitamin D.

On physical examination, the patient appears frail; she has difficulty climbing onto the examination table and requires assistance. Average blood pressure is 152/76 mm Hg based on two measurements, which is consistent with home measurements taken over the past few weeks. Pulse rate is 64/min. BMI is 19. It takes her 20 seconds to walk 6 meters. The remainder of the examination is unremarkable.

Laboratory studies show a normal chemistry panel; a urine dipstick demonstrates no protein.

Which of the following is the most appropriate next step in management?

(A) Add chlorthalidone

(B) Add lisinopril

(C) Obtain 24-hour ambulatory blood pressure monitoring

(D) Continue current regimen

Item 65

A 45-year-old woman was hospitalized 2 days ago after attempting suicide with an overdose of a benzodiazepine. She is now asymptomatic. Medical history is significant for bipolar disorder, treated with lithium for the past 15 years. She has a 45-pack-year history of smoking and drinks 3 to 4 beers daily.

On physical examination, blood pressure is 142/74 mm Hg supine and 140/80 mm Hg standing, pulse rate is 82/min, and respiration rate is 15/min. BMI is 25. Examination of the heart, lungs, and abdomen is normal. There is no peripheral edema.

Laboratory studies:

Electrolytes:

Sodium	125 mEq/L (125 mmol/L)
Potassium	3.5 mEq/L (3.5 mmol/L)
Chloride	85 mEq/L (85 mmol/L)
Bicarbonate	27 mEq/L (27 mmol/L)
Plasma osmolality	263 mOsm/kg H_2O
Urine sodium	42 mEq/L (42 mmol/L)
Urine osmolality	600 mOsm/kg H_2O

Which of the following is the most likely diagnosis?

(A) Beer potomania

(B) Lithium-induced renal toxicity

(C) Primary polydipsia

(D) Syndrome of inappropriate antidiuretic hormone secretion

Item 66

A 34-year-old woman is evaluated for laboratory abnormalities discovered as part of an evaluation for joint pain. She describes the pain as being diffuse and associated with chronically dry eyes and mouth. She also notes recent-onset mild nocturia. Medical history is otherwise negative, and she takes acetaminophen daily for her joint pain.

On physical examination, vital signs are normal. BMI is 23. Mucous membranes and conjunctivae are dry, and mild parotid enlargement is present. There is no evidence of joint inflammation. The remainder of the examination is unremarkable.

Laboratory studies:

Creatinine	0.9 mg/dL (79.6 µmol/L)
Electrolytes:	
Sodium	138 mEq/L (138 mmol/L)
Potassium	3.1 mEq/L (3.1 mmol/L)
Chloride	118 mEq/L (118 mmol/L)
Bicarbonate	12 mEq/L (12 mmol/L)
Glucose	74 mg/dL (4.1 mmol/L)
Urinalysis	pH 7.0; no blood, glucose, protein, erythrocytes, or leukocytes

Which of the following is the most likely cause of this patient's laboratory findings?

(A) Acetaminophen

(B) Type 1 (hypokalemic distal) renal tubular acidosis

(C) Type 2 (proximal) renal tubular acidosis

(D) Type 4 (hyperkalemic distal) renal tubular acidosis

Item 67

A 65-year-old woman is evaluated during a follow-up visit. She has end-stage kidney disease due to IgA nephropathy; she started peritoneal dialysis 3 months ago. She also has a 10-year history of hypertension. She has done well since starting dialysis, is without current complaints, and has recently resumed exercising regularly. She has three adult children who are encouraging her to explore kidney transplantation and are willing to be evaluated as kidney donors; however, the patient feels that she is "too old." Medications are amlodipine, ramipril, calcitriol, epoetin alfa, and calcium acetate.

On physical examination, temperature is 37.0 °C (98.6 °F), blood pressure is 135/75 mm Hg, pulse rate is 72/min, and respiration rate is 14/min. BMI is 27. The peritoneal dialysis catheter site is nontender without induration or exudate. Cardiac examination reveals normal heart sounds. The lungs are clear. The abdomen is nontender. There is no peripheral edema.

Which of the following kidney replacement strategies is most likely to provide this patient with the best long-term survival?

(A) Change from peritoneal dialysis to hemodialysis

(B) Continue peritoneal dialysis

(C) Continue peritoneal dialysis and evaluate for transplant in 2 to 3 years

(D) Refer for transplant evaluation now

Item 68

A 49-year-old woman is evaluated during a follow-up visit for a 5-year history of stage G3b/A2 chronic kidney disease (CKD) and a 15-year history of hypertension. Medical history is otherwise unremarkable. She is a never-smoker. Family history is notable for her mother who developed end-stage kidney disease due to hypertension at age 60 years. Medications are lisinopril, amlodipine, and hydrochlorothiazide.

On physical examination, temperature is 37.0 °C (98.6 °F), blood pressure is 134/85 mm Hg, pulse rate is 73/min, and respiration rate is 12/min. BMI is 24. There is no jugular venous distention. An S_4 gallop is heard. The lungs are clear. There is no peripheral edema. The remainder of the examination is unremarkable.

Laboratory studies are notable for a serum creatinine level of 2.1 mg/dL (185.6 µmol/L), an estimated glomerular filtration rate of 31 mL/min/1.73 m², and a urine albumin-creatinine ratio of 20 mg/g.

Which of the following is the most appropriate management?

(A) Begin a low protein diet
(B) Lower blood pressure to <130/80 mm Hg
(C) Switch hydrochlorothiazide to furosemide
(D) No changes to current therapy

Item 69

A 65-year-old man is evaluated during a follow-up visit for stage G3b/A3 chronic kidney disease due to diabetic nephropathy. He reports doing well with good baseline exercise tolerance and no shortness of breath. Medical history is also significant for type 2 diabetes mellitus and hypertension. Medications are basal bolus insulin and lisinopril.

On physical examination, temperature is normal, blood pressure is 145/75 mm Hg, pulse rate is 82/min, and respiration rate is 16/min. BMI is 28. There is no jugular venous distention. The lungs are clear.

Laboratory studies:

Bicarbonate	Normal
Creatinine	1.9 mg/dL (168 µmol/L)
Potassium	4.0 mEq/L (4.0 mmol/L)
Estimated glomerular filtration rate	42 mL/min/1.73 m²
Urine protein-creatinine ratio	3900 mg/g

Kidney ultrasound shows mildly echogenic kidneys that are of normal size with no obstruction.

Which of the following is the most appropriate treatment?

(A) Add an angiotensin receptor blocker
(B) Increase lisinopril dose
(C) Replace lisinopril with amlodipine
(D) No change in current medications

Item 70

A 43-year-old man is evaluated in the emergency department for abdominal pain. He has a history of alcohol abuse, with repeated episodes of acute intoxication requiring medical therapy. He also has a history of several episodes of acute pancreatitis, but no history of seizure disorder. He takes no medications.

On physical examination, temperature is 37.4 °C (99.3 °F), blood pressure is 112/66 mm Hg, and pulse rate is 76/min. BMI is 20. There is no evidence of trauma or head injury. There is no evidence of ascites. The abdomen is tender to palpation. Neurologic examination reveals normal pupillary and corneal reflexes, normal muscle tone, and a downgoing plantar reflex.

Laboratory studies:

Blood urea nitrogen	28 mg/dL (10 mmol/L)
Calcium	8.6 mg/dL (2.2 mmol/L)
Creatinine	1.2 mg/dL (106.1 µmol/L) (baseline, 0.8 mg/dL [70.7 µmol/L])
Electrolytes:	
Sodium	135 mEq/L (135 mmol/L)
Potassium	4.9 mEq/L (4.9 mmol/L)
Chloride	96 mEq/L (96 mmol/L)
Bicarbonate	12 mEq/L (12 mmol/L)
Ethanol	62 mg/dL (0.062 g/dL)
Glucose	72 mg/dL (4 mmol/L)
Lactate	0.8 mEq/L (0.8 mmol/L)
Plasma osmolality	293 mOsm/kg H₂O
Phosphorus	3.7 mg/dL (1.2 mmol/L)
Urinalysis	pH 5.5; specific gravity 1.020; no blood, ketones, or cells

Which of the following is the most likely cause of this patient's acidosis?

(A) Acute kidney injury
(B) Alcoholic ketoacidosis
(C) D-Lactic acidosis
(D) Rhabdomyolysis

Item 71

A 50-year-old man is evaluated in the hospital for fatigue, joint pain, and skin lesions. His symptoms started 2 weeks ago with fever and sore throat, which subsided in 2 days. Fatigue and joint pain were noted 1 day after the onset of sore throat, which worsened over the subsequent days. Four days after the onset of symptoms, he noted dark red spots on his ankles and shins, which spread to involve his legs, thighs, and buttocks; the skin lesions were not painful or itchy. He also notes intermittent central abdominal pain, crampy in nature and not related to food. He has hypertension that was previously well controlled with lisinopril and hydrochlorothiazide.

On physical examination, temperature is 37.8 °C (100.0 °F), blood pressure is 170/84 mm Hg, pulse rate is 78/min, and respiration rate is 14/min. BMI is 28. Examination of the joints shows tenderness and increased warmth in the knees, ankles, and elbows without effusions. Cardiac and lung examinations are normal. There is mild guarding around the periumbilical area on abdominal examination.

The appearance of the skin is shown (see top of next page).

Laboratory studies:

Albumin	3.1 g/dL (31 g/L)
Complements (C3 and C4)	Normal
Creatinine	1.8 mg/dL (159 µmol/L)
Hepatitis B antibody profile	Negative
Hepatitis C antibody profile	Negative
Urinalysis	3+ blood; 2+ protein; 50-100 erythrocytes/hpf; 10-15 leukocytes/hpf; few erythrocyte casts
Urine protein-creatinine ratio	2200 mg/g

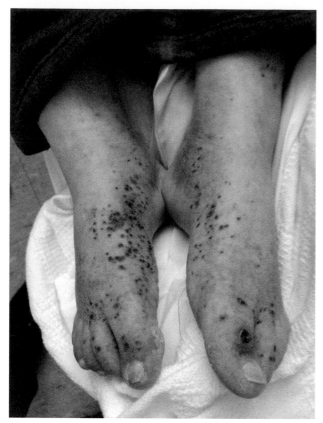

ITEM 71

Lupus serologies, antistreptolysin O antibodies, ANCA, and anti–glomerular basement membrane antibodies are pending. Blood cultures are pending. Stool occult blood test is positive.

Which of the following is the most likely diagnosis?

(A) Cryoglobulinemic vasculitis
(B) Endocarditis
(C) IgA vasculitis
(D) Systemic lupus erythematosus

Item 72

A 23-year-old woman is evaluated in the emergency department for generalized weakness and lightheadedness of 4 hours' duration. She has had no previous contact with the health care system and takes no medications.

On physical examination, blood pressure is 120/80 mm Hg supine and 105/70 mm Hg sitting, and pulse rate is 95/min supine and increases to 108/min upon standing. BMI is 26. Skin turgor is poor. Multiple dental caries are present. There is no jugular venous distention. Cardiac examination reveals a regular rhythm with no murmurs. The lungs are clear. Bowel sounds are hyperactive. The abdomen is soft, nontender, and nondistended.

Laboratory studies:
Electrolytes:

Sodium	138 mEq/L (138 mmol/L)
Potassium	2.8 mEq/L (2.8 mmol/L)
Chloride	90 mEq/L (90 mmol/L)
Bicarbonate	36 mEq/L (36 mmol/L)

Urine studies:

Sodium	45 mEq/L (45 mmol/L)
Potassium	42 mEq/L (42 mmol/L)
Chloride	5.0 mEq/L (5.0 mmol/L)
pH	7.0

Which of the following is the most likely cause of this patient's hypokalemia?

(A) Bartter syndrome
(B) Hypokalemic periodic paralysis
(C) Sjögren syndrome
(D) Vomiting

Item 73

A 35-year-old woman is evaluated in the emergency department for new-onset lower extremity edema. She notes a 1-week history of progressive shortness of breath and fatigue. She attended a picnic 10 days ago and subsequently developed bloody diarrhea, which has largely subsided. Medical history is otherwise unremarkable, and she takes no medications.

On physical examination, temperature is 37.8 °C (100.0 °F), blood pressure is 190/90 mm Hg, pulse rate is 100/min, and respiration rate is 20/min. BMI is 27. There is no skin rash. Cardiopulmonary examination is normal. The abdomen is diffusely tender but without rebound. Bilateral lower extremity edema is noted to the level of the mid calves. On neurologic examination, mental status is normal, and there are no other focal findings.

Laboratory studies:

Hemoglobin	7.0 g/dL (70 g/L)
Platelet count	50,000/µL (50 × 10⁹/L)
Creatinine	7.2 mg/dL (636.5 µmol/L)
Urinalysis	2+ blood; 1+ protein; 0-2 erythrocytes/hpf; 0-2 leukocytes/hpf

Which of the following is the most appropriate next step in diagnosis?

(A) ADAMTS13 activity level
(B) Kidney biopsy
(C) Peripheral blood smear
(D) Urine protein electrophoresis

Item 74

A 28-year-old woman is evaluated in the emergency department for right flank pain of several days' duration and an episode of gross hematuria. She is in her 24th week of pregnancy, which has been uncomplicated, and she has had regular obstetric care. She reports no fevers or chills, abdominal pain, changes in bowel habits, dysuria, or urinary frequency. Family history is notable for her mother with kidney stones. Her only medication is a prenatal vitamin.

On physical examination, the patient is in moderately painful distress localized to the right flank area. Temperature is 37.0 °C (98.6 °F), blood pressure is 118/68 mm Hg, pulse rate is 78/min, and respiration rate is 12/min. BMI is 28. She has a

CONT. gravid uterus, and the abdominal examination is otherwise unremarkable. There is no costovertebral angle or suprapubic tenderness. The remainder of the examination is normal.

Urinalysis shows large blood and >50,000 erythrocytes/hpf but is otherwise normal.

Which of the following is the most appropriate diagnostic test to perform next?

(A) Abdominal MRI
(B) Bilateral kidney ultrasonography
(C) Low-dose noncontrast helical CT
(D) Plain abdominal radiography
(E) Transvaginal ultrasonography

Item 75

A 28-year-old man is evaluated for recurrent nephrolithiasis. Medical history is significant for Crohn disease complicated by multiple small bowel strictures requiring resection. He began developing kidney stones 3 years ago following his last bowel surgery. Analysis of the stones has consistently shown calcium oxalate, and he has been adherent to a low oxalate diet, oral hydration to maintain urine output of at least 2 L/d, and intake of 2 g of calcium carbonate with each meal. However, he has continued to have periodic episodes of kidney stones. Medical history is otherwise unremarkable. Medications are infliximab and calcium carbonate.

On physical examination, temperature is 37.1 °C (98.8 °F), blood pressure is 131/78 mm Hg, pulse rate is 84/min, and respiration rate is 12/min. BMI is 22. The abdominal examination shows healed surgical incisions and is otherwise unremarkable. The remainder of the examination is normal.

Laboratory studies, including complete blood count, electrolytes, and kidney function, are normal. Urinalysis is normal; 24-hour urine chemical analysis shows normal levels of calcium, citrate, and uric acid, but elevated oxalate.

Plain abdominal radiographs show multiple small stones in both kidneys.

Which of the following is the most appropriate additional treatment for this patient?

(A) Cholestyramine
(B) Hydrochlorothiazide
(C) Potassium citrate
(D) Pyridoxine

Item 76

An 80-year-old woman is evaluated in the emergency department for tinnitus, confusion, and unsteady gait. She also has had dry heaves and vomiting for the past few days. Her family notes progressive decline in her overall functional status over the preceding 2 weeks. Medical history is notable for hypertension and osteoarthritis. Medications are lisinopril, hydrochlorothiazide, and aspirin.

On physical examination, temperature is 37.1 °C (98.8 °F), blood pressure is 140/68 mm Hg, pulse rate is 96/min, and respiration rate is 24/min. Estimated central venous pressure is 4.0 cm H_2O. Abdominal examination is unremarkable.

Laboratory studies:
Electrolytes:
Sodium	142 mEq/L (142 mmol/L)
Potassium	3.2 mEq/L (3.2 mmol/L)
Chloride	100 mEq/L (100 mmol/L)
Bicarbonate	20 mEq/L (20 mmol/L)

Arterial blood gases:
pH	7.56
P_{CO_2}	22 mm Hg (2.9 kPa)

Chest radiograph is normal.

Which of the following is the most likely diagnosis?

(A) Respiratory alkalosis with chronic compensation
(B) Respiratory alkalosis and increased anion gap metabolic acidosis
(C) Respiratory alkalosis and metabolic alkalosis
(D) Respiratory alkalosis, increased anion gap metabolic acidosis, and metabolic alkalosis

Item 77

A 53-year-old woman is evaluated during a routine follow-up visit. Medical history is significant for hypertension and chronic active hepatitis B infection. Her hepatitis B infection has been treated with tenofovir for the past 5 years with suppression of her serum hepatitis B DNA levels. She currently notes mild generalized weakness but otherwise feels well. Medications are ramipril and tenofovir.

On physical examination, temperature is 37.0 °C (98.6 °F), blood pressure is 136/79 mm Hg, pulse rate is 70/min, and respiration rate is 14/min. BMI is 22. Abdominal examination shows a normal-sized liver and no splenomegaly. The remainder of the examination is normal.

Laboratory studies:
Bicarbonate	21 mEq/L (21 mmol/L)
Creatinine	1.2 mg/dL (106.1 µmol/L) (3 years ago: 0.8 mg/dL [70.7 µmol/L])
Glucose	87 mg/dL (4.8 mmol/L)
Phosphorus	2.2 mg/dL (0.71 mmol/L)
Urinalysis	1+ protein; 2+ glucose; no cells or casts

Which of the following is the most likely cause of this patient's kidney findings?

(A) Hypertensive nephropathy
(B) Membranoproliferative glomerulonephritis
(C) Membranous glomerulopathy
(D) Tubulointerstitial disease

Item 78

A 37-year-old man is evaluated in the emergency department for nausea and vomiting of 12 hours' duration. The patient states that he has been drinking large amounts of alcohol for several weeks and has eaten very little for the past week. His last alcoholic drink was more than 24 hours ago. He also reports intermittent diarrhea for the past

CONT.

2 months. History is notable for chronic alcoholism. He takes no medications.

On physical examination, the patient is cachectic. Blood pressure is 100/65 mm Hg, and pulse rate is 105/min. BMI is 17. Proximal muscle wasting is noted. There is no evidence of jaundice or ascites. The liver is enlarged and mildly tender. There is no asterixis. Neurologic examination is unremarkable.

While awaiting the results of laboratory studies, the patient is given intravenous saline with dextrose and vitamins. His respiration rate becomes markedly diminished, and he requires intubation. His laboratory studies return and show the following:

Laboratory studies:

Albumin	3.0 g/dL (30 g/L)
Calcium	8.0 mg/dL (2.0 mmol/L)
Electrolytes:	
Sodium	132 mEq/L (132 mmol/L)
Potassium	3.4 mEq/L (3.4 mmol/L)
Chloride	90 mEq/L (90 mmol/L)
Bicarbonate	32 mEq/L (32 mmol/L)
Magnesium	1.7 mg/dL (0.7 mmol/L)
Phosphorus	1.5 mg/dL (0.48 mmol/L)

Which of the following is the most likely cause of this patient's respiratory failure?

(A) Hypocalcemia

(B) Hypokalemia

(C) Hypomagnesemia

(D) Hyponatremia

(E) Hypophosphatemia

Item 79

A 57-year-old woman is evaluated during a preoperative physical examination for a total left knee replacement. Medical history is significant for osteoarthritis; her only medication is over-the-counter ibuprofen, which she takes multiple times daily for pain relief.

On physical examination, blood pressure is 152/90 mm Hg, and pulse rate is 64/min. BMI is 34. Severe osteoarthritic changes are noted in the left knee. Trace pitting edema in the ankles is noted. The remainder of the examination is unremarkable.

Laboratory studies show a serum creatinine level of 1.2 mg/dL (106.1 µmol/L) and a serum potassium level of 5.1 mEq/L (5.1 mmol/L); urine dipstick demonstrates no blood or protein.

Which of the following is the most appropriate next step in the management of this patient's blood pressure?

(A) Begin a low-dose ACE inhibitor

(B) Begin low-dose hydrochlorothiazide

(C) Discontinue ibuprofen

(D) Obtain a plasma aldosterone-plasma renin ratio

Item 80

A 64-year-old man is hospitalized with confusion, nausea, and dizziness. He has not felt well for weeks. Medi-

cal history is notable for hypertension, atrial fibrillation, and hyperlipidemia. He had a superior mesenteric artery embolus 2 years ago and had a resection of a large segment of his small bowel. He has chronic diarrhea. Medications are rosuvastatin, metoprolol, warfarin, and enalapril. His wife confirms that he takes no additional medications, including over-the-counter drugs or supplements.

On physical examination, temperature is 37.2 °C (99.0 °F), blood pressure is 108/60 mm Hg, pulse rate is 96/min, and respiration rate is 18/min. BMI is 22. He is confused to place and time and is easily distractible. The remainder of the physical examination is noncontributory.

Laboratory studies:

Blood urea nitrogen	14 mg/dL (5 mmol/L)
Electrolytes:	
Sodium	140 mEq/L (140 mmol/L)
Potassium	3.8 mEq/L (3.8 mmol/L)
Chloride	106 mEq/L (106 mmol/L)
Bicarbonate	20 mEq/L (20 mmol/L)
Glucose	90 mg/dL (5 mmol/L)
Lactate	Normal
Arterial blood gases:	
pH	7.37
P_{CO_2}	36 mm Hg (4.8 kPa)
Plasma osmolality	296 mOsm/kg H$_2$O

Which of the following is the most likely diagnosis?

(A) D-Lactic acidosis

(B) Ethylene glycol or methanol poisoning

(C) Propylene glycol toxicity

(D) Pyroglutamic acidosis

Item 81

A 70-year-old woman is evaluated in the emergency department for acute-onset fever and rigors that began during hemodialysis. She has end-stage kidney disease due to chronic glomerulonephritis. She started hemodialysis 1 month ago via a right internal jugular tunneled cuffed catheter. A left forearm arteriovenous fistula was placed 1 week ago. Medications are labetalol, sevelamer, epoetin alfa, and calcitriol.

On physical examination, temperature is 37.9 °C (100.2 °F), blood pressure is 145/95 mm Hg, pulse rate is 95/min, and respiration rate is 20/min. BMI is 23. Examination of the right internal jugular catheter site reveals no tenderness, induration, or discharge. The left forearm arteriovenous fistula is nontender with a clean, well-healed surgical incision. There is no heart murmur. The lungs are clear. The remainder of the physical examination is unremarkable.

Laboratory studies are notable for a leukocyte count of 13,000/µL (13 × 10⁹/L) and a plasma lactate level of 1.0 mEq/L (1.0 mmol/L). Blood cultures are pending.

A chest radiograph is normal.

Which of the following is the most appropriate next step in management?

(A) Begin vancomycin

(B) Begin vancomycin and ceftazidime

(C) Exchange dialysis catheter over a wire

(D) Remove dialysis catheter and observe

Item 82

A 66-year-old woman is hospitalized for nausea and vomiting, worsening dyspnea on exertion, and weakness of 4 days' duration. Medical history is notable for heart failure, COPD, and hypertension. Medications are carvedilol, amlodipine, albuterol, and tiotropium inhalers.

On physical examination, blood pressure is 108/65 mm Hg, pulse rate is 98/min, and respiration rate is 20/min. Oxygen saturation is 91% on ambient air. BMI is 36. Cardiovascular examination demonstrates an S_4 and no jugular venous distention. Lung examination demonstrates no wheezing or crackles. There is 1+ pitting edema in the ankles. The remainder of the physical examination is normal.

Laboratory studies:

Bicarbonate	29 mEq/L (29 mmol/L)
Potassium	3.0 mEq/L (3.0 mmol/L)
Arterial blood gas studies:	
pH	7.47
P_{CO_2}	44 mm Hg (5.9 kPa)
P_{O_2}	70 mm Hg (9.3 kPa)

A chest radiograph shows flattened diaphragms and a narrow cardiac silhouette.

Which of the following is the most appropriate next step in management?

(A) Administer 0.9% saline intravenously
(B) Administer furosemide intravenously
(C) Measure urine chloride level
(D) Measure urine sodium level

Item 83

A 42-year-old woman is evaluated in the emergency department for an episode of blood in her urine associated with right-sided abdominal pain. She reports no dysuria, urgency, or frequency. She notes a history of chronic, nonlocalized abdominal discomfort, but has no history of urinary tract infections. She otherwise has been healthy. Family history indicates that her mother and father are both alive without medical problems, as are three brothers and one sister. She is sexually active, and her only medication is an oral contraceptive.

On physical examination, the patient is in mild distress. Temperature is 37.0 °C (98.6 °F), blood pressure is 150/100 mm Hg, pulse rate is 88/min and regular, and respiration rate is 15/min. BMI is 30. Cardiovascular and pulmonary examinations are normal. There is no costovertebral angle tenderness. On abdominal examination, there is diffuse tenderness to moderate palpation without rebound. There are palpable masses in the right and left abdomen, with increased discomfort with palpation on the right.

Laboratory studies:

Hematocrit	42%
Leukocyte count	8500/µL (8.5×10^9/L)
Blood urea nitrogen	25 mg/dL (8.9 mmol/L)
Creatinine	2.0 mg/dL (176.8 µmol/L)
Urinalysis	Too numerous to count erythrocytes/hpf; 3-5 leukocytes/hpf
Human chorionic gonadotropin	Negative

Which of the following is the most likely diagnosis?

(A) Autosomal dominant polycystic kidney disease
(B) Renal cell carcinoma
(C) Renal vein thrombosis
(D) Urinary tract infection

Item 84

A 42-year-old man is hospitalized to begin chemotherapy for recently diagnosed Burkitt-like lymphoma. He is started on aggressive intravenous volume repletion with isotonic sodium chloride and allopurinol. Three days into receiving hyper-CVAD therapy (cyclophosphamide, vincristine, doxorubicin, dexamethasone), he develops decreasing urine output to 0.6 mL/kg/h. His only other medication is as-needed ondansetron.

On physical examination, blood pressure is 130/72 mm Hg. There is lymphadenopathy involving the cervical and submental chains and supraclavicular areas bilaterally, as well as bulky axillary and inguinal lymphadenopathy. Heart rate and rhythm are regular. Lungs are clear. The spleen is palpable approximately 4 cm below the left costal margin. There is no hepatomegaly. There is no edema, cyanosis, or clubbing of the extremities.

Laboratory studies:

Blood urea nitrogen	22 mg/dL (7.9 mmol/L)
Calcium	7.3 mg/dL (1.8 mmol/L) (baseline, 8.7 mg/dL [2.2 mmol/L])
Creatinine	1.3 mg/dL (114.9 µmol/L) (baseline, 0.9 mg/dL [79.6 µmol/L])
Phosphorus	6.5 mg/dL (2.1 mmol/L) (baseline, 3.3 mg/dL [1.1 mmol/L])
Potassium	5.1 mEq/L (5.1 mmol/L) (baseline, 4.3 mEq/L [4.3 mmol/L])
Urate	14 mg/dL (0.83 mmol/L) (pretreatment level, 6.2 mg/dL [0.37 mmol/L])
Urinalysis	pH 5.5; multiple urate crystals

Which of the following is the most appropriate treatment?

(A) Begin hemodialysis
(B) Begin urine alkalinization
(C) Increase allopurinol dose
(D) Substitute rasburicase for allopurinol

Item 85

A 20-year-old woman is seen during a follow-up visit for hematuria. She was evaluated 1 week ago for hematuria of 5 days' duration. She recalled having a sore throat around the time of onset of hematuria, but no fever, dysuria, flank pain, or other symptoms. Urinalysis at that time showed too numerous to count erythrocytes/hpf with a few erythrocyte casts. Laboratory studies at that time showed the following: normal complement levels, a serum creatinine level of 0.7 mg/dL (61.9 µmol/L), negative antinuclear antibodies and ANCA, and a urine protein-creatinine ratio of 1100 mg/g. Kidney ultrasound was normal. She has been healthy, and her only medication is an oral contraceptive pill.

On physical examination, temperature is 37.1 °C (98.7 °F), blood pressure is 130/80 mm Hg, pulse rate is 78/min, and respiration rate is 16/min. BMI is 22. Mild pharyngeal congestion is noted. There is no edema. The remainder of the physical examination, including skin, joints, and nasal and oral mucosa, is normal.

Current laboratory studies show a urinalysis with 5-10 erythrocytes/hpf without casts, a serum creatinine level of 0.6 mg/dL (53 µmol/L), and a urine protein-creatinine ratio of 100 mg/g.

Which of the following is the most appropriate next step in management?

(A) ACE inhibitor therapy

(B) Kidney biopsy

(C) Oral glucocorticoids

(D) Continued observation

Item 86

A 35-year-old woman is evaluated during a follow-up visit. She is at 37 weeks' gestation of her first pregnancy. Preeclampsia was diagnosed at 32 weeks when she was found to be hypertensive with mild proteinuria; she was previously normotensive. Her subsequent prenatal obstetric and laboratory monitoring has remained stable, and she is without symptoms. Medical history is otherwise unremarkable, and her only medication is a prenatal vitamin.

On physical examination, temperature is 36.9 °C (98.4 °F), blood pressure is 148/85 mm Hg, pulse rate is 87/min, and respiration rate is 12/min. BMI is 27. Examination of the lungs and heart is normal. The abdomen shows expected changes of pregnancy but is otherwise normal. There is trace bipedal edema. The remainder of the examination is unremarkable.

Laboratory studies are significant for a normal platelet count, blood urea nitrogen, serum creatinine, electrolyte panel, and liver chemistry studies.

Which of the following is the most appropriate next step in management?

(A) Antihypertensive therapy

(B) Aspirin therapy

(C) Delivery of the baby

(D) Glucocorticoids

(E) Continued monitoring until term

Item 87

A 40-year-old man is seen in follow-up for evaluation of proteinuria detected on urinalysis as part of an insurance physical examination. He is otherwise asymptomatic. Medical history is significant for obesity but is otherwise unremarkable with no prior kidney disease. He takes no medications.

On physical examination, patient is afebrile, blood pressure is 155/105 mm Hg, pulse rate is 74/min, and respiration rate is 14/min. BMI is 38. Cardiopulmonary and abdominal examinations are unremarkable. There is no arthritis, rash, or lower extremity edema.

Laboratory studies:

Albumin	4.2 g/dL (42 g/L)
Complements (C3 and C4)	Normal
Creatinine	1.0 mg/dL (88.4 µmol/L)
Antinuclear antibodies	Negative
Hepatitis B surface antigen	Negative
Hepatitis C antibodies	Negative
HIV antibodies	Negative
Urinalysis	3+ protein; no blood or cells
Urine protein-creatinine ratio	2000 mg/g

Kidney biopsy shows enlarged glomeruli with focal segmental sclerosis; immunofluorescence is nonspecific, and electron microscopy shows mild foot process effacement.

In addition to starting an ACE inhibitor, which of the following is the most appropriate additional next step in management?

(A) Prednisone

(B) Rapid plasma reagin test

(C) Tacrolimus

(D) Weight loss

Item 88

A 77-year-old woman was evaluated in the hospital for worsening kidney function. She presented 14 days ago with substernal chest pain and underwent coronary catheterization that showed left anterior descending arterial thrombosis that was treated with balloon angioplasty and stenting. Hospital course was uneventful, and she was discharged 11 days ago. She now presents for a follow-up evaluation. Medical history is significant for hypertension, type 2 diabetes mellitus, and stage 3A chronic kidney disease. She has a 90-pack-year smoking history and continues to smoke. Current medications are aspirin, lisinopril, atorvastatin, clopidogrel, metoprolol, and insulin.

On physical examination, temperature is 37.6 °C (99.7 °F), blood pressure is 140/86 mm Hg sitting and 134/78 mm Hg standing, and pulse rate is 66/min sitting and 70/min standing. BMI is 28. The lungs are clear, and the heart and abdominal examinations are normal. There is no lower extremity edema.

Skin findings of the lower extremities are shown (see top of next page).

Laboratory studies:

Blood urea nitrogen	48 mg/dL (17.1 mmol/L)
Creatinine	3.1 mg/dL (274 µmol/L) (baseline: 1.3 mg/dL [114.9 µmol/L])
Urinalysis	1+ blood; 2+ protein; positive for leukocyte esterase; 5-10 erythrocytes/hpf; 10-15 leukocytes/hpf with eosinophils; no casts or crystals

Which of the following is the most likely diagnosis?

(A) Acute interstitial nephritis

(B) Atheroembolism

(C) Contrast-induced nephropathy

(D) Polyarteritis nodosa

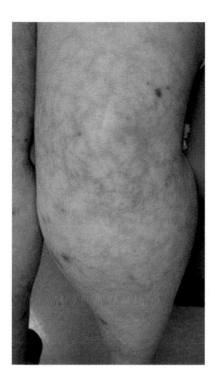

ITEM 88

Item 89

A 57-year-old man is evaluated for treatment of newly diagnosed hypertension. History is notable for hyperlipidemia, which is treated with moderate-dose simvastatin. The patient is black.

On physical examination, blood pressure is 151/94 mm Hg, and pulse rate is 72/min. BMI is 28. The remainder of the examination is unremarkable.

Laboratory studies show a serum creatinine level of 1.0 mg/dL (88.4 µmol/L), a fasting plasma glucose level of 104 mg/dL (5.8 mmol/L), and a serum potassium level of 4.5 mEq/L (4.5 mmol/L); a urine dipstick demonstrates no blood or protein.

In addition to recommending lifestyle modifications, which of the following is the most appropriate initial antihypertensive therapy for this patient?

(A) Amlodipine
(B) Diltiazem
(C) Hydrochlorothiazide
(D) Lisinopril

Item 90

A 24-year-old man is hospitalized following an attempted suicide by overdose.

On physical examination, the patient has trouble staying awake and does not respond to questions. Temperature is 37.0 °C (98.6 °F), blood pressure is 146/96 mm Hg, pulse rate is 112/min, and respiration rate is 22/min. BMI is 28. The general medical examination is normal. On neurologic examination, his pupils react to light and are

symmetric. Deep tendon reflexes are slightly diminished but symmetric.

Laboratory studies:

Blood urea nitrogen	28 mg/dL (10 mmol/L)
Creatinine	2.2 mg/dL (194.5 µmol/L)
Electrolytes:	
Sodium	136 mEq/L (136 mmol/L)
Potassium	4.0 mEq/L (4.0 mmol/L)
Chloride	96 mEq/L (96 mmol/L)
Bicarbonate	12 mEq/L (12 mmol/L)
Glucose	90 mg/dL (5 mmol/L)
Plasma osmolality	314 mOsm/kg H_2O
Serum ethanol	Undetectable
Arterial blood gases:	
pH	7.24
P_{CO_2}	28 mm Hg (3.7 kPa)
P_{O_2}	102 mm Hg (13.6 kPa)

Additional toxicology studies are pending.

Intravenous hydration and fomepizole are administered, and emergent hemodialysis is planned.

Which of the following is the most appropriate additional management intervention in this patient?

(A) Activated charcoal gastric decontamination
(B) Intravenous ethanol
(C) Intravenous sodium bicarbonate
(D) No additional therapy

Item 91

A 61-year-old woman is evaluated during a routine health maintenance visit. She has no symptoms or concerns at this time. She has stage G4/A1 chronic kidney disease due to autosomal dominant polycystic kidney disease and a 22-year history of hypertension. Medications are fosinopril, furosemide, and sodium bicarbonate.

On physical examination, temperature is 37.0 °C (98.6 °F), blood pressure is 129/72 mm Hg, pulse rate is 84/min, and respiration rate is 14/min. BMI is 28. Bilateral flank fullness is noted. The lungs are clear. There is no peripheral edema.

Laboratory studies:

Calcium	9.0 mg/dL (2.3 mmol/L)
Creatinine	2.8 mg/dL (247.5 µmol/L)
Phosphorus	3.5 mg/dL (1.13 mmol/L)
Intact parathyroid hormone	450 pg/mL (450 ng/L)
25-Hydroxy vitamin D	42 ng/mL (104.8 nmol/L)

Which of the following is the most appropriate next step in management?

(A) Bisphosphonate therapy
(B) Dual-energy x-ray absorptiometry scan
(C) Oral calcitriol
(D) Parathyroidectomy

Item 92

A 38-year-old man is evaluated in the emergency department for acute abdominal pain. Medical history

CONT.

is significant for excessive alcohol use and recurrent acute pancreatitis. He drinks six beers daily. He takes no medications.

On physical examination, the patient is in acute distress and indicates epigastric pain. Temperature is 38.0 °C (100.4 °F), blood pressure is 160/88 mm Hg, pulse rate is 88/min, and respiration rate is 20/min. BMI is 25. Chest and heart examinations are normal. The abdomen is slightly distended, with tenderness to minimal palpation in the epigastric area. There is no peripheral edema.

Laboratory studies:

Leukocyte count	10,000/µL (10×10^9/L)
Blood urea nitrogen	15 mg/dL (5.4 mmol/L)
Creatinine	1.2 mg/dL (106.1 µmol/L)
Electrolytes:	
Sodium	128 mEq/L (128 mmol/L)
Potassium	4.0 mEq/L (4.0 mmol/L)
Chloride	99 mEq/L (99 mmol/L)
Bicarbonate	24 mEq/L (24 mmol/L)
Glucose	90 mg/dL (5 mmol/L)
Lipase	620 U/L
Plasma osmolality	290 mOsm/kg H_2O
Urine osmolality	400 mOsm/kg H_2O

Which of the following is the most likely cause of this patient's hyponatremia?

(A) Adrenal insufficiency

(B) Pseudohyponatremia

(C) Psychogenic polydipsia

(D) Syndrome of inappropriate antidiuretic hormone secretion

Item 93

A 25-year-old woman is evaluated for an acute onset of swelling of the lower extremities and a 9.1-kg (20 lb) weight gain over 10 days. She notes that her urine output has diminished and that her urine appears "frothy." Medical history is significant for an unknown kidney problem as a child that resolved with medical therapy. She currently takes no medications.

On physical examination, temperature is normal, blood pressure is 100/70 mm Hg, pulse rate is 74/min, and respiration rate is 14/min. BMI is 22. Anasarca is present. Decreased breath sounds are noted at both lung bases. Cardiac examination is normal. Abdominal distention with edema of the abdominal wall is present. There is no skin rash or joint swelling.

Laboratory studies:

Albumin	1.2 g/dL (12 g/L)
Creatinine	1.1 mg/dL (97.2 µmol/L)
Urinalysis	3+ protein; 0-2 erythrocytes/hpf; 0-2 leukocytes/hpf
Urine protein-creatinine ratio	10,500 mg/g

Kidney biopsy results reveal normal-appearing glomeruli on light microscopy with immunofluorescence staining showing no immune complex deposition; electron microscopy results are pending.

Which of the following is the most appropriate treatment?

(A) Cyclophosphamide

(B) Lisinopril

(C) Prednisone

(D) No pharmacologic treatment

Item 94

A 19-year-old man is evaluated in the emergency department for weakness and inability to walk that began shortly after a 5-mile run. In the morning, he had a related episode of weakness of both lower limbs that lasted for 1 hour and resolved spontaneously. He also notes about a 5.0-kg (11-lb) weight loss over the past 7 months, episodes of palpitations, and heat intolerance. He was previously in good health. He takes no medications.

On physical examination, blood pressure is 150/90 mm Hg, pulse rate is 106/min, and respiration rate is 20/min. BMI is 18. The thyroid is enlarged. There is a fine tremor of the outstretched hands. There is symmetric muscle weakness with areflexia in the lower and upper extremities. The remainder of the examination is unremarkable.

Laboratory studies:

Electrolytes:	
Sodium	142 mEq/L (142 mmol/L)
Potassium	2.0 mEq/L (2.0 mmol/L)
Chloride	104 mEq/L (104 mmol/L)
Bicarbonate	24 mEq/L (24 mmol/L)

Which of the following is the most likely diagnosis?

(A) Bartter syndrome

(B) Hypokalemic periodic paralysis

(C) Primary hyperaldosteronism

(D) Sjögren syndrome

Item 95

A 33-year-old woman seeks preconception counseling. She and her partner plan to conceive a child within the next few months. She stopped taking her oral contraceptive several months ago. She has a 3-year history of hypertension treated successfully with losartan. Her home blood pressure measurements are typically in the range of 110-115/70-75 mm Hg. She feels well and has no specific complaints. Medical history is otherwise normal, and family history is notable for hypertension in her parents. Medications are losartan, 50 mg/d, and a prenatal vitamin.

On physical examination, temperature is 37.1 °C (98.8 °F), blood pressure is 112/71 mm Hg, pulse rate is 87/min, and respiration rate is 16/min. BMI is 23. The remainder of the examination, including neurologic examination, is normal.

Laboratory studies, including complete blood count, liver chemistries, kidney function studies, and urinalysis, are normal.

Which of the following is the most appropriate next step in management?

(A) Continue losartan at current dose
(B) Decrease losartan dose to 25 mg/d
(C) Stop losartan and monitor blood pressure
(D) Switch losartan to labetalol

Item 96

A 45-year-old man is evaluated for increased urination and thirst of several months' duration. He also notes twice-nightly nocturia during this time period. Medical history is significant for bipolar disorder diagnosed 20 years ago that has been successfully treated with lithium.

On physical examination, blood pressure is 110/70 mm Hg supine and 105/65 mm Hg standing, pulse rate is 88/min supine and 95/min standing, and respiration rate is 20/min. BMI is 25. Examination of the lymph nodes, chest, heart, and abdomen is normal.

Laboratory studies:

Blood urea nitrogen	24 mg/dL (8.6 mmol/L)
Creatinine	1.5 mg/dL (132.6 µmol/L)
Electrolytes:	
Sodium	144 mEq/L (144 mmol/L)
Potassium	4.5 mEq/L (4.5 mmol/L)
Chloride	115 mEq/L (115 mmol/L)
Bicarbonate	24 mEq/L (24 mmol/L)
Glucose	90 mg/dL (5 mmol/L)
Plasma osmolality	320 mOsm/kg H_2O
Urine osmolality	240 mOsm/kg H_2O

Which of the following is the most appropriate diagnostic test to perform next?

(A) Cosyntropin stimulation test
(B) Serum thyroid-stimulating hormone measurement
(C) Urine sodium measurement
(D) Water restriction test

Item 97

A 45-year-old man is evaluated in the emergency department for proximal muscle weakness worsening over the course of the day. Medical history is significant for non-anuric end-stage kidney disease, hypertension, and hyperlipidemia. Medications are lisinopril, atorvastatin, amlodipine, aspirin, and sevelamer. He missed his regular hemodialysis session yesterday and has not been dialyzed for 3 days.

On physical examination, blood pressure is 170/90 mm Hg, and pulse rate is 77/min. Estimated central venous pressure is 10 cm H_2O. Cardiac examination reveals a regular rhythm with an S_4 but no murmurs. The lungs are clear. There is 2+ edema of the lower extremities.

Laboratory studies are significant for a plasma glucose level of 110 mg/dL (6.1 mmol/L) and a serum potassium level of 8.0 mEq/L (8.0 mmol/L).

An electrocardiogram shows peaked T waves.

Emergent hemodialysis is planned.

In addition to intravenous calcium gluconate, which of the following is the most appropriate next step in treatment?

(A) Intravenous glucose and insulin
(B) Intravenous high-dose bumetanide
(C) Intravenous sodium bicarbonate
(D) Oral sodium polystyrene sulfonate in sorbitol

Item 98

A 60-year-old woman is evaluated during a follow-up visit for hypertension. History is also notable for hyperlipidemia. She tolerates her medications well except for minor pedal edema since starting her antihypertensive medication. She is active and plays tennis three times per week. Current medications are amlodipine, 5 mg/d, and rosuvastatin.

On physical examination, the average of two blood pressure measurements is 152/86 mm Hg, which is consistent with measurements she has obtained at home over the past 3 months. Pulse rate is 64/min. BMI is 22. Trace pedal edema is noted. The remainder of the examination is unremarkable.

Laboratory studies show a normal chemistry panel; a urine dipstick demonstrates no protein.

Which of the following is the most appropriate next step in management?

(A) Add lisinopril
(B) Add metoprolol
(C) Increase amlodipine to 10 mg/d
(D) Continue current regimen

Item 99

A 54-year-old man is evaluated for elevated blood pressure noted recently at a local health fair. He has no other medical history and takes no medications.

On this visit and on two subsequent nurse visits, the patient's blood pressure measurements are less than 140/90 mm Hg. BMI is 34. Cardiac examination reveals an S_4 gallop. The remainder of the examination is normal.

Laboratory studies show a normal chemistry panel, and a urine dipstick demonstrates no blood or protein.

Electrocardiogram demonstrates evidence of left ventricular hypertrophy.

Which of the following is the most appropriate next step in management?

(A) Ambulatory blood pressure monitoring
(B) Lisinopril
(C) Plasma aldosterone-plasma renin ratio
(D) Repeat blood pressure measurement in 6 months

Item 100

A 46-year-old woman is evaluated in the emergency department for difficulty catching her breath, generalized weakness, and paresthesias of the hands and feet. Medical history is significant for hypertension and generalized anxiety disorder. Medications are hydrochlorothiazide and paroxetine.

On physical examination, the patient appears anxious and is breathing rapidly. Temperature is 36.5 °C (97.7 °F), blood pressure is 108/62 mm Hg, pulse rate is 104/min, and respiration rate is 24/min. Oxygen saturation on ambient air is 99%. BMI is 24. There is no stridor, crackles, or wheezing on lung examination. The remainder of the physical examination is normal.

Laboratory studies:

Bicarbonate	21 mEq/L (21 mmol/L)
Arterial blood gas studies:	
pH	7.58
P_{CO_2}	22 mm Hg (2.9 kPa)
P_{O_2}	103 mm Hg (13.7 kPa)

Which of the following is the most likely acid–base disorder in this patient?

(A) Metabolic alkalosis and acute respiratory compensation

(B) Metabolic alkalosis and chronic respiratory compensation

(C) Respiratory alkalosis and acute metabolic compensation

(D) Respiratory alkalosis and chronic metabolic compensation

Item 101

A 58-year-old woman is evaluated during a follow-up visit for a 5-year history of stage G3b/A1 chronic kidney disease caused by analgesic nephropathy. History is also notable for hypertension. She takes amlodipine and no longer uses analgesics.

On physical examination, temperature is 37.0 °C (98.6 °F), blood pressure is 132/78 mm Hg, pulse rate is 82/min, and respiration rate is 14/min. BMI is 26. Cardiac examination reveals no murmur, rub, or gallop. The lungs are clear.

Laboratory studies:

Creatinine	1.8 mg/dL (159.1 µmol/L)
Electrolytes:	
Sodium	140 mEq/L (140 mmol/L)
Potassium	5.4 mEq/L (5.4 mmol/L)
Chloride	110 mEq/L (110 mmol/L)
Bicarbonate	18 mEq/L (18 mmol/L)
Arterial blood gases:	
pH	7.36
P_{CO_2}	35 mm Hg (4.7 kPa)
Estimated glomerular filtration rate	33 mL/min/1.73 m²

Which of the following is the most appropriate treatment?

(A) Intravenous sodium bicarbonate

(B) Oral potassium citrate

(C) Oral sodium bicarbonate

(D) Continue current therapy

Item 102

A 35-year-old man is evaluated in the hospital for acute kidney injury. He presented with worsening fatigue, decreased urination, and progressive swelling in the ankles occurring over the course of 2 to 3 weeks. Laboratory studies at the time of diagnosis showed a serum creatinine level of 6.7 mg/dL (592.3 µmol/L) (baseline of 0.9 mg/dL [79.6 µmol/L] 1 year ago). Medical history is significant for a 3-year history of inflammatory bowel disease that has been well controlled with daily mesalamine therapy. He does not take any over-the-counter drugs.

On physical examination, temperature is 37.0 °C (98.6 °F), blood pressure is 118/67 mm Hg, pulse rate is 60/min, and respiration rate is 16/min. BMI is 20. Cardiac examination is normal. The lungs show crackles at the bases bilaterally. There is lower extremity edema to the mid calf. The remainder of the examination is normal.

Dipstick urinalysis shows 1+ protein but is otherwise normal. Urine microscopy shows 2-3 erythrocytes/hpf, 5-10 leukocytes/hpf, and leukocyte casts. Urine protein-creatinine ratio is 1060 mg/g. Urine cultures are negative.

Kidney ultrasound shows normal-sized kidneys with mildly increased parenchymal echogenicity, no hydronephrosis, and no renal calculi.

Which of the following is the most likely cause of this patient's acute kidney injury?

(A) Interstitial nephritis

(B) Lupus nephritis

(C) Membranous glomerulopathy

(D) Rapidly progressive glomerulonephritis

Item 103

A 41-year-old woman is evaluated during a routine obstetrics visit. She is in the third trimester of her first pregnancy. Her previous visits have been unremarkable, with blood pressures within the normal range for pregnancy. She has noticed mild shortness of breath with exertion and mild peripheral edema in her lower extremities. She reports no urinary changes. Medical history is notable for type 1 diabetes mellitus; she reports well-controlled blood sugars. Family history is notable for her mother who has hypertension. Medications are insulin and prenatal vitamins.

On physical examination, temperature is 37.1 °C (98.8 °F), blood pressure is 162/112 mm Hg, pulse rate is 87/min, and respiration rate is 16/min. BMI is 28. Cardiac examination reveals a grade 2/6 crescendo-decrescendo murmur at the right upper sternal border and an S_3 gallop. Estimated central venous pressure is 14 cm H_2O. Bibasilar crackles are noted at the lung bases bilaterally. The patient has a gravid uterus and an otherwise unremarkable abdominal examination. There is trace lower extremity edema.

Laboratory studies are significant for a platelet count of 75,000 µL (75 × 10⁹/L); a comprehensive metabolic profile with liver chemistry tests, peripheral blood smear, and urinalysis are normal.

Which of the following is the most likely diagnosis?

(A) Chronic hypertension

(B) HELLP syndrome

(C) Normal changes of pregnancy

(D) Preeclampsia

Item 104

A 69-year-old woman is evaluated during a follow-up visit for stage G4/A1 chronic kidney disease due to hypertensive nephrosclerosis. History is also significant for peripheral arterial disease with right femoral-popliteal bypass 1 year ago. Medications are metoprolol, atorvastatin, aspirin, and calcium acetate.

On physical examination, temperature is 37.0 °C (98.6 °F), blood pressure is 132/89 mm Hg, pulse rate is 61/min, and respiration rate is 13/min. BMI is 27. There is an audible S_4 gallop and reduced pedal pulses. The lungs are clear. The lower extremities are warm with normal capillary refill. There is no peripheral edema.

Laboratory studies:

Albumin	4.2 g/dL (42 g/L)
Calcium	8.3 mg/dL (2.1 mmol/L)
Creatinine	2.6 mg/dL (229.8 µmol/L)
Phosphorus	6.9 mg/dL (2.23 mmol/L)
Intact parathyroid hormone	95 pg/mL (95 ng/L)
Estimated glomerular filtration rate	22 mL/min/1.73 m²

Review of a previous chest radiograph is remarkable for a heavily calcified aorta but is otherwise clear.

In addition to dietary counseling regarding a low phosphate diet, which of the following is the most appropriate treatment?

(A) Calcitriol

(B) Calcium carbonate

(C) Cinacalcet

(D) Sevelamer

Item 105

A 72-year-old man is evaluated for a 3-month history of slowly progressive anemia and fatigue. He has a 3-year history of end-stage kidney disease and receives hemodialysis three times weekly. Prior to starting hemodialysis he was able to maintain adequate iron stores with oral iron therapy. Erythropoietin for symptomatic anemia was initiated 3 years ago with the onset of dialysis; he responded well, with an increase in his hemoglobin level to 11 g/dL (110 g/L) and a decrease in symptoms. There have been no changes in his medications, which consist of erythropoietin, three times weekly; oral iron sulfate, 325 mg three times daily; lisinopril; metoprolol; nifedipine; sevelamer; and aspirin.

On physical examination, the patient is afebrile. Blood pressure is 144/94 mm Hg, pulse rate is 76/min, and respiration rate is 16/min. The lungs are clear. There is no edema.

Laboratory studies:

Hemoglobin	9.8 g/dL (98 g/L)
Ferritin	80 ng/mL (80 µg/L)
Transferrin saturation	12%

Which of the following is the most appropriate management?

(A) Administer intravenous iron

(B) Increase erythropoietin dose

(C) Increase oral iron dose

(D) Measure erythropoietin level

Item 106

A 52-year-old man is evaluated for a recent diagnosis of membranous glomerulopathy (MG). He presented with a 1-month history of increasing lower extremity edema and was found to have nephrotic-range proteinuria. Evaluation included normal serum complement levels; negative serologies for antinuclear antibodies, hepatitis B, and hepatitis C; and negative serum protein electrophoresis. Kidney biopsy showed changes consistent with MG; staining for antibodies to the phospholipase A_2 receptor (PLA$_2$R) was negative. Medical history is otherwise significant for hypertension. He is up-to-date with recommended health maintenance interventions. He has a 25-pack-year smoking history and is a current smoker. His only medication is ramipril.

On physical examination, temperature is 36.7 °C (98.0 °F), blood pressure is 140/80 mm Hg, pulse rate is 68/min, and respiration rate is 14/min. BMI is 31. Pulmonary and abdominal examinations are normal. There is lower extremity edema to the knees bilaterally.

Which of the following is the most appropriate next diagnostic step?

(A) Chest radiography

(B) PET/CT of the chest

(C) Whole body CT

(D) No additional testing

Item 107

A 57-year-old man is hospitalized with *Streptococcus viridans* endocarditis; intravenous ceftriaxone for 6 weeks will be initiated. History is significant for stage G5/A2 chronic kidney disease due to IgA nephropathy and hypertension. Placement of a left forearm arteriovenous fistula occurred 12 days ago. He does not yet require dialysis. Medications are lisinopril, furosemide, and sevelamer.

On physical examination, temperature is 37.0 °C (98.6 °F), blood pressure is 128/84 mm Hg, pulse rate is 77/min, and respiration rate is 17/min. BMI is 25. A grade 3/6 holosystolic murmur is present at the left sternal border. There is no pericardial rub. The arteriovenous fistula has a palpable thrill. The lungs are clear. There is no asterixis. There is no peripheral edema.

Which of the following is the most appropriate vascular access for antibiotic administration?

(A) A peripherally inserted central catheter line

(B) A single-lumen catheter in the left subclavian vein

(C) A single-lumen catheter in the right internal jugular vein

(D) The arteriovenous fistula

Item 108

A 32-year-old woman is evaluated in the emergency department 30 minutes after a motor vehicle accident in which she struck her head on the steering wheel. She is awake and conversant and has no major symptoms aside from a mild headache. She is at 23 weeks' gestation of her second pregnancy. She has been receiving routine prenatal care, and her pregnancy has been uncomplicated. Her only medication is a prenatal vitamin.

On physical examination, the patient is in neck immobilization. Temperature is 37.1 °C (98.7 °F), blood pressure is 111/63 mm Hg, pulse rate is 76/min, and respiration rate is 12/min. BMI is 24. There is a contusion on the upper forehead but no other evidence of trauma. The abdomen shows normal changes of pregnancy but is otherwise normal. The remainder of the physical and neurologic examinations is unremarkable.

Initial laboratory studies show a serum sodium level of 131 mEq/L (131 mmol/L); the remainder of the electrolytes, blood urea nitrogen, and serum creatinine are normal.

Which of the following is the most likely cause of this patient's decrease in her serum sodium level?

(A) Cerebral salt wasting
(B) Normal physiologic changes of pregnancy
(C) Pituitary apoplexy
(D) Syndrome of inappropriate antidiuretic hormone secretion

Answers and Critiques

Item 1   Answer: D

Educational Objective: Manage prehypertension.

In addition to lifestyle modifications, rechecking blood pressure in 1 year is appropriate for this patient with prehypertension. Although the eighth report of the Joint National Committee (JNC) did not address prehypertension, JNC 7 defined prehypertension as a systolic blood pressure of 120-139 mm Hg or a diastolic blood pressure of 80-89 mm Hg in the absence of preexisting end-organ disease (for example, diabetes mellitus, chronic kidney disease, or cardiovascular disease). Lifestyle modifications, including a low salt diet and exercise regimen, can be used to effectively reduce blood pressure in patients with prehypertension. Patients with prehypertension may also adopt the DASH (Dietary Approaches to Stop Hypertension) diet, which emphasizes vegetables, fruits, whole grains, legumes, and low-fat dairy products and limits sweets, red meat, and saturated/total fat, along with dedicated weight loss planning. Appropriate follow-up for those with prehypertension occurs at annual visits. The mean blood pressure in this patient (even accounting for the potential of inaccurate technique upon initial check-in) falls within the prehypertensive range, making lifestyle modifications and follow-up in 1 year the appropriate management. If blood pressures measuring 140/90 mm Hg or greater were documented, this would require repeat measurements for at least three visits over the period of at least 1 week of more to establish a diagnosis of hypertension.

Although there is an increased risk of stroke and cardiovascular disease for every level of blood pressure above 115/75 mm Hg and an increased risk of the development of hypertension, treatment of prehypertension using pharmacologic therapy (such as an ACE inhibitor or diuretic) has not yet been demonstrated to reduce this risk.

Ambulatory blood pressure monitoring records blood pressures periodically during normal activities. It is indicated primarily for diagnosis of suspected white coat hypertension (persistently elevated blood pressure readings in the office without evidence of end-organ damage) or to confirm a poor response to antihypertensive medication. It may also be useful in assessing for masked hypertension (evidence of end-organ damage without apparent elevated blood pressures) or for evaluating episodic or resistant hypertension. It is not indicated for this patient with evidence of prehypertension.

KEY POINT

- Prehypertension is managed with lifestyle modifications and annual follow-up visits to monitor blood pressure.

Bibliography

McInnes G. Pre-hypertension: how low to go and do drugs have a role? Br J Clin Pharmacol. 2012 Feb;73(2):187-93. [PMID: 21883385]

Item 2   Answer: D

Educational Objective: Select the most appropriate imaging modality for a patient with chronic kidney disease.

Ultrasonography of the abdomen and pelvis is appropriate for this patient with chronic kidney disease (CKD). She requires imaging studies to evaluate her kidneys and genitourinary tract through a noninvasive and additional lesions known as the source of gross hematuria. Ultrasonography is an appropriate initial screening test because it can provide necessary information without exposure to the risks associated with the administration of contrast agents in patients with severe CKD who are at increased risk of contrast-induced nephropathy (CIN) and gadolinium-induced nephrogenic systemic fibrosis (NSF).

This patient has risk factors for CIN (older age, elevated serum creatinine, diabetes mellitus); therefore, a contrast-enhanced CT to evaluate for lesions of the kidneys and genitourinary tract as a cause of her hematuria should be performed only if similar information cannot be obtained from tests that entail less risk to the patient.

The use of gadolinium in MRI studies is relatively contraindicated in patients with an estimated glomerular filtration rate of less than 30 mL/min/1.73 m² due to the increased risk of NSF. Although most NSF cases have occurred in patients with end-stage kidney disease, there have been isolated case reports occurring in patients with stage G4 CKD. Gadolinium-enhanced MRI is therefore contraindicated in these patients unless there is a compelling clinical indication and the patient is fully informed of the risk of NSF.

Radiography of the abdomen and pelvis may be a reasonable test to rule out nephrolithiasis. However, the patient does not have symptoms suggestive of nephrolithiasis, and a plain radiograph would not provide information to determine whether there are structural lesions in the kidneys or genitourinary tract.

KEY POINT

- Ultrasonography is an appropriate imaging modality for patients with chronic kidney disease to avoid adverse events such as contrast-induced nephropathy or nephrogenic systemic fibrosis.

Bibliography

Manjunath V, Perazella MA. Imaging patients with kidney disease in the era of NSF: can it be done safely? Clin Nephrol. 2011 Apr;75(4):279-85. [PMID: 21426881]

Item 3   Answer: D

Educational Objective: Identify the increased risk for transitional cell carcinoma in patients with Balkan endemic nephropathy.

This patient has Balkan endemic nephropathy (BEN) and is at increased risk for transitional cell carcinoma. BEN is a slowly progressive tubulointerstitial disease that has recently been linked to aristolochic acid. Aristolochic acid is a nephrotoxic alkaloid from the plant *Aristolochia clematis*, which is endemic to the Balkan region and is sometimes a component of herbal therapies used for weight loss. BEN is believed to be due to exposure to low levels of aristolochic acid over years, compared with more acute toxicity associated with ingestion of herbal preparations. Characteristics of BEN include chronic kidney disease due to tubulointerstitial injury, tubular dysfunction (polyuria and decreased concentrating ability, glucosuria without hyperglycemia, and tubular proteinuria), and anemia. Because aristolochic acid is also mutagenic, patients with BEN are at increased risk for transitional cell carcinomas of the renal pelvis, ureters, and bladder. Therefore, annual surveillance with urine cytology is recommended.

Although this patient has glucosuria, BEN is not associated with an increased incidence of diabetes mellitus. The glucosuria is due to a tubular defect, resulting in glucosuria with normoglycemia.

Intracranial cerebral aneurysms are associated with autosomal dominant polycystic kidney disease, which is characterized by large kidneys with multiple kidney cysts.

Patients with BEN are at higher risk for transitional cell carcinoma, not renal cell carcinoma.

KEY POINT

- Patients with Balkan endemic nephropathy are at increased risk for transitional cell carcinomas of the renal pelvis, ureters, and bladder.

Bibliography
Gökmen MR, Cosyns JP, Arlt VM, et al. The epidemiology, diagnosis, and management of aristolochic acid nephropathy: a narrative review. Ann Intern Med. 2013 Mar 19;158(6):469-77. [PMID: 23552405]

Item 4   Answer: C

Educational Objective: Diagnose hemoglobinuria.

This patient most likely has hemoglobinuria, possibly due to intravascular hemolysis from his mechanical mitral valve, whose dysfunction is suggested by the finding of mitral regurgitation on physical examination. Fragmentation hemolysis in this setting manifests as a microangiopathic hemolytic anemia with thrombocytopenia and is accompanied by the release of free hemoglobin into the circulation. Free hemoglobin is partially bound by haptoglobin but may also be filtered into the urine, producing a red color. Heme reacts with peroxidase in the urine dipstick, causing a false-positive result for blood. Hemoglobinuria is distinguished from true

hematuria by the absence of erythrocytes on urine microscopy. Similar findings on urinalysis will also occur with the release of myoglobin into the circulation, usually from muscle injury (rhabdomyolysis). Myoglobin is a small molecule relative to hemoglobin, is not bound within the circulation by haptoglobin, and is readily filtered through the kidneys, resulting in red-colored urine. It also reacts with peroxidase in the urine dipstick indicating blood, although microscopic examination will also be negative for erythrocytes.

Bladder cancer is a concern in a patient with a significant smoking history presenting with a finding of red urine. However, the urine color change in bladder cancer is due to bleeding into the urinary tract, and erythrocytes would be seen on urinalysis.

Glomerulonephritis may be associated with bleeding into the urine and would be suspected if erythrocytes, particularly acanthocytes (dysmorphic erythrocytes), were found on urine microscopic examination. Proteinuria may also be found in glomerulonephritis, although this patient's proteinuria is relatively mild and may result from tubular damage caused by hemoglobin toxicity.

Nephrolithiasis often presents with true hematuria in association with acute flank pain radiating to the ipsilateral groin, with or without costovertebral angle tenderness. Despite his history of nephrolithiasis, this patient does not have suggestive clinical symptoms and has no evidence of erythrocytes on urinalysis, making this an unlikely diagnosis.

KEY POINT

- Hemoglobinuria is distinguished from true hematuria by the absence of erythrocytes on urine microscopy.

Bibliography
Sharp VJ, Barnes KT, Erickson BA. Assessment of asymptomatic microscopic hematuria in adults. Am Fam Physician. 2013 Dec 1;88(11):747-54. [PMID: 24364522]

Item 5   Answer: A

Educational Objective: Treat a patient with uncontrolled hypertension.

The addition of chlorthalidone is the most appropriate next step in management in this patient who has uncontrolled hypertension with evidence of end-organ damage (left ventricular hypertrophy, chronic kidney disease, and retinopathy) despite being on three medications. However, he does not meet the definition of resistant hypertension, which is defined by blood pressure readings not at target despite three agents, one of which must be a diuretic. Persistent volume expansion, even if not sufficient to produce clinically evident edema, contributes significantly to hypertension; because of this, use of diuretics is almost always required to achieve adequate blood pressure control in patients with resistant blood pressure. Therefore, the addition of a diuretic such as chlorthalidone is appropriate for this patient before other drugs are added. Chlorthalidone is often preferred over other thiazide-type diuretics primarily due to its higher potency and longer duration of action.

Although limited data exist regarding the most effective medication regimen for patients requiring multi-drug therapy, a reasonable approach is to use medications recommended by hypertension treatment guidelines that have different mechanisms of action, with consideration of other agents with an antihypertensive effect indicated for treatment of comorbid conditions (such as a β-blocker for atrial fibrillation). For example, in addition to diuretic therapy, the combination of a long-acting dihydropyridine calcium channel blocker with an ACE inhibitor or angiotensin receptor blocker is often effective and generally well tolerated.

Vasodilator agents (hydralazine or minoxidil) and centrally acting agents (clonidine or guanfacine) may be effective, although side effects are common. Therefore, these medications are more commonly used as add-on therapy to other guideline-recommended agents and would not be an appropriate choice in this patient who is not currently on a diuretic. Additionally, minoxidil promotes sodium retention and is almost always given with a diuretic. Its use in this patient who is not taking a diuretic would not be appropriate.

Switching from nifedipine to amlodipine would not be expected to significantly improve blood pressure because both drugs are in the same class.

KEY POINT

- Diuretics are almost always required to achieve adequate blood pressure control in patients with resistant blood pressure.

Bibliography
Vongpatanasin W. Resistant hypertension: a review of diagnosis and management. JAMA. 2014 Jun 4;311(21):2216-24. [PMID: 24893089]

Item 6   Answer: A

Educational Objective: Diagnose AL amyloidosis with kidney manifestations.

AL amyloidosis secondary to a plasma cell dyscrasia is the most likely diagnosis. Amyloid consists of randomly oriented fibrils composed of various proteins that form organized β-pleated sheets within the tissues; amyloid resulting from monoclonal lambda or kappa light chains is termed *AL amyloid*. AL amyloid may present with nonspecific systemic symptoms such as fatigue or weight loss, but most commonly presents with symptoms associated with infiltration of different organ systems. These may include restrictive cardiomyopathy, peripheral neuropathy, hepatosplenomegaly, and, less commonly, cutaneous purpura and macroglossia. In amyloidosis involving the kidney, glomerular lesions tend to be prominent and present with proteinuria, often in the nephrotic range. However, amyloid deposits may also be found in tubular basement membranes, the interstitial space, and blood vessels. Findings on biopsy show deposits that stain apple green on Congo

red staining under a polarizing microscope; these deposits are also visible on electron microscopy. In this patient, the presence of the nephrotic syndrome, autonomic symptoms (diarrhea and postural hypotension), and sensory neuropathy is highly suggestive of AL amyloidosis.

Although diabetes mellitus may present with similar systemic manifestations, such as autonomic and peripheral neuropathy and the nephrotic syndrome, these manifestations are typically seen after many years of diabetes, and this patient does not have evidence of diabetes on his current laboratory studies or on prior studies.

Myeloma nephropathy results from filtering of myeloma light chains with minimal albumin, with the light chains accumulating in the renal tubule causing tubular injury and typically forming casts (cast nephropathy). Filtered light chains are often not detected on routine dipstick testing and require identification with urine electrophoresis. The degree of albuminuria seen in this patient is less consistent with the findings typically seen in myeloma nephropathy.

Primary focal segmental glomerulosclerosis is a kidney-limited disease and is not associated with the systemic manifestations exhibited in this patient.

KEY POINT

- In amyloidosis involving the kidney, glomerular lesions tend to be prominent and present with proteinuria, often in the nephrotic range.

Bibliography
Leung N, Bridoux F, Hutchison CA, et al; International Kidney and Monoclonal Gammopathy Research Group. Monoclonal gammopathy of renal significance: when MGUS is no longer undetermined or insignificant. Blood. 2012 Nov 22;120(22):4292-5. [PMID: 23047823]

Item 7   Answer: D

Educational Objective: Diagnose type 4 (hyperkalemic distal) renal tubular acidosis.

Type 4 (hyperkalemic distal) renal tubular acidosis (RTA) is the most likely cause of this patient's metabolic findings. Type 4 (hyperkalemic distal) RTA is caused by aldosterone deficiency or resistance. Primary aldosterone deficiency is seen in primary adrenal deficiency (Addison disease), and relative aldosterone deficiency may be seen in the syndrome of hyporeninemic hypoaldosteronism in which there is diminished renin release by the kidney. This occurs most commonly in patients with mild to moderate kidney disease due to diabetic nephropathy (such as this patient) or chronic interstitial nephritis (such as in systemic lupus erythematosus or AIDS). It may also be associated with acute glomerulonephritis, specific drugs that impair renin release (NSAIDs and calcineurin inhibitors), tubulointerstitial disease, and drugs that reduce aldosterone production (ACE inhibitors, cyclooxygenase inhibitors, and heparin). Patients with type 4 (hyperkalemic distal) RTA typically present with hyperkalemia, a normal anion gap metabolic acidosis, and impaired urine acidification, but with the ability to maintain the urine pH to <5.5. The specific cause can be differentiated by measurement of plasma renin activity, serum aldosterone, and serum cortisol. Initial treatment includes correction of the underlying cause if possible, with discontinuation of offending medications. Replacement of mineralocorticoids with fludrocortisone is indicated for patients with documented deficiency and should be considered for those with hyporeninemic hypoaldosteronism unless hypertension or heart failure is present.

Although kidney failure may cause hyperkalemia and metabolic acidosis, the acidosis associated with kidney failure more commonly reflects an increase in the anion gap with impaired organic acid excretion.

Type 1 (hypokalemic distal) RTA results from a defect in urine acidification in the distal tubule with impaired excretion of hydrogen ions and a normal anion gap metabolic acidosis. However, this tubular defect also results in potassium wasting and hypokalemia, which are not present in this patient.

Type 2 (proximal) RTA involves a defect in regenerating bicarbonate in the proximal tubule and is characterized by hypokalemia, glycosuria (in the setting of normal plasma glucose), low-molecular-weight proteinuria, and renal phosphate wasting, none of which is present in this patient.

KEY POINT

- Patients with type 4 (hyperkalemic distal) renal tubular acidosis typically present with hyperkalemia, a normal anion gap metabolic acidosis, and impaired urine acidification, but with the ability to maintain the urine pH to <5.5.

Bibliography

Karet FE. Mechanisms in hyperkalemic renal tubular acidosis. J Am Soc Nephrol. 2009 Feb;20(2):251-4. [PMID: 19193780]

Item 8   Answer: B

Educational Objective: Differentiate between glomerular and nonglomerular hematuria.

Evaluation for glomerular disease is the most appropriate next step for this patient. An initial step in evaluating hematuria is assessing whether the likely source of bleeding is from the glomerulus or elsewhere in the urinary tract. Glomerular hematuria is typically characterized by brown- or tea-colored urine with dysmorphic erythrocytes (or acanthocytes) and/or erythrocyte casts on urine sediment examination, although some glomerular disorders may cause gross hematuria. Other findings suggestive of a glomerular source include proteinuria. Nonglomerular bleeding typically presents with isomorphic erythrocytes in the urine without evidence of glomerular dysfunction. Glomerular causes of hematuria include inflammatory processes such as glomerulonephritis that may lead to rapid declines in kidney function but may also include more benign or indolent diseases such as thin glomerular basement membrane disease, IgA nephropathy, and other forms

of chronic glomerulonephritis. The clinical presentation in this asymptomatic patient with normal kidney function and apparent recurrent episodes of gross hematuria is consistent with IgA nephropathy as a cause of her hematuria.

Cystoscopy is used to evaluate for lower urinary tract causes of nonglomerular bleeding. It is not an appropriate next step in this patient with evidence of glomerular bleeding and no other risk factors for lower urinary tract pathology.

Noncontrast helical abdominal CT can be used to detect kidney stones or other potential causes of nonglomerular hematuria. However, this patient's presentation is not suggestive of nephrolithiasis, and she has evidence of a glomerular source of her hematuria. Additionally, the preferred method of kidney imaging in younger patients, particularly women of childbearing age, is ultrasonography due to decreased radiation exposure.

Measurement of serum creatine kinase levels is useful in evaluating for rhabdomyolysis. This diagnosis should be suspected when dipstick urinalysis is positive for heme with a negative microscopic urinalysis for erythrocytes; however, this patient has evidence of erythrocytes in her urine. Additionally, she does not have a clinical history consistent with rhabdomyolysis, and her urine studies suggest a glomerular cause of her hematuria.

KEY POINT

- Glomerular hematuria typically features brown- or tea-colored urine with dysmorphic erythrocytes (or acanthocytes) and/or erythrocyte casts on urine sediment examination.

Bibliography

Wyatt RJ, Julian BA. IgA nephropathy. N Engl J Med. 2013 Jun 20;368(25):2402-14. [PMID: 23782179]

Item 9   Answer: C

Educational Objective: Diagnose thin glomerular basement membrane disease.

The most likely diagnosis is thin glomerular basement membrane (GBM) disease, an inherited type IV collagen abnormality that causes thinning of the GBM and results in hematuria. The disorder may affect up to 5% of the population, and 30% to 50% of patients report a family history of hematuria. The disease is characterized by microscopic or macroscopic hematuria that may be first discovered in young adults. Diagnosis is usually based on the history of persistent hematuria, normal kidney function, and positive family history of hematuria without kidney failure; biopsy is not typically required. Long-term prognosis for kidney function is excellent, with rare progression to chronic kidney disease (CKD).

Fabry disease is a rare X-linked inherited disorder in which there is deficiency of α-galactosidase A (an enzyme in the glycosphingolipid pathway) that leads to progressive deposit of globotriaosylceramide (Gb3) in lysosomes. This disorder may present as CKD in young adulthood. Other associated clinical features include premature coronary artery disease, severe neuropathic pain, telangiectasias, and angiokeratomas. Because Fabry disease is X-linked and this patient has no other clinical findings of this disorder, it is not a likely diagnostic consideration.

Hereditary nephritis (also known as Alport syndrome), also a heritable disorder of type IV collagen, is a rare cause of end-stage kidney disease with a prevalence of 0.4% among adult U.S. patients. Most cases are X-linked (80%) and are associated with sensorineural hearing loss and lenticonus (conical deformation of the lens), with proteinuria, hypertension, and kidney failure developing over time. The remaining cases are autosomal recessive (15%) or autosomal dominant (5%) and may also be associated with hearing loss. Female carriers variably develop kidney disease depending on activity of the X chromosome in somatic renal cells. The prevalence of this disorder and the patient's gender make this a less likely possibility.

Tuberous sclerosis complex (TSC) results from mutations in genes coding for proteins that have a tumor-suppressing effect. Disruption of these gene products allows abnormal cell proliferation in different tissues, including the skin, brain, lung, liver, and kidney. Mild TSC may be detected in adulthood. Renal angiomyolipomas are a characteristic kidney lesion in TSC and occur in 75% of patients on imaging. The lack of evidence of other lesions suggestive of TSC and her normal kidney ultrasound make this an unlikely diagnosis in this patient.

KEY POINT

- Diagnosis of thin glomerular basement membrane disease is usually based on the history of persistent hematuria, normal kidney function, and positive family history of hematuria without kidney failure.

Bibliography

Tryggvason K, Patrakka J. Thin basement membrane nephropathy. J Am Soc Nephrol. 2006 Mar;17(3):813-22. [PMID: 16467446]

Item 10   Answer: B

Educational Objective: Treat stage 1 hypertension in a patient with diabetes mellitus and chronic kidney disease.

The ACE inhibitor lisinopril is appropriate antihypertensive therapy for this patient. He was recently diagnosed with diabetes mellitus and stage 1 hypertension (defined as a systolic blood pressure of 140-159 mm Hg and/or a diastolic blood pressure of 90-99 mm Hg) and is now noted to have chronic kidney disease (CKD). There is evidence that in patients with hypertension and CKD, regardless of diabetes status, renin-angiotensin system agents (ACE inhibitor or angiotensin receptor blocker [ARB]) have a protective effect on kidney function. Based on this evidence, the eighth report of the Joint National Committee (JNC 8) recommends the use of these agents in patients with hypertension and CKD, with or

without diabetes. The blood pressure goal recommended by the JNC 8 and the American Diabetes Association is <140/90 mm Hg for adult patients with hypertension and diabetes.

Recommendations for more aggressive blood pressure goals of <130/80 mm Hg in this population have recently been tempered by the lack of efficacy in reducing mortality with lower blood pressure goals and an increase in adverse events related to antihypertensive agents. Thus, initial combination therapy is not warranted in this case. Furthermore, the combination of two renin-angiotensin system agents for antihypertensive management in the setting of diabetes and moderately increased albuminuria (formerly known as microalbuminuria) has not been shown to improve outcomes and is associated with higher rates of hyperkalemia and other adverse events.

KEY POINT

- The eighth report of the Joint National Committee recommends an ACE inhibitor or angiotensin receptor blocker for patients with hypertension and chronic kidney disease, with or without diabetes mellitus.

Bibliography

Barnett AH, Bain SC, Bouter P, et al; Diabetics Exposed to Telmisartan and Enalapril Study Group. Angiotensin-receptor blockade versus converting-enzyme inhibition in type 2 diabetes and nephropathy. N Engl J Med. 2004;351(19):1952. [PMID: 15516696]

Item 11   Answer: D

Educational Objective: Recommend lifestyle modifications in a patient with newly diagnosed hypertension.

Lifestyle modification is the most appropriate next step in management for this 73-year-old patient with likely stage 1 hypertension based on consistently elevated blood pressure determinations. He has no evidence of end-organ manifestations on history or physical examination. Therefore, lifestyle modifications, including a low sodium diet; a diet such as DASH (Dietary Approaches to Stop Hypertension) that emphasizes vegetables, fruits, whole grains, legumes, and low-fat dairy products and limits sweets, red meat, and saturated/total fat; weight loss irrespective of diet; and exercise, are the most appropriate initial management strategies. The most effective lifestyle modification is salt restriction to 1500 mg/d, which lowers blood pressure by an average of 7/3 mm Hg. The eighth report of the Joint National Committee (JNC 8) recommends a blood pressure goal of <150/90 mm Hg for those ≥60 years of age. Because his blood pressure measurements have been around 155/85 mm Hg, salt restriction alone as part of lifestyle modifications may be enough to avoid the use of medications to achieve the treatment goal for this 73-year-old patient.

Although the α-blocker doxazosin may be considered for its dual blood pressure–lowering effect and its effect on urinary frequency, its use as first-line therapy for persistent hypertension following lifestyle modification should be decided while considering its adverse effect profile (such as orthostatic hypotension) and its increased incidence of heart failure that was noted in the Antihypertensive and Lipid Lowering Treatment to Prevent Heart Attack Trial (ALLHAT).

This patient may ultimately require medical treatment; because he has gout, the angiotensin receptor blocker (ARB) losartan may be preferred not only for its benefits in lowering blood pressure but also for its uricosuric effect. This is in contrast to thiazide diuretics such as hydrochlorothiazide, which increases serum urate.

β-Blockers such as metoprolol are no longer recommended as primary initial therapy for hypertension given their side-effect profiles, which includes higher cardiovascular-related events and mortality compared with ARBs.

Because this patient has evidence of persistently elevated blood pressures and likely stage 1 hypertension, a 6-month follow-up of his blood pressures without intervention is not appropriate.

KEY POINT

- Lifestyle modifications are indicated for all patients with hypertension, which can produce reductions in blood pressure that are equivalent to antihypertensive agents.

Bibliography

Eckel RH, Jakicic JM, Ard JD, et al. 2013 AHA/ACC guideline on lifestyle management to reduce cardiovascular risk: a report of the American College of Cardiology/American Heart Association Task Force on Practice Guidelines. J Am Coll Cardiol. 2014 Jul 1;63(25 Pt B):2960-84. [PMID: 24239922]

Item 12   Answer: D
Educational Objective: Manage infection-related glomerulonephritis.

The most appropriate management for this patient is to continue current therapy. This patient with methicillin-resistant *Staphylococcus aureus* endocarditis is found to have worsening kidney function since hospitalization. The differential diagnosis includes infection-related glomerulonephritis (IRGN), drug-induced nephrotoxicity, acute interstitial nephritis (AIN), and septic emboli. The finding of a nephritic urine sediment (erythrocytes, erythrocyte casts, and proteinuria) in an azotemic patient with an active infection suggests IRGN. IRGN is an immune complex–mediated disease most frequently associated with nonstreptococcal infections, with the antigen in the immune complex derived from the infectious agent. Immune complexes deposit in the subepithelial area and activate complement with recruitment of inflammatory cells, leading to a proliferative GN. The likelihood of IRGN is high in this patient given the low C3 complement, the absence of cryoglobulins, and the lack of clinical findings suggestive of other causes on the differential diagnosis.

Glucocorticoids are not typically used in IRGN because there is usually improvement with control of the associated infection.

A kidney biopsy is not indicated because the probability of IRGN is high. However, biopsy would be appropriate if this patient's kidney function fails to improve with treatment of the underlying infection.

Drug-induced tubular toxicity (for example, with vancomycin) typically occurs after 7 to 10 days of antibiotic therapy and the urine sediment does not show cells, unlike in this patient. Antibiotic-induced AIN is typically associated with mild proteinuria, erythrocytes, leukocytes, and leukocyte casts on urinalysis. Eosinophiluria, recurrence of fevers, rash, and peripheral eosinophilia may also be seen and typically occur after 7 to 10 days of therapy, none of which is present in this patient. Therefore, switching vancomycin to daptomycin is not appropriate.

KEY POINT

- Management of infection-related glomerulonephritis typically only consists of treatment of the underlying infection.

Bibliography

Nasr SH, Radhakrishnan J, D'Agati VD. Bacterial infection-related glomerulonephritis in adults. Kidney Int. 2013 May;83(5):792-803. [PMID: 23302723]

Item 13   Answer: D
Educational Objective: Treat a patient who has chronic kidney disease and hypertension.

The most appropriate management for this patient with hypertension and chronic kidney disease (CKD) is to continue the current medication regimen. Although hypertension is a common cause of CKD, hypertension is also highly prevalent in patients with CKD not caused by hypertension. The presence of hypertension in CKD promotes progression of underlying kidney disease and increases cardiovascular risk. Therefore, optimal management of hypertension is an important component of evaluating and treating all patients with CKD. For patients with CKD, the eighth report from the Joint National Committee (JNC 8) recommends a blood pressure target goal of <140/90 mm Hg using a medication regimen that includes an ACE inhibitor or angiotensin receptor blocker (ARB). In general, there is insufficient evidence to justify lower blood pressure goals unless patients have severely increased albuminuria, usually defined as >300 mg/g (stage A3), which is not present in this patient. His hypertension is currently at target goal, and he is taking an ACE inhibitor. Therefore, no changes to his medications are needed at this time.

The addition of the ARB losartan is inappropriate because the patient is already at goal blood pressure. Furthermore, studies have demonstrated that combination ACE inhibitor/ARB therapy worsens clinical outcomes and should not be used to treat patients with CKD.

Increasing this patient's lisinopril dose is unnecessary at this time because the patient is already at goal blood pressure.

Replacing lisinopril with amlodipine is not indicated because the JNC 8 guidelines recommend the use of an ACE inhibitor (such as lisinopril) or ARB as first-line therapy for hypertension in patients with CKD, and not dihydropyridine calcium channel blockers, which have a lower renoprotective effect. Additionally, this patient is at the recommended blood pressure goal.

KEY POINT

- For patients with chronic kidney disease, the eighth report from the Joint National Committee recommends a blood pressure target goal of <140/90 mm Hg using a medication regimen that includes an ACE inhibitor or angiotensin receptor blocker.

Bibliography

James PA, Oparil S, Carter BL, et al. 2014 evidence-based guideline for the management of high blood pressure in adults: report from the panel members appointed to the Eighth Joint National Committee (JNC 8). JAMA 2014 Feb 5;311(5):507-20. [PMID: 24352797]

Item 14   Answer: D
Educational Objective: Manage isolated hematuria.

Serial kidney function and urine protein determinations are appropriate for this young patient with asymptomatic microhematuria. The evaluation of asymptomatic hematuria is somewhat different in younger patients as compared with older patients. In the former, hematuria is likely from mild glomerular disease (such as IgA nephropathy and genetic disorders such as collagen mutations). In older patients, structural changes, stones, infection, and cancers predominate. This young patient presents with asymptomatic microhematuria and has a family history of hematuria (without kidney failure) on her mother's side. Serologic and imaging studies are normal, there are no structural abnormalities of the kidney (such as kidney stones), and infection is unlikely based on the urinalysis. She likely has a familial hematuric syndrome, which is typically associated with either X-linked or somatic mutations of type IV collagen. In female carriers of X-linked hereditary nephritis (Alport syndrome), kidney failure may occur later in life. Thus, annual measurements of blood pressure, kidney function, and urine protein are reasonable (although there are no consensus guidelines defining the frequency of testing).

Cystoscopy is usually performed in patients with hematuria who are older than 35 years of age or who have risk factors for lower urinary tract malignancy (such as smoking, aniline dye, or cyclophosphamide exposure). This patient is at low risk for urinary tract malignancy and therefore does not have an indication for cystoscopy or urine cytology. Similarly, an abdominal CT could identify a renal malignancy that might have been missed on kidney ultrasound, which is not indicated in this young patient.

A kidney biopsy is often performed in a patient with unexplained abnormalities on urinalysis (such as hematuria or proteinuria) in the presence of evidence of kidney failure in order to establish the diagnosis and guide therapy. However, this patient has normal kidney function and stable microhematuria without other clear risk factors for progressive kidney disease. Therefore, kidney biopsy is not currently indicated.

KEY POINT

- Patients with isolated hematuria with a family history of hematuria may require serial measurements of kidney function and urine protein because kidney failure may occur later in life.

Bibliography

Davis R, Jones JS, Barocas DA, et al; American Urological Association. J Urol. 2012 Dec;188(6 suppl):2473-81. Diagnosis, evaluation and follow-up of asymptomatic microhematuria (AMH) in adults: AUA guideline. [PMID: 23098784]

Item 15   Answer: A
Educational Objective: Treat a patient with hypertension based on ambulatory blood pressure monitoring.

Initiation of a low-dose ACE inhibitor with follow-up in 2 weeks is appropriate for this patient with hypertension. Lower thresholds for the definition of hypertension exist for measurements obtained in the ambulatory setting. In general, blood pressure averages ≥135/85 mm Hg by ambulatory blood pressure monitoring or home monitoring meet most consensus panels' definition of hypertension, and nighttime hypertension is defined by average values >125/75 mm Hg. This is to reflect the typical blood pressure drop from daytime to nighttime (during sleep) of approximately 15%, noted in both normotensive and hypertensive patients. A lack of blood pressure drop of at least 10% ("non-dipping") is independently associated with left ventricular hypertrophy, cardiovascular events, moderately increased albuminuria (formerly known as microalbuminuria), and a more rapid rate of decline in glomerular filtration rate. This patient has hypertension defined by ambulatory readings and is a non-dipper with nighttime hypertension; therefore, pharmacologic therapy is indicated.

Although it has been shown that melatonin release is diminished in non-dippers and in small studies melatonin can lower nighttime blood pressure, there are no large trials with cardiovascular end points to recommend this therapy.

Observation is appropriate in the setting of prehypertension or white coat hypertension; however, this patient has confirmed hypertension and requires pharmacologic therapy.

KEY POINT

- Blood pressure averages ≥135/85 mm Hg by ambulatory blood pressure monitoring or home monitoring meet most consensus panels' definition of hypertension and should be treated with pharmacologic therapy.

Bibliography

Mancia G, De Backer G, Dominiczak A, et al; Management of Arterial Hypertension of the European Society of Hypertension; European Society of Cardiology. 2007 Guidelines for the Management of Arterial Hypertension: The Task Force for the Management of Arterial Hypertension of the European Society of Hypertension (ESH) and of the European Society of Cardiology (ESC). Erratum in: J Hypertens. 2007 Aug;25(8):1749. J Hypertens. 2007 Jun;25(6):1105-87. [PMID: 17563527]

Item 16   Answer: D

Educational Objective: Manage uric acid nephrolithiasis with adequate urine output and urine alkalinization.

Urine alkalinization is the most appropriate treatment for this patient with uric acid nephrolithiasis not adequately treated with increased urine output. Uric acid is an uncommon cause of nephrolithiasis (approximately 10% of cases). It is more common in hot arid climates where low urine output and acidic urine (low urine pH) are more likely. These two factors, particularly low urine pH, markedly increase the risk of uric acid stones by favoring the development of insoluble uric acid from the relatively soluble urate salt. Elevated serum urate levels, gout, and associated hyperuricosuria are other risk factors, although many patients with uric acid stones do not have these risk factors. Other comorbid risk factors for uric acid stones include diabetes mellitus, the metabolic syndrome, and chronic diarrhea. Oral hydration to maintain a urine output of at least 2 L/d is the mainstay of therapy. If this is inadequate, the next treatment is urine alkalinization (usually with potassium citrate or potassium bicarbonate) to increase the solubility of uric acid.

Treatment with xanthine oxidase inhibitors such as allopurinol to lower uric acid production is usually reserved for patients with refractory disease despite adequate urine output and urine alkalinization or those with very high 24-hour urine uric acid levels (>1000 mg/24 h [5.9 mmol/24 h]). Therefore, allopurinol is not the next treatment of choice in this patient with mild uricosuria who has not undergone a trial of urine alkalinization.

Cholestyramine binds bile salts and oxalate in the gut and is sometimes used as a treatment for kidney stones related to hyperoxaluria but would likely not benefit this patient with uric acid stones.

Thiazide diuretics, such as hydrochlorothiazide, decrease hypercalciuria by increasing proximal sodium reabsorption and passive calcium reabsorption in the kidney. However, this is a strategy for treating calcium-based nephrolithiasis and is not effective for uric acid stones.

KEY POINT

- Management of uric acid nephrolithiasis includes adequate urine output, urine alkalinization, and xanthine oxidase inhibitors if needed to decrease uric acid production.

Bibliography

Wiederkehr MR, Moe OW. Uric acid nephrolithiasis: a systemic metabolic disorder. Clin Rev Bone Miner Metab. 2011 Dec;9(3-4):207-17. [PMID: 25045326]

Item 17   Answer: D

Educational Objective: Treat resistant hypertension by switching a thiazide diuretic to a loop diuretic in a patient with chronic kidney disease.

Switching hydrochlorothiazide to furosemide is the most appropriate next step in this patient. Uncontrolled hypertension in a patient who is already on three drugs, one of which is a diuretic, is defined as resistant hypertension. The approach to patients with resistant hypertension centers around lifestyle changes (particularly salt reduction and optimizing medication adherence) and choosing appropriate drug combinations. In patients with diabetic nephropathy and chronic kidney disease (CKD), ACE inhibitors or angiotensin receptor blockers should be used as an initial therapy given the established benefit of these agents in patients with diabetes mellitus and proteinuria. Most patients will require a second medication, and diuretic therapy is typically used in patients with CKD because persistent volume expansion contributes significantly to hypertension. Although thiazide diuretics are frequently used as initial therapy, they are generally less effective when the glomerular filtration rate drops below 30 mL/min/1.73 m². When this occurs, loop diuretics tend to be more effective and should be used instead of (or added to) thiazide diuretics. The dosage of loop diuretics depends on the sodium intake and the severity of CKD. Generally, furosemide doses of 40 to 80 mg once or twice daily is initiated with a salt-restricted diet and adjusted according to the response.

Adding a second inhibitor of the renin-angiotensin system such as aliskiren increases the risk of acute kidney injury and hyperkalemia without any benefit on renal and cardiovascular end points; therefore, combination therapy with renin-angiotensin inhibitors should not be used.

The centrally acting agent clonidine and the vasodilator minoxidil are potent antihypertensives sometimes used in cases of resistant hypertension if maximal doses of more conventional agents are unsuccessful. However, this patient is not currently on optimal triple therapy, and both agents also increase the risk of orthostatic hypotension in those with autonomic neuropathy, such as this patient. Moreover, the use of minoxidil without adequate diuresis will worsen salt and water retention and should be avoided.

KEY POINT

- In the setting of chronic kidney disease stage 4 and greater (glomerular filtration rate <30 mL/min/1.73 m²), thiazide diuretics lose potency, and loop diuretics may often be required.

Bibliography

Kidney Disease: Improving Global Outcomes (KDIGO) Blood Pressure Work Group. KDIGO clinical practice guideline for the management of blood pressure in chronic kidney disease. Kidney Int Suppl. 2012 2(1):337-414. Available at www.kdigo.org/clinical_practice_guidelines/pdf/KDIGO_BP_GL.pdf. Accessed February 25, 2015.

Item 18   Answer: D

Educational Objective: Recommend non-dialytic therapy for a very elderly patient who has end-stage kidney disease and a high burden of comorbid conditions and poor functional status.

The most appropriate next step in the management of this patient's end-stage kidney disease (ESKD) is to recommend non-dialytic therapy. Dialysis may be beneficial in prolonging life with a good quality in many older patients; therefore, age itself is not always an absolute limiting factor in deciding whether dialysis is appropriate for a specific older patient. However, studies have shown that very elderly patients with a high burden of comorbid conditions and poor functional status may live as long or longer with non-dialytic therapy that is focused on alleviating symptoms and maximizing quality of life. Moreover, most nursing facility residents have a progressive decline in functional status after starting dialysis. Therefore, in this very elderly resident with multiple comorbidities who lives in a nursing facility, pursuing non-dialytic therapy is the most appropriate recommendation. The option of non-dialytic care should not be seen as refusal to provide care or provision of a lower level of care than those receiving dialysis, but rather as an appropriate recommendation based on expected outcomes in these patients. Palliative medicine and hospice services can be helpful in managing patients who choose this mode of therapy.

In older patients who choose to pursue dialysis, there are few definitive data regarding outcomes with hemodialysis versus peritoneal methods, although hemodialysis is typically chosen more frequently by older adults. However, neither modality is appropriate in the patient given his advanced age and other clinical circumstances.

KEY POINT

- Very elderly patients who have end-stage kidney disease with a high burden of comorbid conditions and poor functional status may live as long or longer with non-dialytic therapy that is focused on alleviating symptoms and maximizing quality of life.

Bibliography

Kurella Tamura M, Covinsky KE, Chertow GM, Yaffe K, Landefeld CS, McCulloch CE. Functional status of elderly adults before and after initiation of dialysis. N Engl J Med 2009 Oct 15;361(16):1539-47. [PMID: 19828531]

Item 19   Answer: D

Educational Objective: Treat a patient with stage 2 hypertension using combination therapy.

Combination therapy with the ACE inhibitor lisinopril and the calcium channel blocker (CCB) amlodipine is appropriate for this patient with stage 2 hypertension, which is defined as a systolic blood pressure ≥160 mm Hg and/or a diastolic blood pressure ≥100 mm Hg. There is

general agreement among hypertension societies that a single agent is unlikely to control blood pressure in patients who are >20/10 mm Hg above target blood pressure. In this circumstance, initial therapy may include a combination of two agents either separately or in a fixed-dose pill. A combination of two agents at moderate doses is often more successful at achieving blood pressure goals than one blood pressure agent at maximal dose and minimizes the side effects that are more commonly noted at higher doses. Several combination regimens are appropriate, including the combination of a thiazide diuretic with an ACE inhibitor or angiotensin receptor blocker (ARB), or an ARB with a CCB; these combinations have been supported by both the eighth report from the Joint National Committee (JNC 8) and the European Society of Hypertension as reasonable approaches to management. However, there is evidence from the Avoiding Cardiovascular Events in Combination Therapy in Patients Living with Systolic Hypertension (ACCOMPLISH) trial that a reduced rate of cardiovascular events may occur with the combination of an ACE inhibitor and CCB compared to an ACE inhibitor and thiazide. The combination of a thiazide and CCB is also an effective strategy for blood pressure lowering, although there is less evidence of the effectiveness of this regimen compared with other combination therapies.

There is general consensus that the dual use of renin-angiotensin-aldosterone agents (ACE inhibitor, ARB, or the direct renin inhibitor aliskiren) should not be used because of evidence showing that combining these medications is not associated with improved cardiovascular or renal end points and results in increased adverse events, including hypotension and hyperkalemia.

Given this patient's degree of hypertension (measurement of 160/92 mm Hg at her current visit), it is unlikely that a single agent will achieve her treatment goal of <140/90 mm Hg. Therefore, combination therapy is indicated as initial treatment.

KEY POINT

- Combination antihypertensive therapy is appropriate for patients who are >20/10 mm Hg above their target blood pressure goal.

Bibliography

Jamerson K, Weber MA, Bakris GL, et al; ACCOMPLISH Trial Investigators. Benazepril plus amlodipine or hydrochlorothiazide for hypertension in high-risk patients. N Engl J Med. 2008 Dec 4;359(23):2417-28. [PMID: 19052124]

Item 20   Answer: A

Educational Objective: Diagnose white coat hypertension using ambulatory blood pressure monitoring.

Ambulatory blood pressure monitoring (ABPM) is appropriate to evaluate this patient for white coat hypertension. ABPM is accomplished with a device that typically measures blood pressure every 15 to 20 minutes during the day and every 30 to 60 minutes at night. White coat hypertension is defined as blood pressure readings in the office ≥140/90 mm Hg and out-of-office readings that average <135/85 mm Hg. Prevalence may be as high as 10% to 20% of patients diagnosed with hypertension. This patient's blood pressure measurements have been elevated in the office but normal at home and require further documentation with 24-hour ABPM. If she has normal blood pressure at home, her blood pressure would be classified as white coat hypertension, which does not pose an increased risk of cardiovascular events but does increase her risk of future development of hypertension. Conversely, hypertension documented by ABPM is associated with a higher risk of cardiovascular death compared with hypertension determined in the office or at home. A summary of interpretation of office-based, ABPM, and self-recorded blood pressure readings is **shown**.

Interpretation of Blood Pressure Readings			
Blood Pressure Category	**Office-Based Readings (mm Hg)**	**24-Hour Ambulatory Readings (mm Hg)**	**Self-Recorded (mm Hg)**
Hypertension (Nonelderly)	Systolic ≥140 or diastolic ≥90	≥135/85	≥135/85
White Coat Hypertension	≥140/90	<135/85	<135/85
Masked Hypertension	<140/90	>135/85	>135/85

Urine testing for fractionated metanephrines is used to evaluate for pheochromocytoma as a secondary cause of hypertension. Pheochromocytoma is generally suspected in patients with the symptom triad of episodic headache, sweating, and tachycardia associated with coincident increases in blood pressure. Similar symptoms may be seen with episodes of anxiety and panic attacks, which occur with increased frequency in patients with depression, as is present in this patient. However, these symptoms are not associated with significant blood pressure elevations when caused by anxiety or panic attacks. Documentation of consistent symptoms with accompanying blood pressure elevations would increase consideration of pheochromocytoma; however, testing for this diagnosis would not be indicated in the absence of this relationship, and further assessment for anxiety and panic attacks would be indicated.

Ambulatory electrocardiography or echocardiography would not be the appropriate next steps given the lack of other cardiovascular examination findings; palpitations are common and a nonspecific finding in possible hypertension.

Plasma aldosterone-plasma renin ratio would not be appropriate given this patient's normal laboratory findings and the lack of a firm diagnosis of hypertension.

KEY POINT

- Ambulatory blood pressure monitoring is useful to evaluate patients for white coat hypertension.

Bibliography
Pierdomenico SD, Cuccurullo F. Prognostic value of white-coat and masked hypertension diagnosed by ambulatory monitoring in initially untreated subjects: an updated meta analysis. Am J Hypertens. 2011 Jan;24(1):52-8. [PMID: 20847724]

Item 21   Answer: D   H

Educational Objective: Diagnose aminoglycoside-induced nephrotoxicity.

This patient has developed acute kidney injury (AKI) from gentamicin. Aminoglycoside-induced AKI typically presents as nonoliguric acute tubular necrosis (ATN) with granular casts in the urine sediment and a fractional excretion of sodium >1%. The serum creatinine characteristically rises 5 to 10 days after starting therapy. Hypokalemia and hypomagnesemia can also occur with aminoglycoside toxicity due to kidney potassium and magnesium wasting. Recognizing drug-induced ATN is important because eliminating the nephrotoxic agent often leads to renal recovery. Incidence increases in older patients and in patients with decreased effective blood volume, chronic kidney disease, or concomitant nephrotoxin exposure.

Cephalosporins, such as cefazolin, can cause AKI from acute interstitial nephritis. Urine findings include leukocytes, erythrocytes, and leukocyte casts. Fever, maculopapular rash, peripheral eosinophilia, and eosinophiluria can also occur. Onset of AKI after drug exposure ranges from 3 to 5 days with a second exposure, to as long as several weeks to months with a first exposure. This patient does not have any features of acute interstitial nephritis. Furthermore, cefazolin was discontinued prior to the elevation in serum creatinine.

Cholesterol embolism occurs in patients with atherosclerotic disease after undergoing an invasive vascular procedure or receiving an anticoagulant or thrombolytic agent within the past several months. Emboli from ruptured atheromatous plaques occlude small and medium arterioles, causing ischemia and inflammation with organ dysfunction. Clinical features include rash (livedo reticularis), AKI, purple discoloration of the toes, bowel ischemia, neurologic manifestations, and eosinophilia. This patient does not have findings of embolic phenomena.

Iodinated contrast can induce vasospasm and cause ischemic injury or direct damage to the kidneys. Low osmolar contrast is thought to be safer than high osmolar contrast. Contrast-induced nephropathy (CIN) is defined as either an increase in serum creatinine of 0.5 mg/dL (44.2 µmol/L) or an increase in serum creatinine of 25% from baseline at 48 hours after contrast administration. This patient had no change in the serum creatinine level at 48 hours, making CIN an unlikely diagnosis.

- Aminoglycoside-induced acute kidney injury typically presents as nonoliguric acute tubular necrosis with granular casts in the urine sediment and a fractional excretion of sodium >1%, and the serum creatinine characteristically rises 5 to 10 days after starting therapy.

Bibliography

Pannu N, Nadim MK. An overview of drug-induced acute kidney injury. Crit Care Med. 2008 Apr;36(4 suppl):S216-23. [PMID: 18382197]

Item 22   Answer: D

Educational Objective: Monitor complications of immunosuppressive medications used in kidney transplantation.

New-onset diabetes mellitus and dyslipidemia should be monitored in this patient. Although kidney transplant recipients have improved clinical outcomes compared with patients who remain on dialysis, they require lifelong immunosuppression to prevent rejection of the transplanted kidney. In addition to increasing the risk of hypertension, infection, and certain malignancies, these medications can predispose patients to metabolic complications that should be anticipated by clinicians. Kidney transplant recipients are predisposed to new onset diabetes after transplantation (often referred to as NODAT). Medications that promote development of NODAT include glucocorticoids, tacrolimus, and the mammalian target of rapamycin (mTOR) inhibitors sirolimus and everolimus. Dyslipidemia is also a common complication posttransplantation, and commonly used immunosuppressive medications that promote dyslipidemia include cyclosporine and mTOR inhibitors. Because cardiovascular disease is the leading cause of death among kidney transplant recipients, it is important to aggressively treat modifiable cardiac risk factors, including diabetes and dyslipidemia. It is important to emphasize that many medications, including some statins, can significantly alter the pharmacokinetics of immunosuppressant medications. Clinicians should therefore never change medication regimens in kidney transplant recipients without ensuring that there will be no adverse drug interactions.

Although hypophosphatemia is commonly observed in the posttransplant period, which is due in part to residual secondary hyperparathyroidism, hyperphosphatemia is not commonly observed unless there is severely impaired allograft function.

Hyperthyroidism is not a common complication of kidney transplantation or of immunosuppressive medications typically used in kidney transplant recipients.

Many patients have residual hyperparathyroidism after transplant that can be slow to resolve; hypercalcemia is relatively commonly observed posttransplant but hypocalcemia is uncommon. Therefore, hypoparathyroidism is unlikely in this patient.

- Kidney transplant recipients require lifelong immunosuppression and must be monitored for metabolic complications such as diabetes mellitus and dyslipidemia.

Bibliography

Kidney Disease: Improving Global Outcomes (KDIGO) Transplant Work Group. KDIGO clinical practice guideline for the care of kidney transplant recipients. Am J Transplant. 2009 Nov;9 (suppl 3):S1-S155. [PMID: 19845597]

Item 23   Answer: A

Educational Objective: Recommend mechanical stone removal for a patient with a large (>10 mm) kidney stone.

Mechanical removal is the most appropriate management of this patient's 12-mm kidney stone located in the right renal pelvis. Large (>10 mm) stones are less likely than smaller stones to pass on their own, with or without use of medications to facilitate stone passage. Mechanical stone removal in the renal pelvis is often achieved with shock wave lithotripsy. Stones in the ureter may be addressed with either shock wave lithotripsy or ureteroscopy (often with ureteroscopic lithotripsy), usually depending on the specific location and size of the stone. Percutaneous antegrade ureteroscopy or retroperitoneal laparoscopy is generally reserved for impacted stones or other situations in which less invasive techniques would likely not be successful. Currently, open stone removal is rarely performed. Other indications for mechanical stone removal include stones <10 mm in size that have failed to pass with medical therapy. Involvement of a urologist is recommended for patients with nephrolithiasis who have urosepsis, acute kidney injury, anuria, or refractory pain, as well as those who are at high risk of complications such as having a single kidney, because more invasive interventions may be required in these situations.

Uncomplicated kidney stones <10 mm in size may usually be treated with conservative management (including hydration, analgesia, observation, and periodic re-evaluation) and medical expulsive therapy, which usually consists of either an α-blocker (such as tamsulosin) or calcium channel blocker (such as nifedipine). Although some clinicians may also treat with glucocorticoids in addition to medical expulsive therapy to decrease inflammation and swelling to facilitate stone passage, the effectiveness of this approach has not been documented.

- Mechanical stone removal is appropriate for patients with large (>10 mm) kidney stones or those with smaller stones who have failed medical management or have complicated nephrolithiasis (urosepsis, acute kidney injury, anuria, refractory pain).

Bibliography

Brener ZZ, Winchester JF, Salman H, Bergman M. Nephrolithiasis: evaluation and management. South Med J. 2011 Feb;104(2):133-9. [PMID: 21258231]

Item 24   Answer: C

Educational Objective: Diagnose IgG4-related interstitial nephritis.

The most likely diagnosis is IgG4-related interstitial nephritis. This patient has a history of autoimmune pancreatitis and now presents with acute kidney injury. Her urinalysis is most consistent with a tubulointerstitial pattern, with mild proteinuria and the presence of inflammatory cells. This history and clinical presentation suggest the possibility of IgG4-related interstitial nephritis. Systemic IgG4-related disease is an uncommon disorder characterized by infiltration of different organs by lymphoplasmacytic infiltrates of IgG4-positive plasma cells with resultant fibrosis associated with elevated serum IgG4 levels. Autoimmune pancreatitis is one form of IgG-related disease, although other organs such as the kidney may be affected, most commonly as interstitial nephritis. IgG4-related interstitial nephritis may present with acute or chronic kidney failure as well as renal mass–like lesions on imaging. As with other IgG4-related diseases, almost all patients with IgG4-related kidney disease will have elevated serum IgG4 levels, and the kidneys may be diffusely enlarged on imaging due to cellular infiltration. Definitive diagnosis requires kidney biopsy with staining for IgG4-positive plasma cells. Treatment is similar to other IgG4-related diseases using immunosuppression with glucocorticoids.

ANCA-associated vasculitis and anti–glomerular basement membrane antibody disease typically cause rapidly progressive glomerulonephritis with significant proteinuria and hematuria in the sediment, occasionally with erythrocyte casts, none of which is present in this patient.

Lupus nephritis is primarily a glomerular lesion with significant proteinuria in the context of other clinical findings suggestive of systemic lupus erythematosus. This patient's clinical presentation is therefore less consistent with this diagnosis.

KEY POINT

- IgG4-related disease is characterized by infiltration of different organs by lymphoplasmacytic infiltrates of IgG4-positive plasma cells with resultant fibrosis associated with elevated serum IgG4 levels.

Bibliography

Saeki T, Kawano M. IgG4-related kidney disease. [erratum in: Kidney Int. 2014 Jun;85(6):1472.] Kidney Int. 2014 Feb;85(2):251-7. [PMID: 24107849]

Item 25   Answer: D

Educational Objective: Diagnose diuretic-related metabolic alkalosis.

Urine diuretic screening is appropriate for this patient. The first step when assessing a patient with metabolic alkalosis is to clinically assess the patient's volume status. This patient has metabolic alkalosis as implied by the elevated serum bicarbonate and is hypovolemic as evidenced by the orthostatic blood pressure and pulse changes. Such a patient would be expected to have low urine concentrations of sodium and chloride. However, this patient's urine electrolytes show increased excretion of sodium and chloride despite the evident hypovolemia. These findings suggest the presence of active diuretic use or a renal tubular defect that impairs handling of sodium and chloride, such as Bartter and Gitelman syndromes. These rare autosomal recessive genetic disorders of renal sodium and chloride transporters clinically mimic loop diuretic and thiazide diuretic use, respectively, but should be considered only after diuretic use has been eliminated with negative urine diuretic screening.

Measurement of 24-hour urine free cortisol excretion is a standard test for diagnosing Cushing syndrome, which is characterized by proximal muscle weakness, hypokalemia, hypertension, and diabetes mellitus. These findings are not present in this patient.

Plasma aldosterone-plasma renin ratio is unlikely to be helpful in this situation. Although primary hyperaldosteronism is characterized by hypokalemia and metabolic alkalosis, the absence of hypertension makes this diagnosis unlikely. Finally, diuretics and Gitelman and Bartter syndromes are associated with various degrees of volume contraction and secondary hyperaldosteronism. Plasma aldosterone and renin activity levels will not differentiate these disorders.

Thyroid dysfunction is not associated with acid-base abnormalities and may be associated with hypokalemia only in rare and severe cases such as thyrotoxic periodic paralysis, in which attacks of profound generalized weakness occur suddenly with preserved consciousness.

KEY POINT

- Diuretic use can mimic the metabolic alkalosis findings of inherited kidney disorders of sodium and chloride handling such as Bartter and Gitelman syndromes.

Bibliography

Medford-Davis L, Rafique Z. Derangements of potassium. Emerg Med Clin North Am. 2014 May;32(2):329-47. [PMID: 24766936]

Item 26   Answer: A

Educational Objective: Identify decreased muscle mass as a cause of decreased serum creatinine.

Decreased muscle mass is the most likely cause of this patient's decreased serum creatinine level. She has likely lost significant muscle mass as a consequence of stroke with paralysis, causing immobility and inability to maintain oral protein intake. She has severe protein-calorie malnutrition, as is evidenced by a low BMI and a severely depressed serum albumin level. Because creatinine is derived from the metabolism of creatine, a constituent of skeletal muscle, any condition that results in decreased muscle mass would be expected to cause long-term decreases in the serum creatinine level in the absence of any change in kidney function.

Acute, but transient, decreases in creatinine have also been documented in some patients with chronic kidney disease and diabetes mellitus following ischemic stroke.

Diabetic kidney disease is chronically progressive, with rapidity of kidney function decline dependent on type 1 or 2 status, blood pressure and glycemic control, and reduction in proteinuria through use of renin-angiotensin system blockade. There is no known means of reversing diabetic kidney disease, and spontaneous improvement is unlikely.

Chlorthalidone, a thiazide diuretic, likely decreases blood pressure primarily by its effect on endothelial cells but can also result in volume contraction and mild hypovolemia, which generally results in increased, not decreased, serum creatinine.

Lisinopril, an ACE inhibitor, decreases the production of angiotensin II, resulting in decreased arterial blood pressure (systemic effect) and efferent arteriolar dilation (local effect). Both of these processes decrease pressure across the glomerular vascular bed, and thus the glomerular filtration rate. Consequently, serum creatinine is expected to increase by 25% to 30% with appropriate dosing of an ACE inhibitor.

KEY POINT

- Any condition that results in decreased muscle mass would be expected to cause long-term decreases in the serum creatinine level in the absence of any change in kidney function.

Bibliography

Haider DG, Ferrari J, Mittermayer F, et al. A transient improvement in renal function occurs after ischemic stroke. Ren Fail. 2012;34(1):7-12. [PMID: 22023107]

Item 27   Answer: B

Educational Objective: Provide appropriate pneumococcal vaccinations for a patient with chronic kidney disease.

This patient should receive the pneumococcal conjugate vaccine in 6 months. Because infection is a leading cause of death in patients with chronic kidney disease (CKD) and end-stage kidney disease, proper vaccination to prevent infections should improve patient outcomes. The Advisory Committee on Immunization Practices (ACIP) recommends pneumococcal vaccination for all patients with severe CKD. This patient with stage G4/A3 CKD should receive the 13-valent pneumococcal conjugate vaccine (PCV-13) 1 or more years after the 23-valent pneumococcal polysaccharide vaccine (PPSV-23). A second dose of PPSV-23 should be administered 5 or more years after the first dose. Because this patient was immunized with PPSV-23 6 months ago, he should receive PVC-13 in 6 months and PPSV-23 in 4 years and 6 months.

Other immunocompromising conditions that are indications for pneumococcal vaccination are anatomic and functional asplenia, congenital or acquired immunodefi-

ciency (including B- or T-lymphocyte deficiency, complement deficiencies, and phagocytic disorders excluding chronic granulomatous disease), HIV infection, the nephrotic syndrome, leukemia, lymphoma, Hodgkin lymphoma, generalized malignancy, multiple myeloma, solid-organ transplant, and iatrogenic immunosuppression (including long-term systemic glucocorticoids and radiation therapy).

For patients younger than 65 years of age with CKD who have not been previously immunized against invasive pneumococcal disease, the ACIP recommends that PCV-13 be administered first followed by PPSV-23 no sooner than 8 weeks later.

KEY POINT

- The Advisory Committee on Immunization Practices recommends pneumococcal vaccination with both the 13-valent pneumococcal conjugate and 23-valent pneumococcal polysaccharide vaccines for all patients with severe chronic kidney disease.

Bibliography

Kim DK, Bridges CB, Harriman KH; Advisory Committee on Immunization Practices. Advisory committee on immunization practices recommended immunization schedule for adults aged 19 years or older: United States, 2015. Ann Intern Med. 2015 Feb 3;162(3):214-23. doi:10.7326/M14-2755

Item 28   Answer: C

Educational Objective: Identify laxative abuse as a cause of metabolic acidosis.

Laxative abuse is the most likely cause of this patient's acid-base and electrolyte abnormalities. She has a normal anion gap metabolic acidosis in the setting of physical examination findings consistent with low/normal extracellular fluid status and low/normal blood pressure. The etiology of a normal anion gap metabolic acidosis is typically due to either the inability of the kidney to excrete acid (renal tubular acidosis) or loss of bicarbonate, usually through the gastrointestinal tract. Differentiating the cause of a normal anion gap metabolic acidosis may be accomplished by measurement of the urine anion gap, which is calculated as follows: $(U_{Na} + U_K - U_{Cl})$. The urine anion gap is a surrogate method of estimating the ability of the kidney to excrete an acid load. The normal physiologic response to systemic acidosis is an increase in urine acid excretion resulting in an increase in urine ammonium, which is difficult to measure clinically. However, because ammonium carries a positive charge, chloride is excreted into the urine in equal amounts with ammonium to maintain electrical neutrality. Therefore, the amount of chloride in the urine reflects the amount of ammonium present, with a positive urine anion gap suggesting a kidney source of acid loss, and a negative urine anion gap is consistent with gastrointestinal bicarbonate loss. The negative urine anion gap in this patient (-6 mEq/L [6 mmol/L]) indicates a gastrointestinal cause of her normal anion gap metabolic acidosis, and laxative abuse is a likely explanation. In addition, hypokalemia combined with low urine potassium

Answers and Critiques

indicates appropriate renal compensation to attempt to retain filtered potassium.

The vomiting associated with bulimia nervosa leads to loss of gastric acid with a resulting metabolic alkalosis, not metabolic acidosis.

Active diuretic use leads to kidney potassium wasting and a metabolic alkalosis, as does Gitelman syndrome, a defect that mimics the clinical picture of thiazide diuretic use.

Renal causes of normal anion gap metabolic acidosis are due to specific defects in renal handling of bicarbonate reclamation or in hydrogen ion secretion. Type 1 (hypokalemic distal) renal tubular acidosis is caused by a defect in hydrogen secretion by the distal tubule and is associated with a positive urine anion gap, a high urine potassium secretion, and hypokalemia.

KEY POINT

- Normal anion gap metabolic acidosis can be caused by gastrointestinal bicarbonate loss induced by laxative abuse.

Bibliography

Roerig JL, Steffen KJ, Mitchell JE, Zunker C. Laxative abuse: epidemiology, diagnosis and management. Drugs. 2010 Aug 20;70(12):1487-503. [PMID: 20687617]

Item 29   Answer: D

Educational Objective: Evaluate for malignancy in a kidney transplant recipient.

In addition to age- and sex-appropriate screening, this kidney transplant recipient should be evaluated for skin cancer. Patients who receive kidney transplants are at increased risk of malignancy compared with the general population, and this risk is attributable, at least in part, to the effects of immunosuppressive medications. Kidney transplant patients are at particularly high risk for squamous cell carcinomas (SCC) of the skin and posttransplant lymphoproliferative disease. Unlike in the general population, SCC is more common than basal cell carcinoma and accounts for approximately 90% of skin cancers in organ recipients. Some studies have shown that transplant recipients have more than a 200-fold increased risk of SCC compared with the general population. Moreover, SCC occurring in a transplant recipient is much more likely to metastasize than in non-transplant patients. Transplant recipients, particularly those with fair skin, should therefore be closely monitored for the development of precancerous or cancerous lesions and promptly treated.

Although kidney transplant recipients are at moderately increased risk for colon and lung cancer, insufficient data support more aggressive screening for these cancers than in the general population. Similarly, male kidney transplant recipients are not at increased of prostate cancer, so risk versus harm of screening should be approached as for the general population.

KEY POINT

- Kidney transplant patients are at particularly high risk for squamous cell carcinomas of the skin and posttransplant lymphoproliferative disease and should be evaluated for these diseases, in addition to age- and sex-appropriate screening.

Bibliography

Engels EA, Pfeiffer RM, Fraumeni JF Jr, et al. Spectrum of cancer risk among US solid organ transplant recipients. JAMA. 2011 Nov 2;306(17):1891-901. [PMID: 22045767]

Item 30   Answer: A

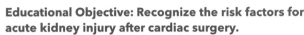

Educational Objective: Recognize the risk factors for acute kidney injury after cardiac surgery.

This patient's baseline estimated glomerular filtration rate (eGFR) is considered the strongest predictor of the development of acute kidney injury (AKI) in the perioperative period. An elevated preoperative serum creatinine level and the presence of chronic kidney disease (CKD) are the strongest nonmodifiable predictors of the development of AKI after cardiac surgery. This patient has severe kidney disease with an elevated baseline serum creatinine level of 2.3 mg/dL (203.3 μmol/L), with an eGFR of 25 mL/min/1.73 m² and stage 4 CKD. Other nonmodifiable risk factors for post–cardiac surgery AKI include advanced age, female gender, reduced left ventricular function or the presence of heart failure, insulin-dependent diabetes mellitus, peripheral vascular disease, and COPD.

Some observational studies have shown a BMI >30 to be a predictor of AKI post–cardiac surgery. However, the strength of the data is weak, and this patient has a BMI of 25.

Hypertension has not been shown to be a strong predictor for the development of AKI post–cardiac surgery.

Lisinopril and simvastatin have not been established as medications that increase the risk of AKI post–cardiac surgery. In fact, some observational studies indicate that they may have renoprotective properties and should be continued in the perioperative setting.

KEY POINT

- Preexisting chronic kidney disease is the strongest nonmodifiable predictor of the development of acute kidney injury after cardiac surgery.

Bibliography

Thakar CV. Perioperative acute kidney injury. Adv Chronic Kidney Dis. 2013 Jan;20(1):67-75. [PMID: 23265598]

Item 31   Answer: B

Educational Objective: Diagnose oncogenic osteomalacia.

This patient's findings of bone pain and hypophosphatemia with kidney phosphate wasting in the setting of inappropriately low serum concentration of 1,25-dihydroxy vitamin D, normal 25-hydroxy vitamin D concentration, and elevated alkaline phosphatase are consistent with oncogenic osteomalacia. The swelling of the finger is consistent with a mesenchymal tumor. Oncogenic osteomalacia is typically caused by benign mesenchymal tumors of vascular or skeletal origin. Overexpression of fibroblast growth factor–23 by these tumors is associated with decreased resorption of phosphate in the renal tubules with resultant hypophosphatemia and hyperphosphaturia. The tubular defect also impairs calcitriol synthesis. Chronic hypophosphatemia causes abnormal mineralization of bone, increased alkaline phosphatase, and, in the longer term, osteomalacia and associated fractures. Removal of the tumor leads to reversal of the biochemical abnormalities and healing of the bone disease.

Nutritional vitamin D deficiency results in low serum calcium levels and low 25-hydroxy vitamin D concentration, and it does not cause kidney phosphate wasting as seen in this patient.

Primary hyperparathyroidism is defined by an elevated parathyroid hormone level, elevated serum calcium level, and increased 1,25-dihydroxy vitamin D, all of which are absent in this patient.

X-Linked hypophosphatemic rickets can present with the same biochemical markers as noted in this case. However, it usually presents with typical signs of rickets in young children, and clinical expression of this condition in adulthood would not be expected.

KEY POINT

- Oncogenic osteomalacia is characterized by bone pain and hypophosphatemia with kidney phosphate wasting in the setting of low 1,25-dihydroxy vitamin D and normal 25-hydroxy vitamin D concentrations.

Bibliography

Imel EA, Econs MJ. Approach to the hypophosphatemic patient. J Clin Endocrinol Metab. 2012 Mar;97(3):696-706. [PMID: 22392950]

Item 32   Answer: A

Educational Objective: Treat acute kidney injury with continuous renal replacement therapy.

Continuous renal replacement therapy (CRRT) is the most appropriate treatment for this patient who has hemodynamic instability and oliguric acute kidney injury (AKI) with laboratory and urinary findings consistent with acute tubular necrosis (ATN). CRRT is indicated for treatment of electrolyte abnormalities (hyperkalemia, hyperphosphatemia), metabolic acidosis, and volume overload as seen in this patient. CRRT represents a spectrum of dialysis modalities specifically developed for the management of critically ill patients with AKI who cannot tolerate traditional intermittent hemodialysis due to hemodynamic instability, or in whom intermittent hemodialysis cannot control volume or metabolic derangement. CRRT is performed continuously (24 hours/day) through a venovenous access. Venous access is obtained by placing a large double-lumen catheter into either the internal jugular, femoral, or subclavian vein, as would be done for hemodialysis. There are several variations of CRRT that may involve diffusion-based solute removal (dialysis) or convection-based solute and water removal (filtration).

The major advantage of CRRT over intermittent hemodialysis is its slower rate of solute and fluid removal per unit of time, resulting in better hemodynamic tolerance. Therefore, CRRT is the preferred method of renal replacement therapy for critically ill unstable patients such as the patient in this case. Furthermore, the continuous nature of the therapy allows for better control of volume, acid-base, electrolytes, and azotemia.

Slow continuous ultrafiltration is a type of extracorporeal therapy by which plasma water is removed continuously. Although this therapy will help with fluid overload, it will not correct the azotemia or electrolyte and acid-base abnormalities in this patient.

Starting a furosemide infusion in this patient will not correct the electrolyte or acid-base abnormalities. Furthermore, in the setting of ATN with oliguria, furosemide is unlikely to be effective in volume removal.

KEY POINT

- Continuous renal replacement therapy is preferred for critically ill, unstable patients with acute kidney injury because it provides a slower rate of solute and fluid removal per unit of time, resulting in better hemodynamic tolerance.

Bibliography

Tolwani A. Continuous renal replacement therapy for AKI. N Engl J Med. 2012 Dec 27;367(26):2505-14. [PMID: 23268665]

Item 33   Answer: A

Educational Objective: Diagnose anti–glomerular basement membrane antibody disease.

The most likely diagnosis is anti–glomerular basement membrane (GBM) antibody disease. This 50-year-old patient has pulmonary-renal syndrome, including hemoptysis followed by hypoxic respiratory failure and kidney failure with an active urine sediment with protein, erythrocytes, and leukocytes, suggesting an underlying glomerulonephritis. The differential diagnosis of pulmonary-renal syndrome includes small-vessel vasculitis (ANCA associated), anti-GBM antibody disease (Goodpasture syndrome), and rarely, other autoimmune diseases such as cryoglobulinemic vasculitis, systemic lupus erythematosus, and IgA vasculitis. Anti-GBM antibody disease is an autoimmune disease caused by antibodies directed against the noncollagenous domain of type IV collagen that bind to the GBM, inciting an inflammatory response resulting in damage to the GBM and the formation of a proliferative

CONT.

and often crescentic glomerulonephritis. The same process occurs with the basement membrane of pulmonary capillaries, leading to pulmonary hemorrhage. Serologies show normal complement levels and elevated levels of anti-GBM antibodies in the serum. On kidney biopsy, there is a proliferative glomerulonephritis, often with many crescents (shown, left panel). There is linear deposition of immunoglobulin along the GBM by immunofluorescence, but no electron-dense deposits on electron microscopy (shown, right panel). Treatment is immunosuppressive therapy with cyclophosphamide and glucocorticoids, combined with daily plasmapheresis to remove circulating anti-GBM antibodies.

Although heart failure can be associated with pulmonary edema and hemoptysis with acute kidney injury (cardiorenal syndrome), such patients typically show signs of severe volume overload and normal urine sediment, unlike this patient.

Membranous nephropathy is associated with the nephrotic syndrome with a low serum albumin level, which is not seen in this patient. The nephrotic syndrome alone is not typically associated with pulmonary disease, although it can be complicated with venous thromboembolic manifestations such as pulmonary embolism. However, this patient's pulmonary presentation with significant hemoptysis and infiltrates on chest radiograph is not consistent with pulmonary emboli as the cause of his respiratory failure.

Microscopic polyangiitis is the most common cause of pulmonary-renal syndrome. However, in the absence of a serum ANCA level or evidence of peripheral vasculitic lesions (for example, palpable purpura), it is not possible to clinically differentiate this disease from anti-GBM antibody disease. A kidney biopsy is diagnostic, showing little or no immune deposits in microscopic polyangiitis ("pauci-immune glomerulonephritis"). In this patient, extensive linear deposition of IgG along the GBM is noted, which is classic of anti-GBM antibody disease.

Bibliography

Hellmark T, Segelmark M. Diagnosis and classification of Goodpasture's disease (anti-GBM). J Autoimmun. 2014 Feb-Mar;48-49:108-12. [PMID: 24456936]

Item 34   Answer: D

Educational Objective: Manage elevated serum creatinine due to trimethoprim.

Continuing this patient's current antibiotic therapy is the most appropriate management. Creatinine is normally filtered by the kidney from the serum, although a smaller amount is also secreted by the proximal tubule. In patients with more advanced chronic kidney disease (CKD), such as this patient, up to 50% of urine creatinine may be secreted instead of being filtered through the glomerulus. Trimethoprim is known to interfere with creatinine secretion without affecting the glomerular filtration rate (GFR) and can cause increases in serum creatinine of up to 0.5 mg/dL (44.2 µmol/L); this rise in serum creatinine therefore does not reflect a drop in actual kidney function. This effect is reversible upon discontinuation of the medication. Trimethoprim also inhibits the epithelial sodium channel in the collecting tubule, effectively acting as a potassium-sparing diuretic and potentially increasing the serum potassium level. The risk of hyperkalemia is therefore increased when using trimethoprim-containing antibiotics, particularly in patients who are on high-dose trimethoprim, who have underlying CKD that may predispose to hyperkalemia, or who are taking a medication with a potassium-sparing effect (such as an ACE inhibitor or angiotensin receptor blocker). Because of this, trimethoprim should be used with caution

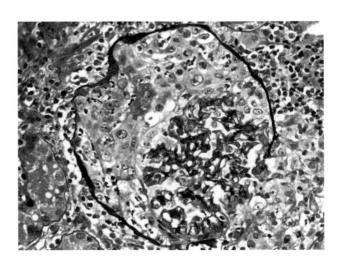

ITEM 33

and with close monitoring in patients with any of these underlying risk factors who require its use for treating infection. This patient's potassium level is within the normal range, and continued close monitoring during her antibiotic therapy is indicated.

Rifampin may cause red or orange discoloration of the urine but is not associated with a decreased GFR, an increase in serum creatinine, or hyperkalemia.

Urine eosinophil testing by means of special stains has been used classically to diagnose acute interstitial nephritis, which is a diagnostic consideration in a patient taking sulfa drugs. However, testing for urine eosinophils is neither sensitive nor specific for this diagnosis, which recent literature suggests may only be definitively made on the basis of kidney biopsy.

KEY POINT

- Trimethoprim is known to interfere with creatinine secretion without affecting the glomerular filtration rate and can cause increases in serum creatinine of up to 0.5 mg/dL (44.2 µmol/L); this rise therefore does not reflect a drop in actual kidney function.

Bibliography

Gentry CA, Nguyen AT. An evaluation of hyperkalemia and serum creatinine elevation associated with different dosage levels of outpatient trimethoprim-sulfamethoxazole with and without concomitant medications. Ann Pharmacother. 2013 Dec;47(12):1618-26. [PMID: 24259630]

Item 35   Answer: C

Educational Objective: Evaluate a patient with suspected nephrolithiasis using noncontrast helical abdominal CT.

Noncontrast helical abdominal CT is the most appropriate diagnostic test to perform next in this patient with a clinical presentation consistent with nephrolithiasis. The findings of unilateral pain combined with hematuria without inflammation on urinalysis suggest nephrolithiasis, and the location of the pain in the inguinal region suggests that the stone may be in the distal ureter. Ultrasonography is increasingly used as an initial study for evaluation of suspected nephrolithiasis because of increased availability, lack of radiation exposure, and lower cost than CT; it is also the study of choice in pregnant patients. However, ultrasonography is less sensitive than CT for detecting kidney stones in the distal ureter or for evaluating other potential nonurologic conditions that may be responsible for the pain. Given this patient's clinical picture that is consistent with nephrolithiasis but with a negative ultrasound for kidney stones, further imaging with noncontrast helical abdominal CT is indicated. Additionally, the absence of hydronephrosis on ultrasound does not rule out nephrolithiasis.

Although renal vein thrombosis can cause hematuria, this diagnosis is less likely given the location of this patient's pain, normal kidney function, and lack of proteinuria. Therefore, Doppler ultrasonography of the renal veins is inappropriate.

Kidney biopsy may be appropriate for patients with suspected glomerulonephritis. Glomerulonephritis typically presents with evidence of decreased kidney function with inflammation and glomerular damage seen as variable proteinuria, hematuria, and possibly dysmorphic erythrocytes and erythrocyte casts on urinalysis. However, this patient's clinical history and laboratory findings are not consistent with glomerulonephritis, and kidney biopsy is not indicated.

Urine cultures are appropriate to diagnose a urinary tract infection or pyelonephritis. However, a urinary tract infection is unlikely in this patient given the absence of dysuria and a urinalysis negative for significant leukocytes, leukocyte esterase, or nitrites.

KEY POINT

- Ultrasonography and noncontrast helical CT of the abdomen are testing options for evaluation of suspected nephrolithiasis; CT is indicated if initial ultrasound testing is negative in a patient with a high clinical suspicion for kidney stones.

Bibliography

Fulgham PF, Assimos DG, Pearle MS, Preminger GM. Clinical effectiveness protocols for imaging in the management of ureteral calculous disease: AUA technology assessment. J Urol. 2013 Apr;189(4):1203-13. [PMID: 23085059]

Item 36   Answer: D

Educational Objective: Diagnose prerenal acute kidney injury in a patient taking diuretics.

The most likely diagnosis is prerenal acute kidney injury (AKI). AKI occurs most commonly in the setting of true volume depletion or decreased effective blood volume as seen in this patient with decreased cardiac output. In patients with AKI and oliguria, the fractional excretion of sodium (FE_{Na}) may be helpful in differentiating between prerenal AKI and AKI from renal tubular cell damage or acute tubular necrosis (ATN). The FE_{Na} measures the percent of filtered sodium excreted in the urine and is calculated as $(U_{Sodium} \times P_{Cr})/(U_{Cr} \times P_{Sodium}) \times 100$. It is considered a more accurate measurement of kidney sodium avidity in prerenal states than the urine sodium concentration because these individuals are both sodium and water avid, which may cause an elevated urine sodium concentration despite kidney sodium retention. However, the FE_{Na} is less reliable when diuretics are being used because the urine sodium may not accurately reflect attempts by the kidney to retain sodium. Because urea is less sensitive to the effects of diuretics, the fractional excretion of urea (FE_{Urea}) may be more useful in this setting. The FE_{Urea} is calculated as $(U_{Urea} \times P_{Cr})/(U_{Cr} \times P_{Urea}) \times 100$, with values <35% suggesting a prerenal state. In this patient, the FE_{Na} is higher than expected in a prerenal state at 1.9%, but the FE_{Urea} is only 8.8%, suggesting an underlying prerenal state.

The urine sediment of a patient with acute interstitial nephritis will typically reflect inflammation with leukocytes, erythrocytes, or leukocyte casts, none of which is seen in this patient's urine sediment.

The urine sediment in patients with ATN will usually show evidence of tubular damage with sloughed tubular epithelial cells or coarse granular casts. These are not present in this patient, making ATN less likely.

Although this patient has a history of benign prostatic hyperplasia, postrenal obstruction is unlikely due to the presence of an indwelling urinary catheter.

KEY POINT

- Because urea is less sensitive to the effects of diuretics, the fractional excretion of urea may be more useful in this setting to identify the cause of acute kidney injury.

Bibliography

Gotfried J, Wiesen J, Raina R, Nally JV Jr. Finding the cause of acute kidney injury: which index of fractional excretion is better? Cleve Clin J Med. 2012 Feb;79(2):121-6. [PMID: 22301562]

Item 37   Answer: B

Educational Objective: Treat lupus nephritis with combination immunosuppressive therapy.

Increasing prednisone and adding mycophenolate mofetil are indicated for this patient with class IV lupus nephritis (LN). LN occurs in up to 70% of patients with systemic lupus erythematosus (SLE), with the presence of anti–double-stranded DNA antibodies being a marker for risk. All patients with SLE should be evaluated for possible nephritis at the time of diagnosis, with individualized surveillance based on the presence and degree of kidney abnormalities on laboratory studies. Patients who develop LN typically present with extrarenal symptoms of SLE at the time of diagnosis of LN. Glomerular disorders associated with SLE are classified into six different patterns based upon kidney biopsy histopathology, although there may be some overlap between classes in an individual patient, and some patients may evolve from one class to another. Patients with class I or II LN may have minimal or no kidney findings, and those with classes III and IV present with varying degrees of the nephritic syndrome. Patients with class V LN present predominantly with proteinuria. Class VI is the end stage of long-standing LN. This patient is experiencing a major lupus flare with arthritis, rash, fevers, and class IV LN on kidney biopsy. Class IV LN represents diffuse glomerular involvement and is the most common and severe form of nephritis associated with lupus. It is also associated with elevated anti–double stranded DNA antibody levels and hypocomplementemia, particularly during periods of active disease. Most patients with class III and all patients with class IV LN benefit from aggressive combination immunosuppressive therapy. The optimal initial therapy is to increase glucocorticoid doses (typically an intravenous pulse followed by a tapering oral dose), which is accompanied by either intravenous cyclophosphamide or mycophenolate mofetil.

The use of glucocorticoids alone has been associated with an inferior outcome compared with alkylating agents or antimetabolites in combination with glucocorticoids for patients with LN requiring treatment.

The addition of plasmapheresis to immunosuppressive therapy has not been shown to improve outcomes in patients with LN.

The patient has a high probability of worsening kidney function if not aggressively treated in view of the class IV LN, and any delay engenders the risk of irreversible kidney failure.

KEY POINT

- Most patients with class III lupus nephritis and all patients with class IV lupus nephritis benefit from aggressive combination immunosuppressive therapy.

Bibliography

Bertsias GK, Tektonidou M, Amoura Z, et al. Joint European League Against Rheumatism and European Renal Association-European Dialysis and Transplant Association (EULAR/ERA-EDTA) recommendations for the management of adult and pediatric lupus nephritis. Ann Rheum Dis. 2012 Nov;71(11):1771-82. [PMID: 22851469]

Item 38   Answer: D

Educational Objective: Manage elevated blood pressure in an older patient.

Continued clinical observation is appropriate for this older patient with elevated blood pressure measurements. The eighth report of the Joint National Committee (JNC 8) recommends that pharmacologic treatment be initiated to lower blood pressure in patients aged ≥60 years who have systolic blood pressure persistently ≥150 mm Hg or diastolic blood pressure ≥90 mm Hg, and treat to a goal of systolic <150 mm Hg and diastolic <90 mm Hg. This recommendation is based on good-quality evidence that a blood pressure goal of <150/90 mm Hg reduces the risk of cardiovascular events, but there appears to be no added benefit with lower targets (140-149 mm Hg). Therefore, in this 70-year-old patient in whom multiple readings have not shown blood pressure above this threshold for treatment, continued clinical observation with periodic blood pressure determinations and evaluation for potential end-organ damage associated with hypertension is recommended.

Pharmacologic treatment, such as a thiazide diuretic or an ACE inhibitor, is not indicated at this time.

Although echocardiography is more sensitive for detecting left ventricular hypertrophy than electrocardiography, it is not indicated for evaluation of possible hypertension or as an initial study in patients with documented hypertension in the absence of another indication (such as clinical evidence of heart failure).

KEY POINT

- The eighth report of the Joint National Committee recommends a treatment goal of <150/90 mm Hg for patients with hypertension who are ≥60 years.

Bibliography

James PA, Oparil S, Carter BL. 2014 evidence-based guideline for the management of high blood pressure in adults: report from the panel members appointed to the Eighth Joint National Committee (JNC 8). JAMA. 2014 Feb 5;311(5):507-20. [PMID: 24352797]

Item 39   Answer: B

Educational Objective: Diagnose infection-related glomerulonephritis.

This patient likely has infection-related glomerulonephritis (IRGN) following a streptococcal infection. Supportive evidence includes preceding symptoms of an upper respiratory tract infection suggestive of streptococci (rapid streptococcal antigen test is positive and antistreptolysin O antibodies are elevated), followed by the nephritic syndrome in 1 week, and low C3 levels with normal C4 levels (suggesting an alternative pathway of complement activation, which is typical of IRGN). Most patients will show spontaneous resolution of nephritis with conservative management (antibiotics, blood pressure management, and diuretics).

IgA nephropathy (IgAN) is the most common form of glomerulonephritis. Asymptomatic microscopic hematuria with or without proteinuria is the most common presentation of IgAN, and episodic gross hematuria following an upper respiratory tract infection is a classic presentation. Kidney manifestations usually occur concomitantly with the respiratory infection in IgAN ("synpharyngitic" nephritis), as opposed to the typical 7- to 10-day latent period with IRGN. Moreover, complement levels are typically normal in IgAN, whereas C3 is typically low and C4 is normal in IRGN.

Lupus nephritis may occasionally be precipitated by infections. Patients with lupus typically experience systemic manifestations such as rash and arthritis, although kidney-limited disease is sometimes seen. Both C3 and C4 complement levels are depressed in this condition due to the classical pathway of complement being activated. In IRGN, C3 is typically depleted, with normal levels of C4 due to activation of the alternative pathway of complement.

Small-vessel vasculitis is also associated with glomerulonephritis. However, there are frequently other clinical findings of vasculitis present, and complement levels are typically normal.

KEY POINT

- Infection-related glomerulonephritis is characterized by preceding symptoms of an upper respiratory tract infection suggestive of streptococci, followed by the nephritic syndrome and low C3 levels with normal C4 levels.

Bibliography

Nasr SH, Radhakrishnan J, D'Agati VD. Bacterial infection-related glomerulonephritis in adults. Kidney Int. 2013 May;83(5):792-803. [PMID: 23302723]

Item 40   Answer: C

Educational Objective: Identify orlistat as a cause of acute kidney injury.

This patient has acute oxalate nephropathy most likely caused by orlistat. Orlistat is thought to cause acute kidney injury (AKI) through enteric hyperoxaluria. Orlistat blocks fat uptake and results in the production of calcium soaps from unabsorbed fat in the small bowel. Calcium soaps reduce the availability of free enteric calcium, preventing binding of oxalate in the gut by calcium, and allowing for increased intestinal uptake of oxalate and subsequent renal oxalate excretion. Excessive renal oxalate excretion predisposes to development of oxalate crystals within the tubules and interstitium as seen in this patient, causing intratubular obstruction and acute kidney injury. Volume depletion and preexisting kidney disease appear to increase the risk of developing orlistat-associated nephropathy.

Aristolochic acid is present in some herbal preparations and weight loss supplements and can cause nephropathy. This condition is characterized by extensive, primarily interstitial, fibrosis with tubular loss, which is not seen on this patient's kidney biopsy. Patients with this condition are also at increased risk for urothelial malignancies.

Ephedrine is associated with nephrolithiasis, and analysis of the stones reveals the presence of ephedrine, norephedrine, and pseudoephedrine. Patients may also have rhabdomyolysis. These findings are not found in this patient, making this an unlikely cause of her AKI.

Phentermine is not known to cause AKI or other kidney disorders.

KEY POINT

- Orlistat may be a cause of acute kidney injury by triggering acute oxalate nephropathy, particularly in patients with volume depletion or chronic kidney disease.

Bibliography

Weir MA, Beyea MM, Gomes T, et al. Orlistat and acute kidney injury: an analysis of 953 patients. Arch Intern Med. 2011 Apr 11;171(7):703-4. [PMID: 21482850]

Item 41   Answer: B

Educational Objective: Diagnose membranous glomerulopathy.

The most likely diagnosis is membranous glomerulopathy (MG). This patient has evidence of the nephrotic syndrome, with significant protein loss in the urine, hypoalbuminemia, and edema. He also has a pulmonary embolism, a common complication of the nephrotic syndrome. The clinical presentation of MG is indistinguishable from other causes of the nephrotic syndrome, although the propensity for venous thromboembolism, and particularly renal vein thrombosis, is much higher in MG than other disorders associated with the nephrotic syndrome, such as focal

CONT.

segmental glomerulosclerosis or minimal change glomerulopathy. The pathophysiology of hypercoagulability in the nephrotic syndrome is not well understood, nor has the mechanism underlying the higher propensity for thromboembolism in MG been well defined. The risk appears to be inversely related to the serum albumin level in MG, and prophylactic anticoagulation is frequently given to patients with MG with a serum albumin level of ≤2.8 g/dL (28 g/L). MG is the most common cause of idiopathic nephrotic syndrome in adult white persons but may also be associated with infections, systemic lupus erythematosus, medications, and certain malignancies. Definitive diagnosis is by kidney biopsy.

The hypercoagulable state is associated with the nephrotic syndrome only, not other kidney syndromes such as acute interstitial nephritis or poststreptococcal glomerulonephritis. Additionally, these disorders typically present with evidence of inflammation on urinalysis and kidney failure, neither of which is present in this patient.

The site of thrombosis in thrombotic microangiopathy is the microvasculature, leading to clinical manifestations such as microangiopathic hemolytic anemia, thrombocytopenia, and organ dysfunction (including kidney failure). Large-vessel thrombosis does not occur as is present in this case.

KEY POINT

- Although the clinical presentation of membranous glomerulopathy is indistinguishable from other causes of the nephrotic syndrome, the propensity for thromboembolic events is much higher.

Bibliography

Mirrakhimov AE, Ali AM, Barbaryan A, Prueksaritanond S, Hussain N. Primary nephrotic syndrome in adults as a risk factor for pulmonary embolism: an up-to-date review of the literature. Int J Nephrol. 2014;2014:916760. [PMID: 24829800]

Item 42   Answer: D

Educational Objective: Manage white coat hypertension.

Continued clinical follow-up is appropriate for this patient with white coat hypertension. He has high blood pressure readings in the clinic; however, his ambulatory blood pressure monitor (ABPM) readings do not meet the definition of hypertension. The diagnosis of white coat hypertension is applied to patients with average blood pressure readings ≥140/90 mm Hg in the office and average readings <135/85 mm Hg as determined by ABPM. Daytime (awake) average above 140/90 mm Hg and nighttime (asleep) average above 125/75 mm Hg are also used to diagnose hypertension on ABPM. Analysis of nocturnal readings compared to daytime reading is also helpful. Compared with daytime readings, nocturnal readings are approximately 15% lower ("dipping"). A non-dipping status (failure to drop nocturnal blood pressure by <10%) is associated with more cardiovascular events

compared with dipping. This patient dips appropriately at night. Patients with white coat hypertension may have an elevated cardiovascular risk compared with normotensive patients. Moreover, such patients are also at a higher risk for sustained hypertension. Therefore, close observation for sustained hypertension and end-organ damage is recommended in patients with white coat hypertension.

Echocardiography is more sensitive than electrocardiography in detecting evidence of left ventricular hypertrophy. However, it is not used for the diagnosis of hypertension unless there is evidence of end-organ damage or if the information would help guide subsequent treatment. In this patient with a normal ABPM study without evidence of cardiac disease, echocardiography is not indicated.

Evaluation for secondary causes of hypertension such as primary hyperaldosteronism is not indicated in this patient without evidence of sustained hypertension and a normal serum potassium level.

Drug therapy is not recommended unless sustained hypertension or evidence of end-organ damage is present.

KEY POINT

- In patients with white coat hypertension, close observation for the emergence of sustained hypertension or end-organ damage is recommended; drug therapy is not usually required.

Bibliography

Piper MA, Evans CV, Burda BU, Margolis KL, O'Connor E, Whitlock EP. Diagnostic and predictive accuracy of blood pressure screening methods with consideration of rescreening intervals: a systematic review for the U.S. Preventive Services Task Force. Ann Intern Med. 2015 Feb 3;162(3): 192-204. [PMID: 25531400]

Item 43   Answer: B

Educational Objective: Diagnose thrombotic microangiopathy caused by chemotherapy.

Bevacizumab is the most likely cause of this patient's clinical picture. This patient presents with classic features of thrombotic microangiopathy (TMA), including microangiopathic hemolytic anemia, a low platelet count, and kidney dysfunction. Chemotherapeutic agents known to be associated with TMA include mitomycin C, gemcitabine, tyrosine kinase inhibitors, mammalian target of rapamycin (mTOR) inhibitors (sirolimus, everolimus), and anti-vascular endothelial growth factor (VEGF) inhibitors. VEGF inhibitors are an important class of drugs used in treating metastatic cancer, and they are able to induce a form of microangiopathy very similar to preeclampsia/eclampsia that is associated with severe hypertension and kidney failure. VEGF inhibition by endogenous factors is thought to play a key role in development of preeclampsia/eclampsia, and two VEGF inhibitors, bevacizumab and sunitinib, have been linked to TMA, which typically subsides after stopping the drug. Patients typically present with an insidious onset of kidney failure and hypertension (new or exacerbated). There tends to be a variable amount of proteinuria and a relatively bland urine sediment. The cancer is not typically overt (to differentiate from cancer-associated TMA, in which there are widely metastatic lesions at the time of diagnosis of TMA). Plasmapheresis is not usually effective for treatment of VEGF inhibitor–associated TMA and is not indicated.

The other chemotherapeutic agents (5-fluorouracil, leucovorin, oxaliplatin) being administered are not associated with TMA.

KEY POINT

- Two anti-vascular endothelial growth factor inhibitors, bevacizumab and sunitinib, have been linked to thrombotic microangiopathy, which typically subsides after stopping the drug.

Bibliography
Usui J, Glezerman IG, Salvatore SP. Clinicopathological spectrum of kidney diseases in cancer patients treated with vascular endothelial growth factor inhibitors: a report of 5 cases and review of literature. Hum Pathol 2014 Sep;45(9):1918-27. [PMID: 25087655]

Item 44   Answer: A
Educational Objective: Appropriately time the referral of a patient with chronic kidney disease to a nephrologist.

Nephrologist referral and kidney transplant evaluation should occur now. This patient has severe chronic kidney disease (CKD) and will likely require dialysis within the next 1 to 2 years. All patients with stage G4 or G5 CKD should be referred to a nephrologist for evaluation and optimization of metabolic parameters and preparation for dialysis. Because proper preparation for dialysis can take many months, especially if an arteriovenous fistula must be created for hemodialysis, timely referral is important. Hemodialysis and peritoneal dialysis have similar clinical outcomes; choice of modality should be guided by patient preference, willingness, and ability to participate in self-care. All patients who are willing to consider kidney transplant and do not have absolute medical contraindications should be referred for transplant evaluation once their estimated glomerular filtration rate is below 20 mL/min/1.73 m² because they are then eligible to be placed on a waiting list for a transplant. This is especially important because the waiting list is several years long in most parts of the United States, and early listing maximizes the chances of surviving until transplant. Also, if a living donor is identified, it is possible that the patient may receive a preemptive transplant before requiring dialysis. It is important to refer patients with CKD to a nephrologist early in the course of the disease for evaluation because late referral is associated with increased mortality.

Waiting to refer to a nephrologist for 6 months will delay proper preparation for dialysis therapy, dialysis access placement, and transplant evaluation.

Rechecking serum creatinine in 2 weeks is not indicated because this patient has long-standing CKD that is unlikely to be significantly improved after 2 weeks, and this approach will unnecessarily delay referral to a nephrologist.

Continuing current management is incorrect because the patient requires timely preparation for renal replacement therapy and transplant referral, and delays in nephrology referral for patients with severe CKD are associated with increased risk of mortality.

KEY POINT

- All patients with stage G4 or G5 chronic kidney disease should be referred to a nephrologist for management, and referral for transplant evaluation is indicated once the estimated glomerular filtration rate is below 20 mL/min/1.73 m².

Bibliography
Smart NA, Titus TT. Outcomes of early versus late nephrology referral in chronic kidney disease: a systematic review. Am J Med. 2011 Nov;124(11):1073-80.e2. [PMID: 22017785]

Item 45   Answer: D
Educational Objective: Manage diabetic nephropathy.

Continuing this patient's current therapy is the most appropriate management. This patient has long-standing type 2 diabetes mellitus complicated by proliferative retinopathy and neuropathy. She has worsening proteinuria accompanied by a slow decline in kidney function over several years. Her blood pressure is within the desired range, and she is receiving an ACE inhibitor. Continued management is therefore appropriate. With adequate blood pressure control and use of an ACE inhibitor (or angiotensin receptor blocker [ARB]), progression of diabetic nephropathy is slowed but not eliminated. A maximally tolerated dose of an ACE inhibitor or ARB should be tried in an attempt to lower proteinuria as much as possible.

Calcium channel blockers are effective antihypertensive medications in patients with diabetic nephropathy and hypertension, although they do not have the same degree of renoprotection as either ACE inhibitors or ARBs. Because this patient's blood pressure is well controlled and she is already on an ACE inhibitor, there is no indication for the addition of amlodipine.

Adding an ARB (such as losartan) to an ACE inhibitor has not been shown to improve kidney outcomes, and dual angiotensin system inhibition increases the risk of hyperkalemia and acute kidney injury. It is therefore not recommended, even in patients with significant proteinuria on monotherapy with an ACE inhibitor or ARB.

Both ACE inhibitors and ARBs exert their renoprotective effect by decreasing glomerular hyperfiltration by reducing the glomerular filtration rate (GFR). In most patients with normal to moderately impaired kidney function, this medication-induced decrease in GFR is well tolerated, although this may result in a slight increase in the serum creatinine. Given this patient's mild increase in serum creatinine and normal serum electrolytes, there is no indication for reducing the dose of her ACE inhibitor lisinopril, which is beneficial in treating her hypertension and proteinuria.

- Adequate blood pressure control and use of an ACE inhibitor or angiotensin receptor blocker has been shown to slow the progression of diabetic nephropathy.

Bibliography

Makani H, Bangalore S, Desouza KA, Shah A, Messerli FH. Efficacy and safety of dual blockade of the renin-angiotensin system: meta-analysis of randomised trials. BMJ. 2013 Jan 28;346:f360. [PMID: 23358488]

Item 46   Answer: A

Educational Objective: Diagnose abdominal compartment syndrome.

Bladder pressure measurement is the most appropriate next step in management. Abdominal compartment syndrome (ACS) should be suspected in patients with oliguria or increasing serum creatinine levels who have had abdominal surgery, who have received massive fluid resuscitation, who have a tense abdomen, or who have liver or pancreatic disease with ascites. ACS is typically defined as new organ dysfunction with an intra-abdominal pressure >20 mm Hg. This patient is developing ACS manifested by increased hemodynamic instability, worsening respiratory failure with increased airway pressures and increasing difficulty with oxygenation, a tense abdomen on examination, and oliguric kidney failure. Diagnosis of intra-abdominal hypertension and ACS is accomplished by transduction of bladder pressure. Although medical treatment (diuresis, dialysis, management of ascites) can be tried, surgical decompression of the abdomen is often necessary to definitively treat ACS.

There are no data to support that transfusing patients with severe sepsis to a hemoglobin level above 10 g/dL (100 g/L) improves outcomes. The current Surviving Sepsis Guidelines recommend that, once tissue hypoperfusion has resolved and in the absence of serious comorbidities, erythrocytes should only be transfused when hemoglobin decreases to <7.0 g/dL (70 g/L).

Although this patient's urine sodium is <10 mEq/L (10 mmol/L), clinically he is not intravascularly volume depleted. Therefore, further volume resuscitation is not indicated because it may contribute to worsening organ dysfunction by increasing intra-abdominal pressure.

There is no evidence that hemodynamic monitoring with a pulmonary artery catheter improves clinical outcomes in patients with acute respiratory distress syndrome, and it may be associated with harm.

- Abdominal compartment syndrome should be suspected in patients with oliguria or increasing serum creatinine levels who have had abdominal surgery, who have received massive fluid resuscitation, who have a tense abdomen, or who have liver or pancreatic disease with ascites.

Bibliography

Mohmand H, Goldfarb S. Renal dysfunction associated with intra-abdominal hypertension and the abdominal compartment syndrome. J Am Soc Nephrol. 2011 Apr;22(4):615-21. [PMID: 21310818]

Item 47   Answer: A

Educational Objective: Diagnose statin-induced rhabdomyolysis.

The most likely diagnosis is statin-induced rhabdomyolysis associated with atorvastatin therapy as a cause of this patient's acute kidney injury (AKI). This is supported by her symptoms of muscle weakness, physical examination findings, AKI, and urinalysis with blood but no erythrocytes. Myoglobin released from damaged muscle cause renal tubular obstruction, direct nephrotoxicity, intrarenal vasoconstriction, and AKI. Statin-induced rhabdomyolysis is a rare occurrence, and routine testing of muscle enzymes following initiation of statin therapy is not recommended. However, further evaluation is indicated in patients presenting with suggestive symptoms and clinical findings, as in this patient. Risk factors for development of statin-induced myositis include advanced age, female gender, preexisting chronic kidney disease (CKD), diabetes mellitus, hypothyroidism, high-dose statin therapy, and use of medications metabolized through cytochrome P450 3A4, which may increase serum levels of statins (lovastatin, simvastatin, atorvastatin) metabolized through this pathway. Treatment includes discontinuation of the statin, hydration, and management of any associated electrolyte abnormalities.

Hydrochlorothiazide can cause symptoms of weakness from volume depletion, hyponatremia, or hypokalemia. This patient has no evidence of volume depletion on examination, and her serum potassium level is elevated. Although she has hyponatremia, it is mild and does not explain her symptoms or urinalysis findings.

Although hypothyroidism may be associated with myalgia and elevations of serum muscle enzymes, rhabdomyolysis is rare, and initiation of levothyroxine therapy is not associated with worsening muscle symptoms. This patient's lack of myalgia at the time of hospitalization and mild degree of hypothyroidism make hypothyroid myopathy an unlikely diagnosis.

ACE inhibitors such as lisinopril can cause AKI in certain settings such as hypovolemia or renal artery stenosis. However, this patient's clinical presentation and laboratory findings are not consistent with AKI associated with ACE inhibitor therapy.

- Risk factors for the development of statin-induced rhabdomyolysis include advanced age, female gender, preexisting chronic kidney disease, diabetes mellitus, hypothyroidism, high-dose statin therapy, and use of medications metabolized through cytochrome P450 3A4.

Bibliography
Joy TR, Hegele RA. Narrative review: statin-related myopathy. Ann Intern Med. 2009 Jun 16;150(12):858-68. [PMID:19528564]

Item 48   Answer: C

Educational Objective: Diagnose acquired cystic kidney disease and renal cell carcinoma in a patient with end-stage kidney disease.

The most likely diagnosis is renal cell carcinoma. The patient has acquired cystic kidney disease (ACKD), which becomes more common and progresses during the course of end-stage kidney disease (ESKD); the incidence of ACKD rises dramatically as time on dialysis increases. Patients with ACKD typically have a large number of small bilateral kidney cysts and reduced kidney size. For unclear reasons, patients with ACKD have an approximately 30-fold increased risk for developing renal cell carcinoma, despite this, routine screening for this malignancy is not recommended. However, clinicians should have a high level of suspicion for renal cell carcinoma in patients with ESKD who have flank pain or hematuria that may be suggestive of the diagnosis. Despite the relatively high prevalence of renal cell carcinoma in patients with ACKD, it is an uncommon cause of death in patients with ESKD.

The hallmark of autosomal dominant polycystic kidney disease (ADPKD) is large kidneys with multiple kidney cysts, usually originating in the renal collecting duct. Most patients with ADPKD have a positive family history for cystic kidney disease and/or chronic kidney disease. Diagnosis may be complicated by the fact that a hemorrhagic kidney cyst is usually indistinguishable from a solid renal mass on ultrasound. However, in this patient without a family history, small kidneys on ultrasound, and cysts scattered throughout the renal parenchyma, ADPKD with a hemorrhagic renal cyst is unlikely.

Renal angiomyolipomas and bilateral renal cysts are associated with tuberous sclerosis complex (TSC). However, because this is an autosomal dominant disease, there is almost always a positive family history. Additionally, TSC is a systemic disorder with lesions typically present in various organs and tissues and would be a far less common cause of kidney tumors in a patient with ESKD.

Transitional cell or urothelial carcinomas arise from the mucosal surfaces of the urethra, bladder, and ureters and may also occur in the renal pelvis and calyces; in the upper urinary tract, transitional cell carcinomas also tend to be multifocal and only uncommonly form mass lesions within the kidney. This patient's mass is located in the renal parenchyma, and there is not an increased risk of transitional cell carcinoma with ACKD, making this a less likely diagnosis.

KEY POINT

- Acquired cystic kidney disease is associated with a large number of small bilateral kidney cysts, reduced kidney size, and a markedly increased risk for developing renal cell carcinoma.

Bibliography
Singanamala S, Brewster UC. Should screening for acquired cystic disease and renal malignancy be undertaken in dialysis patients? Semin Dial. 2011 Jul-Aug;24(4):365-6. [PMID: 21851390]

Item 49   Answer: A

Educational Objective: Screen a patient with risk factors for chronic kidney disease.

Urine albumin excretion measurement is appropriate for this patient with risk factors for chronic kidney disease (CKD). Patients with diabetes mellitus are at a markedly increased risk of CKD, and treatment of patients with diabetes and moderately increased albuminuria (formerly known as microalbuminuria) using ACE inhibitors or angiotensin receptor blockers (ARBs) can reduce the risk of progression to overt nephropathy. Moreover, determining the level of albuminuria and estimated glomerular filtration rate is important for detecting the presence of CKD and accurately staging CKD if present. CKD staging has important implications with regard to clinical prognosis. Guidelines differ among several medical organizations regarding the optimal approach to CKD screening. Whereas the American College of Physicians guidelines state that there is insufficient evidence to support or discourage screening for CKD in persons with CKD risk factors such as diabetes, the National Kidney Foundation and the American Diabetes Association support screening for kidney disease in all patients with diabetes.

There is no evidence to support the value of kidney ultrasonography in persons who have no clinical evidence of kidney disease and no family history of genetic kidney disease such as autosomal dominant polycystic kidney disease.

Dipstick urinalysis is not sufficiently sensitive to detect the presence of moderately increased albuminuria; the results are semiquantitative, and estimations of proteinuria can be significantly affected by urine concentration.

Although ARBs have been demonstrated to reduce the risk of progression from moderately increased albuminuria to overt diabetic nephropathy, no studies have demonstrated a beneficial effect of these medications in patients who do not have increased urine albumin excretion or existing hypertension. It remains unknown whether ARBs or ACE inhibitors are protective in patients with moderately increased albuminuria due to etiologies other than diabetic nephropathy.

KEY POINT

- Patients with risk factors for chronic kidney disease should be screened using laboratory studies, most commonly determining the estimated glomerular filtration rate and urine testing for protein or albumin.

Bibliography
Kidney Disease: Improving Global Outcomes (KDIGO) CKD Work Group. KDIGO 2012 Clinical Practice Guideline for the Evaluation and Management of Chronic Kidney Disease. Kidney Int Suppl. 2013;3:1-150.

Item 50   Answer: A

Educational Objective: Treat interstitial nephritis by discontinuing a medication.

Discontinuing omeprazole is appropriate in this patient who may have interstitial nephritis as a cause of chronic tubulointerstitial disease. In contrast to acute kidney injury, chronic tubulointerstitial disease develops over months to years and is a cause of slowly declining kidney function. Chronic tubulointerstitial disease most commonly results from previous injury due to an episode of acute interstitial nephritis, but it can also result from ongoing, subacute interstitial nephritis and other glomerular, vascular, or obstructive diseases that may cause irreversible injury to the tubules and interstitium, even with treatment or resolution of the initial disease process. Symptoms and physical examination findings in patients with chronic tubulointerstitial disease can be minimal or absent unless an active associated disease is present; therefore, the diagnosis is often discovered by abnormalities detected on laboratory testing done for other purposes. This patient was noted to have progressively worsening kidney function, with the only abnormality being mild leukocytosis on urinalysis and subnephrotic-range proteinuria. Evaluation of chronic tubulointerstitial disease is focused on identification of potentially treatable causes. Because proton pump inhibitors are associated with interstitial nephritis, discontinuation of omeprazole is appropriate in this patient.

Although any drug may cause interstitial nephritis, there are no case reports of tamsulosin-induced interstitial nephritis. Stopping tamsulosin may exacerbate the benign prostatic hyperplasia, which could lead to postrenal acute kidney injury.

A 24-hour urine collection may be useful for measuring kidney function and quantifying proteinuria but would not be helpful in establishing the cause of this patient's declining kidney function.

Duplex ultrasonography can be useful for diagnosing renal artery stenosis, but this patient's clinical features of pyuria, mild proteinuria, normal blood pressure, and symmetric kidney size are not consistent with renal artery disease, making this study unnecessary.

KEY POINT

- Proton pump inhibitors are a potentially treatable cause of chronic tubulointerstitial disease.

Bibliography

Chang YS. Hypersensitivity reactions to proton pump inhibitors. Curr Opin Allergy Clin Immunol. 2012 Aug;12(4):348-53. [PMID: 22744268]

Item 51   Answer: B

Educational Objective: Treat a patient with cardiorenal syndrome.

Continuing intravenous diuretic therapy is the most appropriate next step in management. In acute decompensated heart failure, elevated renal venous pressure can cause distended renal venules with increased tubular fluid pressure and backleak, leading to venous congestion and cardiorenal syndrome (CRS). This patient has CRS, defined as a change in function of either the heart or kidneys that may influence the function of the other organ system. CRS is categorized into five types: 1) acute heart failure leading to acute kidney injury (AKI) (CRS1), 2) chronic heart failure leading to chronic kidney disease (CKD), 3) AKI leading to acute heart failure, 4) CKD leading to cardiac dysfunction (heart failure, coronary artery disease, arrhythmias), and 5) systemic conditions leading to simultaneous heart and kidney dysfunction (such as sepsis). Management of CRS may be challenging because treatment of one organ system may cause worsening of the other. In patients with heart failure–related CRS, treatment is directed toward improving cardiac function and fluid balance, which may optimize kidney function. However, it is common to see mild to moderate worsening of kidney function associated with treatment of volume overload until fluid balance is achieved. In general, diuresis in heart failure should be maintained until fluid retention (as seen by elevated central venous pressure and peripheral edema) is resolved, even if this results in asymptomatic mild to moderate decreases in kidney function that are followed closely.

Nesiritide, a recombinant human B-type natriuretic peptide that acts as a vasodilator, is available for treatment of selected patients with acute decompensated heart failure. However, there is no evidence that nesiritide improves kidney function when used in this setting and is therefore an inappropriate addition to therapy for this purpose.

Ultrafiltration, or the removal of plasma water through an extracorporeal circuit, has been used in patients unresponsive to diuretics; however, this patient has responded to diuretic therapy, and ultrafiltration is not indicated at present.

Excessive concern about precipitating kidney failure can lead to underutilization of diuretics and persistent volume overload, which may reduce the efficacy of ACE inhibitors and increase the risk of carvedilol-induced decompensated heart failure.

KEY POINT

- In patients with heart failure–related cardiorenal syndrome, treatment is directed toward improving cardiac function and fluid balance, which may optimize kidney function.

Bibliography

Yancy CW, Jessup M, Bozkurt B, et al. American College of Cardiology Foundation/American Heart Association Task Force on Practice Guidelines. 2013 ACCF/AHA guideline for the management of heart failure: a report of the American College of Cardiology Foundation/American Heart Association Task Force on practice guidelines. Circulation. 2013;128(16):e240-327. [PMID: 23741058]

Item 52   Answer: A

Educational Objective: Diagnose chronic hypertension in a pregnant patient.

Chronic hypertension is the most likely diagnosis. Hypertension prior to the 20th week of gestation is most consistent with previously undiagnosed chronic hypertension, which may go undetected in healthy women because of a minimal need for medical evaluation prior to pregnancy. As in nonpregnant patients, chronic hypertension may be primary (formerly known as essential) or secondary. This patient presents at the 12th week of gestation with persistently elevated blood pressures since her pregnancy was discovered, suggesting that her hypertension predated her pregnancy, and is likely primary because she has no other clinical features or laboratory study results to suggest a different cause. The 2013 American College of Obstetricians and Gynecologists (ACOG) guidelines recommend treating persistent blood pressure elevations of >160/105 mm Hg in women with chronic hypertension, with a goal blood pressure with medical therapy in these patients being 120-160/80-105 mm Hg.

The diagnosis of gestational hypertension requires consistent hypertension after the 20th week of gestation without preexisting hypertension or features of preeclampsia and must resolve within 12 weeks of delivery. Because this patient is persistently hypertensive early in her pregnancy, gestational hypertension is not likely.

Normal physiologic changes associated with pregnancy include increased cardiac output and decreased systemic vascular resistance and blood pressure. Blood pressure elevations to the level seen in this patient are not normally seen in pregnancy, when blood pressures are usually much lower.

Preeclampsia requires the combination of new-onset hypertension after 20 weeks of pregnancy and end-organ damage such as proteinuria, kidney dysfunction, thrombocytopenia, abnormal liver chemistry tests, pulmonary edema, and cerebral or visual symptoms.

KEY POINT

- Hypertension prior to the 20th week of gestation is most consistent with previously undiagnosed chronic hypertension, which may go undetected in healthy women because of a minimal need for medical evaluation prior to pregnancy.

Bibliography

Seely EW, Ecker J. Chronic hypertension in pregnancy. Circulation. 2014 Mar 18;129(11):1254-61. [PMID: 24637432]

Item 53   Answer: B

Educational Objective: Diagnose hyperosmolar hyponatremia.

The most likely diagnosis is hyperosmolar hyponatremia, caused by this patient's significantly elevated plasma glucose level. The patient's elevated plasma osmolality indicates the presence of a hyperosmolar state. Hyperglycemia causes the osmotic translocation of water from the intracellular to the extracellular fluid compartment, which results in a decrease in the serum sodium level by approximately 1.6 mEq/L (1.6 mmol/L) for every 100 mg/dL (5.6 mmol/L) increase in the plasma glucose above 100 mg/dL

(5.6 mmol/L). Hyperosmolar hyponatremia can also be the result of exogenously administered solutes such as mannitol or sucrose.

Pseudohyponatremia is caused by significant hyperlipidemia or the presence of paraproteins in the serum. In these situations, the laboratory measurement of plasma glucose is erroneously low, and the plasma osmolality is normal. This patient has a high plasma osmolality, which is not seen in pseudohyponatremia.

Hypothyroidism, adrenal insufficiency, and the syndrome of inappropriate antidiuretic hormone secretion (SIADH) are associated with hypo-osmolar hyponatremia caused by a decrease in the excretion of free water and are not compatible with the patient's hyperosmolality. Although lung cancer is a common cause of SIADH and may be present in this patient with a lung mass, his laboratory studies are not consistent with this being the cause of his hyponatremia.

Reset osmostat refers to a downward setting of the level at which sensors of plasma osmolality trigger the release of antidiuretic hormone and is associated with quadriplegia, tuberculosis, advanced age, pregnancy, psychiatric disorders, and chronic malnutrition. This lowered setpoint leads to stable, mild hypo-osmolar hyponatremia, which is inconsistent with this patient's findings.

KEY POINT

- Hyperglycemia causes the osmotic translocation of water from the intracellular to the extracellular fluid compartment, which results in a decrease in the serum sodium level by approximately 1.6 mEq/L (1.6 mmol/L) for every 100 mg/dL (5.6 mmol/L) increase in the plasma glucose above 100 mg/dL (5.6 mmol/L).

Bibliography

Sterns RH. Disorders of plasma sodium–causes, consequences, and correction. N Engl J Med. 2015 Jan 1;372(1):55-65. [PMID: 25551526]

Item 54   Answer: D

Educational Objective: Identify tramadol overdose as a cause of respiratory acidosis.

Tramadol, a weak opioid agonist, is the most likely cause of this patient's respiratory findings. She has primary respiratory acidosis characterized by an elevation in P_{CO_2}, a decrease in pH, and a slight increase in bicarbonate. This patient has laboratory findings that suggest an acute onset. For each 10 mm Hg (1.3 kPa) increase in P_{CO_2}, serum bicarbonate increases acutely by 1.0 to 2.0 mEq/L (1.0-2.0 mmol/L) due to the extracellular-to-intracellular shift of hydrogen ions as an immediate compensatory mechanism. Later, renal compensation leads to increased bicarbonate generation, and, after 24 to 48 hours, leads to an increase in serum bicarbonate of 3.0 to 4.0 mEq/L (3.0-4.0 mmol/L) for every 10 mm Hg (1.3 kPa) increase in P_{CO_2}. Primary respiratory acidosis is due to decreased effective ventilation, often noted with opioid overdose, leading to hypercapnia and retention of hydrogen

CONT.

ions. Respiratory acidosis can also result from intrinsic lung pathology or from processes that impede ventilation.

The early phase of acetaminophen overdose is often not associated with any acid-base abnormality. After 72 to 96 hours, patients will often develop an increased anion gap metabolic acidosis related to lactic acidosis. This patient's anion gap is only 11 with no evidence of a metabolic acidosis, making acetaminophen overdose an unlikely cause of her acid-base disorder.

Although decreased respiratory drive can occur in the setting of salicylate intoxication in the later stages, it is more commonly associated with a mixed acid-base abnormality, including an increased anion gap acidosis and respiratory alkalosis, making this an unlikely diagnosis for this patient.

NSAID overdose typically presents with azotemia and hyperkalemia in addition to an increased anion gap metabolic acidosis (primarily a lactic acidosis), making this diagnosis unlikely in this patient.

KEY POINT

- Primary respiratory acidosis is due to decreased effective ventilation, often noted with opioid overdose, leading to hypercapnia and retention of hydrogen ions.

Bibliography

Adrogué HJ, Madias NE. Secondary responses to altered acid-base status: the rules of engagement. J Am Soc Nephrol. 2010 Jun;21(6):920-3. [PMID: 20431042]

Item 55   Answer: B

Educational Objective: Identify hydroxyethyl starch as a cause of acute kidney injury and increased mortality.

Resuscitation therapy with hydroxyethyl starch (HES) is most likely to lead to the development of acute kidney injury (AKI). This patient has septic shock and requires fluid resuscitation to prevent or limit multi-organ failure and reduce mortality. Repetitive fluid challenges are performed by giving a 500- to 1000-mL bolus of crystalloid over short intervals while assessing response to target central venous pressure. Most patients need 4 to 6 L of fluid in the first 6 hours, and a frequent error is underestimating the intravascular volume deficit and the amount of fluid required. The fluid input is typically greater than output owing to vasodilation and capillary leak. HES is a synthetic colloid that is associated with an increased risk of AKI, increased requirement of renal replacement therapy, a trend toward increased blood product transfusion, and increased mortality. HES accumulates in the proximal renal tubular epithelial cell, resulting in vacuolization and swelling of the proximal renal tubular cell, tubular obstruction and injury, and an osmotic nephrosis. As a result, the 2013 Surviving Sepsis Campaign recommends against using any HES in patients with severe sepsis.

Volume resuscitation can be achieved with either crystalloid or colloid solutions. The crystalloid solutions are lactated Ringer solution and 0.9% sodium chloride; the colloid solutions include albumin. Evidence from randomized trials and meta-analyses have found no convincing difference between using crystalloid solutions such as normal saline and lactated Ringer and albumin solutions in the treatment of severe sepsis or septic shock; however, colloid is far more expensive.

KEY POINT

- Hydroxyethyl starch is associated with an increased risk of acute kidney injury, increased requirement of renal replacement therapy, a trend toward increased blood product transfusion, and increased mortality and is not recommended in patients with severe sepsis.

Bibliography

Perner A, Haase N, Guttormsen AB, et al; 6S Trial Group, Scandinavian Critical Care Trials Group. Hydroxyethyl starch 130/0.42 versus Ringer's acetate in severe sepsis. N Engl J Med. 2012 Jul 12;367(2):124. [PMID: 22738085]

Item 56   Answer: A

Educational Objective: Manage a patient at risk for contrast-induced nephropathy.

In addition to discontinuing diuretic therapy, the most appropriate periprocedural management for this patient is to begin intravenous isotonic saline. She is at risk for contrast-induced nephropathy (CIN), and administration of intravenous isotonic saline (1-1.5 mL/kg/h) 3 to 12 hours before the procedure and continued for 6 to 24 hours afterward has been shown to decrease the incidence of CIN in high-risk patients. Risk factors include age older than 75 years, diabetes mellitus, chronic kidney disease, conditions of decreased renal perfusion, and concurrent use of nephrotoxic drugs. Therefore, this patient is at high risk for CIN. In addition to intravenous isotonic saline, other strategies to minimize the risk for CIN include discontinuation of potentially nephrotoxic medications, minimization of contrast volume, and use of low- or iso-osmolal contrast media. The benefit of hydration regimens utilizing isotonic sodium bicarbonate is comparable to isotonic sodium chloride and is not considered to be of significant benefit relative to normal saline.

The benefit of *N*-acetylcysteine in patients at risk for CIN remains controversial, and results from trials are inconsistent. It is therefore not recommended as routine treatment to prevent CIN.

Prophylactic hemodialysis has not been shown to provide benefit compared with medical therapy alone for patients at risk for CIN.

Discontinuation of ACE inhibitors or angiotensin receptor blockers has not been clearly shown to decrease the risk of CIN. Although ACE inhibitors should be discontinued in most cases of acute kidney injury, they can be continued in patients with stable kidney function.

KEY POINT

- Administration of intravenous isotonic saline is appropriate for patients at risk for contrast-induced nephropathy.

Bibliography

Seeliger E, Sendeski M, Rihal CS, Persson PB. Contrast-induced kidney injury: mechanisms, risk factors, and prevention. Eur Heart J. 2012 Aug;33(16):2007-15. [PMID: 22267241]

Item 57　　Answer:　C

Educational Objective: Evaluate kidney function in a patient with acute interstitial nephritis.

In addition to discontinuing omeprazole, repeat kidney function testing in 5 to 7 days is the most appropriate management for this patient with acute interstitial nephritis (AIN). AIN is a condition in which kidney dysfunction results from infiltration of inflammatory cells into the kidney interstitium. It may be associated with drugs, infection, autoimmune diseases, and malignancy, with drug-induced AIN being the most common. Many patients with AIN may be asymptomatic or present with mild, nonspecific symptoms; only 10% to 30% have the classic triad of fever, rash, and eosinophilia. Urinalysis may reveal mild proteinuria, leukocytes, erythrocytes, and leukocyte casts. Drug-induced AIN should be considered in any patient exposed to a potentially offending drug who presents with unexplained acute kidney injury (AKI). Drug-induced AIN is characterized by a slowly increasing serum creatinine 7 to 10 days after exposure; however, it can occur within 1 day of exposure if the patient has been exposed previously. Drug-induced AIN can also occur months after exposure, often with NSAIDs and proton pump inhibitors (PPIs). This patient has a clinical picture consistent with AIN based on clinical and laboratory evidence of kidney injury and urinalysis showing erythrocytes, leukocytes, and leukocyte casts after recently being started on the PPI omeprazole. Discontinuation of the offending agent is the mainstay of therapy. In patients with mild elevations of serum creatinine and minimal clinical findings, stopping the causative drug with close follow-up is usually adequate therapy.

Kidney biopsy is usually not necessary to diagnose AIN, particularly in patients with a consistent clinical and laboratory picture, as seen in this patient. However, kidney biopsy may be indicated in situations where there are inconsistent clinical and laboratory findings, or if kidney function does not improve immediately upon stopping the offending agent.

The role of glucocorticoids in AIN is controversial, with conflicting evidence of benefit in clinical studies. Glucocorticoids are therefore generally reserved for patients who have not responded to discontinuation of the offending agent.

The presence of urine eosinophils detected by Hansel staining of the urine sediment has been classically associated with the diagnosis of AIN but is not specific because they may be associated with other causes of AKI (such as glomerulonephritis), and the absence of urine eosinophils does not exclude AIN. Therefore, this testing is not clinically useful in this patient.

KEY POINT

- Discontinuation of the offending agent is the mainstay of therapy for drug-induced acute interstitial nephritis.

Bibliography

Brewster UC, Perazella MA. Proton pump inhibitors and the kidney: critical review. Clin Nephrol. 2007 Aug;68(2):65-72. [PMID: 17722704]

Item 58　　Answer:　C

Educational Objective: Treat a patient with struvite nephrolithiasis by removing the stone.

The most appropriate next step in management is to remove the struvite stone in the left renal pelvis. Struvite stones are composed of magnesium ammonium phosphate and occur only when ammonium production is increased, which elevates the urine pH and decreases the solubility of phosphate. This is most commonly a consequence of chronic upper urinary tract infection (UTI) with a urease-producing organism, such as *Proteus* or *Klebsiella*. Struvite stones can grow rapidly and become large, filling the entire renal pelvis and taking on a characteristic "staghorn" shape. Although struvite stones affect less than 10% of patients with kidney stones, they occur more commonly in women and in patients predisposed to chronic or recurrent UTI, including those with urologic diversions or neurogenic bladder.

Although treatment of the initial upper UTI is important to prevent struvite stone development, once struvite stones are formed, they are difficult to treat medically, including with chronic antibiotics. Antibiotics may not penetrate the stone, and colonizing bacteria may create an alkaline environment within the stone that promotes continued or recurrent UTI, stone growth, and chronic inflammatory damage to the kidney. Because of this, stone removal is indicated in most cases, and kidney outcomes have been shown to be improved when struvite stones are removed compared with medical therapy. Removal is commonly by percutaneous nephrolithotomy, shock wave lithotripsy, or a combination of both procedures.

Dietary phosphate reduction and urine acidification would be expected to discourage struvite stone formation but are of minimal effectiveness once struvite stones have developed.

KEY POINT

- In most patients with known struvite stones, removal of the stones is indicated.

Bibliography

Frassetto L, Kohlstadt I. Treatment and prevention of kidney stones: an update. Am Fam Physician. 2011 Dec 1;84(11):1234-42. [PMID: 22150656]

Item 59   Answer: B

Educational Objective: Evaluate for HIV infection in a patient with focal segmental glomerulosclerosis.

The most appropriate test to perform is an HIV antibody test in this patient with focal segmental glomerulosclerosis (FSGS). FSGS is the cause of idiopathic nephrotic syndrome in 25% of cases. FSGS may also be secondary to another process, including hyperfiltration injury to the glomerulus as may occur in chronic hypertension, diabetes mellitus, and conditions in which kidney mass is reduced (progressive kidney disease, obesity, sickle cell disease, reflux nephropathy, or after nephrectomy). Direct injury to podocytes may also cause FSGS as seen with certain drugs (pamidronate, interferon) and infections, including HIV. This patient's kidney biopsy results are indicative of the collapsing variant of FSGS, which is classic for HIV-associated glomerulopathy. Therefore, evaluation for HIV infection as a cause of this patient's FSGS is the most appropriate next diagnostic step. In the early stages of HIV-associated glomerulopathy, antiretroviral therapy and angiotensin system blockers may halt disease progression, thus an early diagnosis is important.

Hepatitis B is typically associated with membranous glomerulopathy, and hepatitis C with cryoglobulinemic glomerulonephritis. Serum and urine electrophoresis can be used to test for monoclonal gammopathies. The treponemal antibody test is used to test for syphilis, which is typically associated with membranous nephropathy. None of these disorders is associated with the collapsing glomerulopathy seen on this patient's kidney biopsy.

KEY POINT

- HIV infection is typically associated with the collapsing form of focal segmental glomerulosclerosis; in the early stages, antiretroviral therapy and angiotensin system blockers may halt disease progression.

Bibliography
Hartle PM, Carlo ME, Dwyer JP, Fogo AB. AKI in an HIV patient. J Am Soc Nephrol. 2013 Jul;24(8):1204-8. [PMID: 23559580]

Item 60   Answer: C

Educational Objective: Diagnose glomerulonephritis.

Kidney biopsy is the most appropriate next step in management. This patient has worsening kidney function and new hypertension associated with significant abnormalities on urinalysis, including proteinuria, leukocytes indicating inflammation, hematuria with dysmorphic erythrocytes (acanthocytes), and erythrocyte casts on microscopy. These findings strongly suggest glomerulonephritis. Constitutional symptoms such as fever and arthralgia, as well as non-blanching rash (palpable purpura) and weight loss, further suggest vasculitis as the most likely etiology. Urgent serologic evaluation and kidney biopsy are indicated to diagnose the cause of glomerulonephritis and guide management.

Although this patient has a history of urinary tract infection (UTI), reports fever, and has leukocytes on her urinalysis, her specific lack of symptoms of UTI or other findings consistent with this diagnosis (no costovertebral angle tenderness or bacteria on microscopic urinalysis) make this a less likely diagnosis. UTI would also not be expected to lead to development of hypertension or kidney failure. Therefore, antibiotics are not indicated.

Cystoscopy is typically used to evaluate for hematuria due to a bladder source, such as bladder cancer. The hematuria associated with a bladder source of bleeding is usually structurally normal compared with the dysmorphic erythrocytes seen in this patient; acanthocytes suggest a glomerular source of bleeding. Also, a bladder source of bleeding, such as a malignancy, would not explain the other findings seen on her urinalysis (significant proteinuria, leukocytosis) or her new hypertension and kidney failure, making cystoscopy an inappropriate next step in management.

Kidney ultrasonography can identify structural abnormalities, including nephrolithiasis. However, in this patient with a clinical picture consistent with acute glomerulonephritis, kidney imaging would not be of high diagnostic yield.

KEY POINT

- Urgent serologic evaluation and kidney biopsy are indicated to diagnose the cause of glomerulonephritis and guide management.

Bibliography
Moroni G, Ponticelli C. Rapidly progressive crescentic glomerulonephritis: early treatment is a must. Autoimmune Rev. 2014 Jul;13(7):723-9. [PMID: 24657897]

Item 61   Answer: B

Educational Objective: Manage overcorrection of sodium in a patient with severe asymptomatic hyponatremia at risk for osmotic demyelination syndrome.

Desmopressin intravenously with 5% dextrose is the most appropriate treatment. The patient presented with a 5-day history of gastroenteritis symptoms and severe hyponatremia with a normal neurologic examination. She has chronic asymptomatic hyponatremia that was likely from volume depletion, causing an appropriate elevation in antidiuretic hormone (ADH) secretion, which caused the hyponatremia by retaining the free water she was drinking to maintain hydration. Volume repletion in the hospital led to suppression of ADH production with a subsequent water diuresis, leading to rapid correction. Rapid correction in chronic asymptomatic hyponatremia increases the risk for osmotic demyelination syndrome (ODS), especially in women, which may be delayed for a few days after overcorrection. Overcorrection is considered to be an increase of >8.0 mEq/L (8.0 mmol/L) of

CONT.

the serum sodium within the first 24 hours or >16 mEq/L (16 mmol/L) within the first 48 hours. Desmopressin will terminate the water diuresis, and if given alone will maintain the serum sodium around the current level of 128 mEq/L (128 mmol/L), which still represents overcorrection. Desmopressin intravenously with 5% dextrose will stop the water diuresis and further lower the serum sodium. The 5% dextrose should be given in sufficient volume to reverse the serum sodium level to 120 mEq/L (120 mmol/L) over the first 24 hours and then allowing slow correction.

Fluid restriction alone is inappropriate because the serum sodium will continue correction toward normal and increase the risk of ODS, as will fluid restriction with salt tablets, which will increase the rate of correction.

Providing no further intervention would not reverse the overcorrection, and the patient's serum sodium would likely continue to return to normal, further increasing her risk for ODS.

KEY POINT

- Overcorrection of chronic asymptomatic hyponatremia is associated with the development of osmotic demyelination syndrome and should be reversed using desmopressin with 5% dextrose.

Bibliography

Perianayagam A, Sterns RH, Silver SM, et al. DDAVP is effective in preventing and reversing inadvertent overcorrection of hyponatremia. Clin J Am Soc Nephrol 2008 Mar;3(2):331-6. [PMID: 18235152]

Item 62   Answer: D

Educational Objective: Manage intracranial cerebral aneurysm screening in a patient with autosomal dominant polycystic kidney disease.

No screening is necessary for this asymptomatic patient with autosomal dominant polycystic kidney disease (ADPKD). Intracranial cerebral aneurysms (ICAs) can be detected in 10% to 12% of patients with ADPKD, and a ruptured ICA resulting in a subarachnoid or intracerebral hemorrhage is the most serious extrarenal complication of ADPKD. The prevalence of ICA is higher in patients with ADPKD who have a family history of known ICA or hemorrhagic stroke. Therefore, screening using MR angiography is currently only recommended for patients with ADPKD thought to be at high risk, including those with a family history of aneurysm or subarachnoid hemorrhage or those with a previous rupture. In addition, patients with ADPKD who have high-risk occupations in which a rupture would affect the lives of others (such as driving a school bus) should be screened. There are no differences in screening recommendations based on age. Therefore, there is no indication for screening for ICA in this patient with no symptoms suggestive of possible ICA, no family history of known ICA or hemorrhage, and a low-risk occupation.

KEY POINT

- For patients with autosomal dominant polycystic kidney disease, screening for intracranial cerebral aneurysms using MR angiography is only recommended for those with a family history of aneurysm or subarachnoid hemorrhage, those with a previous rupture, or those with high-risk occupations in which a rupture would affect the lives of others.

Bibliography

Grantham JJ. Clinical practice. Autosomal dominant polycystic kidney disease. N Engl J Med 2008 Oct 2;359(14):1477-85. [PMID: 18832246]

Item 63   Answer: A

Educational Objective: Treat chronic hyponatremia.

In addition to discontinuing fluoxetine, fluid restriction is the appropriate treatment for this patient. She is euvolemic and has hyponatremia with a decreased plasma osmolality and an inappropriately increased urine osmolality. This clinical and laboratory presentation is highly suggestive of the syndrome of inappropriate antidiuretic hormone secretion (SIADH). SIADH has many causes, including various drugs such as selective serotonin reuptake inhibitors like fluoxetine. The initial treatment of asymptomatic patients with SIADH includes management of the underlying cause if possible and free water restriction (in practical terms, fluid restriction) without limiting sodium intake. Discontinuation of fluoxetine should result in resolution of the SIADH with normalization of the serum sodium. In the interim, fluid restriction with a decrease in intake less than urine output will result in a gradual increase in the serum sodium.

Although the serum sodium is significantly decreased, she has no specific neurologic symptoms, which suggests that the hyponatremia is chronic. Rapid normalization of this patient's serum sodium with hypertonic saline would place her at risk for osmotic demyelination syndrome, which may result in severe neurologic symptoms such as paraplegia, dysarthria, dysphagia, diplopia, and locked-in syndrome. Because of this risk, treatment with hypertonic saline is usually limited to patients with severely symptomatic hyponatremia (such as mental status changes or seizures) to rapidly increase the serum sodium.

Treatment with isotonic saline may correct hyponatremia if it is secondary to hypovolemia, but this patient is euvolemic and most likely has SIADH. In this patient, isotonic saline alone, without concomitant fluid restriction, results in volume expansion but may not correct and may possibly worsen the hyponatremia because of inappropriate retention of the water associated with the infusion.

Oral demeclocycline results in renal resistance to antidiuretic hormone and can be effective in treating patients with SIADH. However, it has been associated with acute kidney injury and is generally reserved for patients who have failed other therapies. It should be used with caution in patients with preexisting kidney or liver disease.

CONT.

Tolvaptan, a vasopressin receptor antagonist, results in the excretion of electrolyte free water and is effective in raising the serum sodium in patients with SIADH. It should be used with caution in the treatment of severe, symptomatic hyponatremia, which is not seen in this patient, and as a last resort when other treatments have failed. Because severe liver injury has been reported with its use, the FDA recommends that it not be used in patients with liver disease and that it be used for no more than 30 days.

KEY POINT

- The initial treatment of asymptomatic patients with syndrome of inappropriate antidiuretic hormone secretion includes management of the underlying cause if possible and fluid restriction without limiting sodium intake.

Bibliography

Verbalis JG, Goldsmith SR, Greenberg A, et al. Diagnosis, evaluation, and treatment of hyponatremia: expert panel recommendations. Am J Med. 2013;126(10 suppl 1):S1-42. [PMID: 24074529]

Item 64   Answer: D

Educational Objective: Manage stage 1 hypertension in an older, frail patient.

Continuing the current treatment regimen with the calcium channel blocker amlodipine is appropriate. This 76-year-old patient has stage 1 hypertension and systolic blood pressure measurements in the range of 140 to 150 mm Hg. The treatment goal recommended in the eighth report of the Joint National Committee (JNC 8) for patients with hypertension who are ≥60 years is <150/90 mm Hg. Although she is near this goal, the benefits of further blood pressure reduction must be balanced with the potential risks of increasing a dose, changing the antihypertensive agent, or adding additional antihypertensive agents. Importantly, a recent study defining frailty as the inability to walk 6 meters in less than 8 seconds demonstrated no association with hypertension and mortality, and, in those who were unable to complete the walk test, a reduction in mortality was noted with increased blood pressure. This suggests that the risk of complications, morbidity, and mortality related to lower blood pressure in frail individuals may supersede the potential benefit of lower blood pressure goals.

Although 24-hour ambulatory blood pressure monitoring may be more accurate in defining this patient's blood pressure, home blood pressure monitoring is a reasonable alternative because it is less expensive. Furthermore, additional information is not likely to influence therapy.

KEY POINT

- The risk of complications, morbidity, and mortality related to lower blood pressure in frail individuals may supersede the potential benefit of lower blood pressure goals.

Bibliography

Odden MC, Peralta CA, Haan MN, Covinsky KE. Rethinking the association of high blood pressure with mortality in elderly adults: the impact of frailty. Arch Intern Med. 2012 Aug 13;172(15):1162-8. [PMID: 22801930]

Item 65   Answer: D

Educational Objective: Diagnose the syndrome of inappropriate antidiuretic hormone secretion.

This patient's history and clinical presentation are most consistent with the syndrome of inappropriate antidiuretic hormone secretion (SIADH). On physical examination, she is clinically euvolemic. The appropriate physiologic response to hypo-osmolality in a euvolemic patient is suppression of antidiuretic hormone (ADH) with resultant increase in free water clearance, with urine osmolality less than plasma osmolality. In contrast, this patient demonstrates evidence for increased ADH with hyponatremia and urine osmolality significantly and inappropriately greater than plasma osmolality in spite of her euvolemic status and no apparent stimulus for ADH release.

Because water excretion is, in part, solute dependent, severe limitations in solute intake decrease free water excretion, and hyponatremia may develop in this setting with only modest increases in fluid intake. This syndrome is termed *beer potomania* when observed in patients with chronic alcohol abuse and low solute intake. This patient's relatively high urine osmolality makes beer potomania an unlikely diagnosis.

The most common renal consequence of chronic lithium ingestion is nephrogenic diabetes insipidus; this disorder presents with polyuria and hypernatremia, which are not seen in this patient.

Primary polydipsia should always be considered in the differential diagnosis of patients with mental illness and hyponatremia, particularly those with schizophrenia who are taking psychotropic drugs. Primary polydipsia presents with hyponatremia, decreased plasma osmolality, and decreased urine osmolality, reflecting suppressed ADH levels in response to water overload. Patients with primary polydipsia may also present with abnormalities of ADH regulation such as transient stimulation of ADH release during psychotic episodes and increased renal response to ADH so that at the same levels of ADH, patients who are psychotic may have higher urine osmolalities and a downward resetting of the osmostat that regulates ADH release. Thus, the urine of patients who are psychotic and have primary polydipsia may not be as dilute as would be expected. The significant elevation in urine osmolality makes SIADH the more likely diagnosis in this patient.

KEY POINT

- The syndrome of inappropriate antidiuretic hormone secretion is associated with clinical euvolemia, hypo-osmolar hyponatremia, and urine osmolality inappropriately greater than plasma osmolality.

Bibliography

Verbalis JG, Goldsmith SR, Greenberg A, et al. Diagnosis, evaluation, and treatment of hyponatremia: expert panel recommendations. Am J Med. 2013 Oct;126(10 suppl 1):S1-42. [PMID: 24074529]

Item 66   Answer: B

Educational Objective: Diagnose type 1 (hypokalemic distal) renal tubular acidosis.

The most likely diagnosis is type 1 (hypokalemic distal) renal tubular acidosis (RTA), which results from a defect in urine acidification in the distal tubule with impaired excretion of hydrogen ions, most commonly caused by decreased activity of the proton pump in distal tubular cells. Because of the inability to excrete hydrogen ions, patients develop a metabolic acidosis with compensatory hyperchloremia, resulting in a normal anion gap (8 mEq/L [8 mmol/L] in this patient) and the inability to acidify urine below a pH of 6.0, even after an acid load. The urine pH is therefore almost always inappropriately elevated for the degree of acidemia, and there is a positive urine anion gap. The same defects also cause potassium wasting, and the increased proximal resorption of citrate that occurs with metabolic acidosis leads to hypocitraturia and increased risk of calcium phosphate kidney stones and nephrocalcinosis. Type 1 (hypokalemic distal) RTA is associated with genetic causes, autoimmune disorders, nephrocalcinosis/hypercalciuria, dysproteinemias, drugs/toxins, and tubulointerstitial disease; this patient likely has sicca complex secondary to Sjögren syndrome and kidney involvement with interstitial nephritis.

Acetaminophen is associated with pyroglutamic acidosis (also known as 5-oxoprolinuria), which causes an increased anion gap metabolic acidosis and is less likely to cause a pure normal anion gap metabolic acidosis.

Type 2 (proximal) RTA involves a defect in regenerating bicarbonate in the proximal tubule and is characterized by a normal anion gap metabolic acidosis, hypokalemia, glycosuria (without hyperglycemia), low-molecular-weight proteinuria, and renal phosphate wasting. However, distal urine acidification mechanisms are intact, and the urine pH is usually less than 5.5 without alkali therapy. This patient's high urine pH, absence of glycosuria, and normal urinalysis are inconsistent with type 2 (proximal) RTA.

Type 4 (hyperkalemic distal) RTA is associated with a urine pH <5.5 and hyperkalemia as a result of hypoaldosteronism, neither of which is seen in this patient.

KEY POINT

- Type 1 (hypokalemic distal) renal tubular acidosis results from a defect in urine acidification in the distal tubule with impaired excretion of hydrogen ions.

Bibliography

Duffles Amarante GB, Zotin MC, Rocha E, et al. Renal tubular dysfunction in patients with primary Sjögren syndrome. Clin Nephrol. 2014 Mar;81(3):185-91. [PMID: 24424087]

Item 67   Answer: D

Educational Objective: Understand the risks and benefits of kidney transplantation.

Kidney transplantation would be the most likely strategy to provide this patient with the best long-term survival. Although there is an increase in short-term morbidity and mortality following transplantation, there is strong evidence that kidney transplantation decreases mortality and improves quality of life over the long term. Even though increased recipient age is also associated with reduced patient and allograft survival than younger patients after transplant, carefully selected older patients also benefit from kidney transplantation, and many centers therefore do not have an absolute age cutoff for transplant recipients. Moreover, this patient has family members who are willing to be evaluated as living kidney donors, and kidneys from living donors have superior outcomes compared with kidneys from deceased donors. Therefore, referral for possible kidney transplant in this otherwise healthy patient would be most likely to improve her long-term survival.

There is no clinical indication for this patient to change from peritoneal dialysis to hemodialysis, and clinical outcomes, including mortality and quality of life, are approximately equivalent between these modalities. The choice between peritoneal dialysis and hemodialysis should therefore be driven by patient-specific factors and patient preference if dialysis is pursued.

There is evidence that risk of graft loss and overall mortality are increased in patients who have been treated with dialysis prior to transplant, and that this risk of graft loss and overall mortality increase with the length of dialysis prior to transplant. Therefore, continuing dialysis and reevaluating for possible transplant in 2 to 3 years would not be an optimal management strategy in this otherwise good candidate for transplantation.

KEY POINT

- Kidney transplantation decreases long-term mortality and improves quality of life compared with dialysis.

Bibliography

Tonelli M, Wiebe N, Knoll G, et al. Systematic review: kidney transplantation compared with dialysis in clinically relevant outcomes. Am J Transplant. 2011 Oct;11(10):2093-109. [PMID: 21883901]

Item 68   Answer: D

Educational Objective: Manage blood pressure and diet to slow progression of chronic kidney disease.

Maintaining the current antihypertensive regimen and a standard protein diet is appropriate in this patient to help slow progression of her chronic kidney disease (CKD).

Although earlier, small studies suggested that low protein diets may slow CKD progression, the landmark Modification of Diet in Renal Disease study did not detect a significant protective effect of protein-restricted diets in preventing progression of kidney disease. However, low protein diets may delay onset of symptomatic uremia in patients with late-stage CKD (stage G4/G5).

The eighth report from the Joint National Committee (JNC 8) recommends a target blood pressure of <140/90 mm Hg with ACE inhibitors or angiotensin receptor blockers as first-line agents for treatment of hypertension in patients with CKD. This patient currently meets this recommended goal with an ACE inhibitor as part of her regimen. Although previously recommended by several organizations, there are currently insufficient data to support targeting blood pressures lower than 140/90 mm Hg to prevent progression of kidney disease with the possible exception of patients with severe proteinuria (stage A3 or an albumin-creatinine ratio >300 mg/g), in which some randomized controlled trials have suggested the benefit of a lower blood pressure goal of <130/80 mm Hg.

Volume expansion may contribute to hypertension in CKD; therefore, maintaining normal volume status is important for long-term blood pressure control. Although the diuretic effect of thiazides becomes less effective as the glomerular filtration rate drops, often requiring a switch to a loop diuretic, this patient is clinically euvolemic and with adequate blood pressure control. Additionally, diuretics themselves do not alter progression of proteinuria or CKD. Therefore, there is no indication for switching diuretic therapy in this patient.

KEY POINT

- The eighth report from the Joint National Committee recommends a target blood pressure of <140/90 mm Hg and ACE inhibitors or angiotensin receptor blockers as first-line agents for treatment of hypertension in patients with chronic kidney disease.

Bibliography

Upadhyay A, Earley A, Haynes SM, Uhlig K. Systematic review: blood pressure target in chronic kidney disease and proteinuria as an effect modifier. Ann Intern Med. 2011 Apr 19;154(8):541-8. [PMID: 21403055]

Item 69   Answer: B

Educational Objective: Treat a patient who has chronic kidney disease and proteinuria.

The most appropriate treatment for this patient is to increase the dose of the ACE inhibitor lisinopril. He has chronic kidney disease (CKD) with nephrotic-range proteinuria (urine protein-creatinine ratio >3500 mg/g or a urine protein excretion >3500 mg/24 h) and inadequately controlled hypertension. Increasing lisinopril should decrease his blood pressure and result in some decrease in proteinuria. Although many clinicians are hesitant to escalate the dose of an ACE inhibitor or angiotensin receptor blocker (ARB) in patients with significant CKD, careful upward titration is generally well tolerated with close clinical follow-up. The eighth report from the Joint National Committee (JNC 8) recommends lowering blood pressure

to <140/90 mm Hg, although some experts recommend a lower blood pressure goal of <130/80 mm Hg in patients with heavy proteinuria.

Recent studies have demonstrated that although adding an ARB to an ACE inhibitor usually decreases proteinuria, combination therapy does not improve clinical outcomes and increases the risk of acute kidney injury and hyperkalemia.

Most patients with CKD, and those with CKD and proteinuria in particular, should be treated with an ACE inhibitor or ARB as preferred initial medications due to their demonstrated ability to slow CKD progression. Therefore, replacing lisinopril with the calcium channel blocker amlodipine is not appropriate in this case.

Continuing this patient's current therapy would not improve blood pressure control or decrease proteinuria.

KEY POINT

- Blood pressure control using an ACE inhibitor or angiotensin receptor blocker is the therapy of choice in patients with chronic kidney disease.

Bibliography

Fried LF, Emanuele N, Zhang JH, et al; VA NEPHRON-D Investigators. Combined angiotensin inhibition for the treatment of diabetic nephropathy. N Engl J Med. 2013 Nov 14;369(20):1892-903. [PMID: 24206457]

Item 70   Answer: B   H

Educational Objective: Diagnose alcoholic ketoacidosis.

The most likely diagnosis is alcoholic ketoacidosis. This patient has an increased anion gap metabolic acidosis of 27, and ketoacidosis due to acute ethanol intoxication is the most likely cause. Alcoholic ketoacidosis occurs in patients with chronic ethanol abuse and liver disease and develops following an episode of acute intoxication, at which time the ingested ethanol may have already been extensively metabolized, leading to low or normal serum ethanol levels. Ethanol is oxidized to acetaldehyde and then to acetic acid, during which process the electron-carrier coenzyme nicotinamide adenine dinucleotide (NAD^+) is reduced to NADH in increasing amounts. Simultaneously, rising catecholamine levels cause lipolysis with subsequent generation of free fatty acids and ketone bodies, such as acetoacetate. The high ratio of NADH to NAD^+ leads to increased reduction of acetoacetate to β-hydroxybutyrate. Because the nitroprusside reagent in the serum and urine ketone assays detects only acetoacetate, these tests may be falsely negative due to decreased acetoacetate levels despite the presence of increased levels of the ketone β-hydroxybutyrate, as in this case. Definitive diagnosis may require direct measurement of β-hydroxybutyrate levels in the serum, which is available in some laboratories.

Acute kidney injury can lead to an increased anion gap metabolic acidosis due to the accumulation of acidic

CONT. metabolic by-products and phosphates and sulfates. However, this degree of anion gap would not be expected in this patient who is mildly prerenal with a normal serum phosphorus level.

D-Lactic acidosis is an uncommon cause of increased anion gap metabolic acidosis that is typically identified in patients with small-bowel bacterial overgrowth. Bacterial production of D-lactic acid is undetectable by the serum lactate assay, which recognizes only the L enantiomer. However, this disorder is not associated with chronic alcohol use and would not be a likely diagnostic consideration in this patient.

Rhabdomyolysis is a diagnostic consideration in a patient with a history of alcohol abuse and an anion gap metabolic acidosis, but this condition is frequently associated with hyperkalemia, hyperphosphatemia, hypocalcemia, and a urinalysis positive for blood with no erythrocytes visible on urine microscopy.

KEY POINT

- Alcoholic ketoacidosis occurs in patients with chronic ethanol abuse, frequently with associated liver disease, and develops following an episode of acute intoxication.

Bibliography
Allison MG, McCurdy MT. Alcoholic metabolic emergencies. Emerg Med Clin North Am. 2014 May;32(2):293-301. [PMID: 24766933]

Item 71   Answer: C
Educational Objective: Diagnose IgA vasculitis.

The most likely diagnosis is IgA vasculitis (Henoch-Schönlein purpura). This patient presents with fatigue, joint pain, abdominal pain, petechial/purpural skin lesions, and glomerulonephritis following an upper respiratory tract infection. The differential diagnosis of vasculitis with glomerulonephritis includes infection-related vasculitis (such as endocarditis), cryoglobulinemia, systemic lupus erythematosus, ANCA-associated vasculitis, and IgA vasculitis. Although serologic tests and blood cultures are pending, the patient most likely has IgA vasculitis based on the presence of the tetrad of palpable purpura, arthralgia, abdominal pain, and glomerulonephritis. Although no diagnostic serologic tests for this condition exist, normal complement levels support this diagnosis. Diagnosis is confirmed with biopsy of the affected organ.

Infection-related glomerulonephritis such as endocarditis activates the alternative pathway of complement with low C3 and normal C4 levels. The classical pathway of complement is activated with cryoglobulinemic vasculitis (C4, and sometimes C3, is depressed) and systemic lupus erythematosus (both C3 and C4 are low). In this patient, complement levels are normal, making these diseases less likely. Additionally, cryoglobulinemic vasculitis is associated with hepatitis C virus infection, which is not present in this patient.

KEY POINT

- IgA vasculitis is associated with abdominal pain, palpable purpura, arthralgia, and glomerulonephritis, with normal complement levels.

Bibliography
Jennette JC, Falk RJ, Bacon PA, et al. 2012 revised International Chapel Hill Consensus Conference Nomenclature of Vasculitides. Arthritis Rheum. 2013 Jan;65(1):1-11. [PMID: 23045170]

Item 72   Answer: D
Educational Objective: Identify vomiting as a cause of hypokalemia.

Vomiting is the most likely cause of this patient's hypokalemia. She presents with hypokalemic metabolic alkalosis with extracellular volume depletion. Hypokalemia, defined as a serum potassium concentration <3.5 mEq/L (3.5 mmol/L), can be life-threatening when severe. Patients usually have minimal symptoms unless serum potassium levels are <3.0 mEq/L (3.0 mmol/L); symptoms correlate with the rapidity of the decrease, ranging from generalized weakness and malaise to paralysis, depending on the serum potassium level. This patient's history (generalized weakness and lightheadedness), physical examination findings (volume contraction and dental caries), and urine electrolyte levels are most consistent with vomiting from bulimia nervosa. Vomiting results in loss of hydrogen chloride and fluid from gastric secretions, and, if persistent, results in volume contraction. Hypovolemia activates the renin-angiotensin system with an increase in sodium-hydrogen exchange and increased bicarbonate reabsorption in the proximal tubule due to increased luminal hydrogen ion, and exacerbated by decreased chloride available for reabsorption with sodium. Increased aldosterone secretion stimulates sodium-potassium exchange in the distal tubule. The urine electrolytes in this patient reflect these physiologic changes. With volume depletion, the urine sodium concentration is generally low (<20 mEq/L [20 mmol/L]) due to the kidney's conservation of sodium. However, in this case, excess filtered bicarbonate associated with the alkalosis is excreted through the renal tubule, and sodium is lost in the urine as an obligatory cation with bicarbonate necessary to maintain electroneutrality; this results in increased urine sodium excretion. Because of this, the urine chloride is a more accurate determination of volume status than the urine sodium in metabolic alkalosis. The urine chloride concentration is low (<20 mEq/L [20 mmol/L]), reflecting gastrointestinal losses and prolonged volume contraction that leads to avid reabsorption of chloride with sodium. The urine potassium concentration in this patient is elevated (>40 mEq/L [40 mmol/L]) due to increased aldosterone production and distal nephron bicarbonate delivery that promote potassium loss through the kidney. Treatment of these abnormalities is to treat the vomiting and provide volume expansion with normal saline and potassium replacement, which will reverse these changes and correct the acid-base and electrolyte abnormalities.

Bartter syndrome mimics the effect of a loop diuretic and is accompanied by increased urine sodium (>40 mEq/L [40 mmol/L]), urine potassium (>40 mEq/L [40 mmol/L]), and chloride excretion (>40 mEq/L [40 mmol/L]).

Hypokalemic periodic paralysis is due to a shift of potassium into cells and is not associated with a metabolic alkalosis; furthermore, urine potassium would be low (<20 mEq/L [20 mmol/L]) and not increased.

Hypokalemia from Sjögren syndrome occurs in the setting of renal tubular acidosis, and a hyperchloremic metabolic acidosis would occur, which is not seen in this patient.

KEY POINT

- Hypokalemia due to vomiting is associated with metabolic alkalosis, increased urine potassium excretion, and decreased urine chloride excretion.

Bibliography

Unwin RJ, Luft FC, Shirley DG. Pathophysiology and management of hypokalemia: a clinical perspective. Nat Rev Nephrol. 2011 Feb;7(2): 75-84. [PMID: 21278718]

Item 73   Answer: C

Educational Objective: Diagnose thrombotic microangiopathy.

The next step in diagnosis is a peripheral blood smear. This patient has findings suggestive of Shiga toxin–associated hemolytic uremic syndrome (HUS). This is a diarrhea-associated syndrome of microangiopathic hemolytic anemia, thrombocytopenia, and kidney failure caused by Shiga toxin–producing *Escherichia coli*, typically with serotypes O157:H7, O104:H4, and, less commonly, *Shigella dysenteriae*. Shiga toxin binds to endothelial cells, triggering thrombosis and resulting in a thrombotic microangiopathy. It also binds to renal mesangial cells, podocytes, and renal tubular cells, causing direct damage. These actions lead to acute kidney injury (AKI). Although this patient has a consistent clinical history, a peripheral blood smear is essential to determine whether the anemia is caused by a microangiopathic hemolytic process as indicated by the presence of schistocytes. Stool cultures may reveal the offending organism. Treatment is primarily supportive, and many patients require dialysis.

ADAMTS13 is a metalloprotease enzyme that cleaves von Willebrand factor; low activity levels are supportive of a diagnosis of thrombotic thrombocytopenic purpura (TTP). Although this would be a reasonable study in this patient if a likely diagnosis of Shiga toxin–associated HUS were less clear to assess for the possibility of TTP, confirmation of true thrombocytopenia and microangiopathic hemolytic anemia would be an initial diagnostic step before additional testing.

Kidney biopsy would show evidence of capillary thrombosis as well as glomerular and tubular damage, but it is not necessary to establish the diagnosis of Shiga toxin–associated HUS.

Urine protein electrophoresis may be useful in evaluating AKI due to monoclonal urine immunoglobulin light chains (Bence Jones proteins). Although a plasma cell disorder may cause anemia and AKI due to precipitation of light chains in the renal tubule (myeloma kidney), it is not a cause of microangiopathic hemolytic anemia or thrombocytopenia as seen in this patient.

KEY POINT

- Shiga toxin–associated hemolytic uremic syndrome is a diarrhea-associated syndrome of microangiopathic hemolytic anemia, thrombocytopenia, and kidney failure caused by Shiga toxin–producing *Escherichia coli*.

Bibliography

George JN, Nester CM. Syndromes of thrombotic microangiopathy. N Engl J Med. 2014 Aug 14;371(7):654-66. [PMID: 25119611]

Item 74   Answer: B

Educational Objective: Evaluate a pregnant patient for suspected nephrolithiasis using ultrasonography.

Bilateral kidney ultrasonography is the most appropriate diagnostic study for this pregnant patient with suspected nephrolithiasis. Although noncontrast helical CT has traditionally been the most commonly used imaging technique for suspected nephrolithiasis because it detects most stones, provides helpful anatomic information, visualizes the entire urinary tract, and may potentially provide alternative diagnoses if nephrolithiasis is not detected, it is associated with significant radiation exposure and is therefore contraindicated in pregnant women. Kidney ultrasonography is increasingly being used as an initial diagnostic study for nonpregnant patients with suspected nephrolithiasis, particularly younger patients, to avoid significant radiation exposure, and it is the study of choice for pregnant women with possible kidney stones. Although it is less sensitive than CT for kidney stones, particularly for small stones or those in the distal urinary tract, a positive study for nephrolithiasis can exclude complications such as hydronephrosis and remove the need for more extensive additional testing.

Abdominal MRI can be used during pregnancy, but it is not optimal for imaging kidney stones. Ultrasonography is preferred, although MRI may be a diagnostic option if additional imaging is required for diagnosis.

Low-dose CT is both sensitive and specific for detecting kidney stones but is also associated with significant radiation exposure, similar to conventional stone protocol CT. Low-dose CT is absolutely contraindicated in the first trimester of pregnancy and is used only in specific situations in pregnant women in the second or third trimesters. It is not an appropriate study for this patient.

Plain abdominal radiography has limited utility for suspected nephrolithiasis due to its inability to detect

CONT.

radiolucent stones and the limited anatomic information it provides. It also involves radiation exposure and is not an appropriate next test in this patient.

Transvaginal ultrasonography may be used to detect distal ureteral stones in pregnant women with suspected nephrolithiasis and an unrevealing kidney ultrasound. However, it is not an appropriate next test for this patient.

KEY POINT

- Ultrasonography is the preferred diagnostic imaging modality for pregnant patients with suspected nephrolithiasis because it does not expose patients to radiation.

Bibliography
Semins MJ, Matlaga BR. Kidney stones and pregnancy. Adv Chronic Kidney Dis. 2013 May;20(3):260-4. [PMID: 23928391]

Item 75   Answer: A
Educational Objective: Treat calcium oxalate nephrolithiasis with bile salt binders in a patient with enteric hyperoxaluria.

Treatment with cholestyramine is an appropriate additional therapy for this patient with enteric hyperoxaluria. Hyperoxaluria predisposes to calcium oxalate stone formation. Excessive oxalate in the urine may result from excessive intake (from foods such as chocolate, spinach, rhubarb, or green and black tea) or in situations in which there is significant restriction in dietary calcium intake, which decreases binding of calcium to dietary oxalate in the gut and increases oxalate absorption. Enteric hyperoxaluria results from malabsorption when excessive free fatty acids in the gastrointestinal lumen bind calcium, increasing free oxalate absorption in the colon as may be seen in patients with small bowel disease or bowel resection. In addition to maintaining an adequate urine output of at least 2 L/d and ensuring adequate dietary calcium intake, patients with enteric hyperoxaluria may benefit from the bile salt binder cholestyramine, which also binds oxalate in the gut. This therapy is indicated in this patient with recurrent calcium oxalate nephrolithiasis following small bowel resection unresponsive to other treatments.

Thiazide diuretics, such as hydrochlorothiazide, are used in patients with idiopathic hypercalciuria to reduce calcium excretion in the urine by inducing mild hypovolemia that results in increased sodium reabsorption and passive calcium reabsorption in the proximal tubule. However, this patient does not have evidence of hypercalciuria, and thiazide therapy would not decrease the excessive oxalate in the urine.

Urine citrate inhibits stone formation by binding calcium in the tubular lumen, preventing it from precipitating with oxalate. Citrate excretion can be enhanced in patients with low urine citrate levels by alkalinizing the serum with potassium citrate, which decreases uptake of filtered citrate

from the tubular lumen. However, this patient does not have evidence of hypocitraturia and would not be expected to benefit from additional urine citrate.

Pyridoxine is indicated in some patients with primary hyperoxaluria to improve glyoxylate metabolism and reduce overproduction of oxalate. However, this would not be effective in this patient with enteric hyperoxaluria.

KEY POINT

- Patients with enteric hyperoxaluria and calcium oxalate nephrolithiasis may benefit from treatment with bile salt binders to decrease intestinal oxalate absorption.

Bibliography
Heilberg IP, Goldfarb DS. Optimum nutrition for kidney stone disease. Adv Chronic Kidney Dis. 2013 Mar;20(2):165-74. [PMID: 23439376]

Item 76   Answer: D

Educational Objective: Diagnose a complex mixed acid-base disorder.

The most likely diagnosis is a complex mixed acid-base disorder consisting of respiratory alkalosis, increased anion gap metabolic acidosis, and metabolic alkalosis. Analysis of acid-base disorders requires the identification of the likely dominant acid-base disorder, followed by an assessment of the secondary, compensatory response. When measured values fall outside the range of the predicted secondary response, a mixed acid-base disorder is present; multiple acid-base disturbances may coexist in a single patient. This patient's dominant acid-base disorder is alkalosis, as indicated by the blood pH of 7.56. The low P_{CO_2} indicates a respiratory component to the alkalosis. The expected compensation for chronic respiratory alkalosis is a decrease in the serum bicarbonate of 4 to 5 mEq/L (4-5 mmol/L) for each 10 mm Hg (1.3 kPa) decrease in the P_{CO_2}. The expected serum bicarbonate concentration in this patient is calculated to be 14 to 16 mEq/L (14-16 mmol/L), and the measured serum bicarbonate of 20 mEq/L (20 mmol/L) suggests coexistence of a metabolic alkalosis. This patient also has an elevated anion gap indicating the presence of an increased anion gap metabolic acidosis. The change of the anion gap from normal is 10 mEq/L (10 mmol/L). Calculating the ratio of the change in the anion gap (Δ anion gap) to the change in bicarbonate level (Δ bicarbonate), or the "Δ-Δ ratio," can help confirm if there is a coexisting acid-base disturbance. A ratio of <1 may reflect the presence of concurrent normal anion gap metabolic acidosis, whereas a ratio of >2 may indicate the presence of metabolic alkalosis. This patient's Δ-Δ ratio is 2.5, confirming the coexistence of a metabolic alkalosis. The clinical scenario most likely responsible for this complex acid-base disorder is salicylate toxicity with central hyperventilation from the salicylate, anion gap metabolic acidosis from the salicylate, and metabolic alkalosis from gastritis and vomiting.

KEY POINT

- Analysis of acid-base disorders requires the identification of the likely dominant acid-base disorder, followed by an assessment of the secondary, compensatory response; when measured values fall outside the range of the predicted secondary response, a mixed acid-base disorder is present.

Bibliography

Seifter JL. Integration of acid-base and electrolyte disorders. N Engl J Med. 2014 Nov 6;371(19):1821-31. [PMID: 25372090]

Item 77   Answer: D

Educational Objective: Diagnose drug-induced tubulointerstitial disease presenting as Fanconi syndrome.

This patient has tubulointerstitial disease, likely due to long-standing exposure to tenofovir. Evidence for a tubulointerstitial process includes a slowly progressive course without a clear inciting event, subnephrotic proteinuria, bland urine sediment, and a kidney ultrasound showing atrophic kidneys. History and physical examination should focus on conditions associated with tubulointerstitial disease and a careful review of medications, because numerous medications may induce tubulointerstitial disease. An associated characteristic that may be present with tubulointerstitial disease is abnormal tubular handling of glucose, amino acids, uric acid, phosphate, and bicarbonate (termed *Fanconi syndrome*); renal tubular acidosis is also common. Patients may also have concentrating defects and may present with nocturia and polyuria. With more advanced disease, anemia may be present due to the destruction of erythropoietin-producing cells in the kidney. This patient's findings are consistent with tubulointerstitial disease with Fanconi syndrome, indicated by glucosuria in the context of normoglycemia, trace proteinuria, and hypophosphatemia. Because tenofovir has been associated with tubulointerstitial disease, it is the likely cause in this patient.

Hypertensive nephropathy involves damage to the vascular structures, glomeruli, and tubulointerstitial regions of the kidney. It may cause progressive kidney failure, often with elevated protein excretion (less than 1000 mg/24 h). However, the rapid progression of kidney dysfunction and the presence of tubular dysfunction (Fanconi syndrome) characteristic of tubulointerstitial disease make hypertensive nephropathy less likely in this patient.

Membranoproliferative glomerulonephritis may also be associated with chronic hepatitis B infection and involves immune complex deposition in the glomeruli. It typically presents with hematuria (often with dysmorphic erythrocytes and/or erythrocyte casts), variable degrees of proteinuria, and a reduced glomerular filtration rate. This would not be a consistent finding in this patient with a bland urine sediment.

Membranous glomerulopathy is common in patients with chronic hepatitis B infection and appears to be related to subendothelial and mesangial immune deposits in the glomeruli. Because it primarily affects the glomeruli, it is associated with high levels of proteinuria, usually in the nephrotic range, and would not be expected to present with tubular dysfunction and Fanconi syndrome as seen in this patient.

KEY POINT

- Kidney disease with a tubulointerstitial process is characterized by a slowly progressive course without a clear inciting event, subnephrotic proteinuria, bland urine sediment, and a kidney ultrasound showing atrophic kidneys.

Bibliography

Tourret J, Deray G, Isnard-Bagnis C. Tenofovir effect on the kidneys of HIV-infected patients: a double-edged sword? J Am Soc Nephrol. 2013 Oct;24(10):1519-27. [PMID: 24052632]

Item 78   Answer: E

Educational Objective: Diagnose hypophosphatemia due to refeeding syndrome.

The most likely cause of this patient's respiratory failure is hypophosphatemia, which occurs in patients with chronic alcohol use, malnutrition, or critical illness. Symptoms rarely occur unless the serum phosphate concentration is <2.0 mg/dL (0.65 mmol/L); severe symptoms occur with a serum phosphate concentration <1.0 mg/dL (0.32 mmol/L). Symptoms include weakness, myalgia, rhabdomyolysis, arrhythmias, heart failure, respiratory failure, seizures, coma, and hemolysis. This patient has chronic alcoholism with moderate hypophosphatemia on presentation. Factors that contribute to hypophosphatemia in the patient with chronic alcohol use include decreased dietary intake of phosphate and vitamin D, chronic diarrhea, and a direct toxic effect of alcohol on the proximal tubule. Intravenous dextrose-containing fluids can exacerbate the hypophosphatemia by causing a refeeding syndrome. Glucose stimulates insulin release, which promotes phosphate uptake by the cells and worsening hypophosphatemia. Severe hypophosphatemia can cause respiratory failure from impaired diaphragmatic contractility.

In general, total calcium declines by 0.8 mg/dL (0.2 mmol/L) for each 1.0 g/dL (10 g/L) decrement in serum albumin concentration. This patient's calcium correction for hypoalbuminemia is 8.8 mg/dL (2.2 mmol/L), which is not low and does not explain the respiratory failure.

This patient has mild hypokalemia. Although severe hypokalemia can cause profound muscle weakness, it is unlikely that his serum potassium would decrease to such critically low levels to cause paralysis based on his current treatment.

The patient's magnesium level is within the lower limits of normal range and unlikely to be the cause of his respiratory failure.

Although the patient does have hyponatremia, it is not severe and would not result in respiratory failure. Symptoms

CONT.

of acute hyponatremia are caused by cerebral edema and usually do not manifest until the sodium concentration is lower than 125 mEq/L (125 mmol/L).

KEY POINT

- Intravenous dextrose-containing fluids can exacerbate hypophosphatemia by stimulating insulin release, which promotes phosphate uptake by the cells and worsening hypophosphatemia.

Bibliography
Imel EA, Econs MJ. Approach to the hypophosphatemic patient. J Clin Endocrinol Metab. 2012 Mar;97(3):696-706. [PMID: 22392950]

Item 79   Answer: C

Educational Objective: Identify NSAIDs as a cause of elevated blood pressure

Discontinuing ibuprofen is an appropriate next step in managing this patient's blood pressure. She has elevated blood pressure not yet defined as hypertension, a diagnosis that requires a systolic blood pressure ≥140 mm Hg and/or a diastolic blood pressure ≥90 mm Hg documented during three separate office visits over a period of 1 week or longer. In this case, a review of medications, including over-the-counter and herbal medications, is important because a number of these agents can contribute to elevated blood pressure. This patient is taking an NSAID, ibuprofen, for osteoarthritis. All NSAIDs contribute to hypertension by inhibition of cyclooxygenase-2 in the kidneys, promoting sodium retention and increased intravascular volume. Additional effects of NSAIDs include hyperkalemia, which is mild in this case. NSAIDs lower renal renin secretion and angiotensin II–induced aldosterone release, reducing urine potassium excretion. Therefore, discontinuing the ibuprofen is appropriate for this patient. Reassessing her blood pressure when not taking an NSAID will provide a more accurate measure of her baseline blood pressure status.

Beginning antihypertensive therapy at this point is not indicated; in particular, ACE inhibitor use would be contraindicated because further inhibition of the renin-angiotensin system could exacerbate this patient's hyperkalemia.

Similarly, hydrochlorothiazide is an effective antihypertensive agent, but initiating treatment is not indicated prior to establishing a diagnosis of hypertension.

A plasma aldosterone-plasma renin ratio is used to evaluate patients with hypertension and a high suspicion for hyperaldosteronism (for example, evidence of resistant hypertension and a low serum potassium level). Testing is therefore not indicated in this patient without a clear diagnosis of hypertension and who has hyperkalemia.

KEY POINT

- Identification of medications that contribute to blood pressure elevation is necessary in patients with elevated blood pressure not yet defined as hypertension.

Bibliography
Sudano I, Flammer AJ, Roas S, Enseleit F, Noll G, Ruschitzka F. Nonsteroidal antiinflammatory drugs, acetaminophen, and hypertension. Curr Hypertens Rep. 2012 Aug;14(4):304-9. [PMID: 22610476]

Item 80   Answer: A

Educational Objective: Diagnose D-lactic acidosis.

This patient has an increased anion gap metabolic acidosis, and the most likely cause is D-lactic acidosis. Accumulation of the D-isomer of lactate can occur in patients with short-bowel syndrome following jejunoileal bypass or small-bowel resection. In these patients, excess carbohydrates that reach the colon are metabolized to D-lactate. Symptoms include intermittent confusion, slurred speech, and ataxia. Laboratory studies show increased anion gap metabolic acidosis with normal plasma lactate levels, because the D-isomer is not measured by conventional laboratory assays for lactate. Diagnosis should be considered in patients with an unexplained increased anion gap metabolic acidosis in the appropriate clinical context; it is confirmed by specifically measuring D-lactate.

Ethylene glycol or methanol intoxication should be suspected in patients with an increased anion gap metabolic acidosis associated with a serum bicarbonate level <10 mEq/L (10 mmol/L) and a plasma osmolal gap >10 mOsm/kg H_2O. This patient's serum bicarbonate level is 20 mEq/L (20 mmol/L) and the calculated osmolal gap is 6 mOsm/kg H_2O, making alcohol poisoning a less likely diagnosis.

Propylene glycol is a solvent used as a vehicle for numerous intravenously administered medications. In propylene glycol toxicity, laboratory findings include increased anion gap metabolic acidosis and concomitant increased osmolal gap. The metabolic acidosis is principally due to L-lactic and D-lactic acidosis, the acid metabolites of propylene glycol. This patient's clinical history and osmolal gap are not consistent with propylene glycol toxicity.

Pyroglutamic acidosis is a cause of increased anion gap metabolic acidosis in patients receiving therapeutic doses of acetaminophen on a chronic basis. Clinical manifestations are limited to mental status changes and increased anion gap metabolic acidosis. The syndrome most commonly occurs in patients with critical illness, poor nutrition, liver disease, or chronic kidney disease as well as in persons on a vegetarian diet. Diagnosis can be confirmed by measuring urine levels of pyroglutamic acid. This patient's history is most compatible with D-lactic acidosis and does not support acetaminophen ingestion.

KEY POINT

- Manifestations of D-lactic acidosis include intermittent confusion, slurred speech, ataxia, and an increased anion gap metabolic acidosis with a normal plasma lactate level.

Bibliography
Kraut JA, Madias NE. Lactic acidosis. N Engl J Med. 2014 Dec 11;371(24):2309-19. [PMID: 25494270]

Item 81   **Answer:**   **B**

Educational Objective: Treat suspected catheter-related bacteremia in a patient with end-stage kidney disease.

The most appropriate next step in management is to begin broad-spectrum antibiotic coverage, such as vancomycin plus ceftazidime. This patient with end-stage kidney disease (ESKD) who is receiving dialysis via a catheter is at high risk for catheter-related bacteremia. Infection is the second most common cause of death in patients with ESKD (after cardiovascular disease), and catheter-related infections are an important cause of morbidity and mortality. It is therefore important to provide immediate empiric broad-spectrum antibiotics in patients dialyzing via a catheter who exhibit evidence of infection unless there is another obvious source of fever. Most dialysis-related bacteremias are caused by gram-positive bacteria, and empiric coverage must include therapy that takes into account the local resistance patterns of *Staphylococcus aureus*. Additionally, gram-negative organisms should also be covered until culture results are known and appropriate, focused antimicrobial therapy is prescribed.

If blood cultures remain negative, empiric antibiotics may be stopped if symptoms have resolved and no other potential source of infection has been identified. If blood cultures return positive, it is usually advisable to remove the catheter because success rates for catheter salvage are low for most organisms. If there is no evidence of infection of the catheter tunnel, dialysis catheters can be safely exchanged over a wire in patients who have been asymptomatic on appropriate antibiotic therapy for at least 48 hours. However, either removing or exchanging the dialysis catheter in the setting of possible infection without antibiotic therapy is not appropriate.

KEY POINT

- Immediate empiric broad-spectrum antibiotics must be initiated in patients with end-stage kidney disease who are on dialysis and have suspected catheter-related infection.

Bibliography

Mermel LA, Allon M, Bouza E, et al. Clinical practice guidelines for the diagnosis and management of intravascular catheter-related infection: 2009 Update by the Infectious Diseases Society of America. Clin Infect Dis. 2009 Jul 1;49(1):1-45. [PMID: 19489710]

 Item 82   **Answer:**   **C**

Educational Objective: Measure urine chloride levels to determine the cause of metabolic alkalosis.

Measurement of this patient's urine chloride level is the most appropriate next step in management. She has a metabolic alkalosis as evidenced by the elevated blood pH and elevated serum bicarbonate level. Metabolic alkalosis is caused by net loss of acid or retention of serum bicarbonate. Metabolic alkalosis can be classified as either occurring with normal extracellular fluid volume, hypovolemia, or decreased effective arterial blood volume and increased extracellular fluid volume (heart failure, cirrhosis, nephrosis), or occurring with increased extracellular fluid volume and hypertension. This patient's clinical volume status is equivocal; blood pressure is slightly low and pulse rate is slightly high, yet there is peripheral edema, which could be explained by either cardiac or noncardiac causes (for example, a side effect of amlodipine), and mild hypoxia, which could be cardiac or pulmonary in etiology, given her medical history. Urine chloride measurement can help determine the cause of metabolic alkalosis, particularly if it is difficult to clinically assess volume status. In such patients, a low (<15 mEq/L [15 mmol/L]) urine chloride suggests reduction in extracellular volume and the presence of saline-responsive metabolic alkalosis. Conditions that are associated with saline-responsive metabolic alkalosis include vomiting, remote use of diuretics, and post-hypercapnic metabolic alkalosis. If the urine chloride is high (>15 mEq/L [15 mmol/L]), the metabolic alkalosis is saline resistant and can be caused by active diuretic use, stimulant laxative abuse, and rare renal tubular disorders such as Gitelman and Bartter syndromes. In this case, the patient's metabolic alkalosis is due to vomiting, and a low urine chloride would direct appropriate management to saline infusion.

Saline infusion without first categorizing the nature of the metabolic alkalosis is inappropriate and potentially dangerous in patients with limited cardiac reserve or hypoxia.

There is no clear evidence of volume overload that requires administration of a loop diuretic such as furosemide. Loop diuretic therapy is likely to worsen metabolic alkalosis by increasing the secretion of aldosterone and distal delivery of sodium, resulting in urine potassium and hydrogen loss.

In patients with metabolic alkalosis, measurement of urine chloride rather than urine sodium is used to determine volume status and saline responsiveness because urine sodium can be artificially high during periods of appropriate compensatory urine bicarbonate excretion (sodium is the primary cation excreted in an obligatory fashion with bicarbonate).

KEY POINT

- Measurement of urine chloride levels can be useful to determine volume status and saline responsiveness in patients with metabolic alkalosis.

Bibliography

Soifer JT, Kim HT. Approach to metabolic alkalosis. Emerg Med Clin North Am. 2014 May;32(2):453-63. [PMID: 24766943]

Item 83   **Answer:**   **A**

Educational Objective: Diagnose autosomal dominant polycystic kidney disease.

The most likely diagnosis is autosomal dominant polycystic kidney disease (ADPKD). The hallmark of ADPKD is

CONT.

large kidneys with multiple kidney cysts, and patients may have resulting chronic, mild abdominal discomfort; in some cases, palpable abdominal masses occur, as in this patient. Patients with ADPKD may also present acutely with severe pain and hematuria resulting from bleeding of a cyst, as seen in this patient. ADPKD is the most common inherited kidney disorder, occurring in 1 of 400 to 1 of 1000 live births. Although transmitted in an autosomal dominant manner, a negative family history does not necessarily exclude ADPKD. Approximately 15% of patients with ADPKD have spontaneous mutations that result in the disease. Alternatively, one of the patient's parents may have a less severe phenotype without clinical manifestations.

Renal cell carcinoma does not occur with greater frequency in patients with ADPKD than in the general population and does not present with bilateral abdominal masses.

Renal vein thrombosis may present with acute-onset flank pain and macroscopic hematuria and may show enlargement of the involved kidney. However, renal vein thrombosis does not result in bilateral abdominal masses and is more commonly seen in hypercoagulable states, such as the nephrotic syndrome or the antiphospholipid antibody syndrome. This patient has no evidence of hypercoagulability.

Gross hematuria often occurs in patients with urinary tract infection. However, this patient has no accompanying urinary symptoms, and the leukocytes in her urine are likely the result of gross bleeding into the urinary tract. Additionally, urinary tract infection would not explain the abdominal masses seen in this patient.

KEY POINT

- A negative family history does not exclude autosomal dominant polycystic kidney disease (ADPKD)– approximately 15% of patients with ADPKD have spontaneous mutations that result in the disease.

Bibliography
Grantham JJ. Clinical practice. Autosomal dominant polycystic kidney disease. N Engl J Med 2008 Oct 2;359(14):1477-85. [PMID: 18832246]

Item 84   Answer: D
Educational Objective: Treat tumor lysis syndrome.

Rasburicase is appropriate to treat hyperuricemia in this patient with tumor lysis syndrome (TLS). TLS is characterized by the massive release of uric acid, potassium, and phosphate into the blood from rapid lysis of malignant cells. It typically occurs after initiation of cytotoxic therapy for hematologic malignancies with large tumor burden (such as high-grade lymphomas) or high cell counts (such as acute lymphoblastic leukemia), but TLS can also occur spontaneously. Acute kidney injury (AKI) results from intratubular precipitation of urate and calcium phosphate crystals. Clinical features include hyperuricemia, hyperkalemia, hyperphosphatemia, and hypocalcemia. General principles for the management of patients at high or inter-

mediate risk or presenting with TLS are aggressive volume expansion, management of hyperkalemia, and preventive therapy for hyperuricemia. This patient has TLS with evidence of uric acid nephropathy and requires rasburicase to reduce serum urate levels. Rasburicase rapidly converts uric acid to allantoin, which is 5 to 10 times more soluble than uric acid and readily excreted through the kidney. Rasburicase has a much faster action than allopurinol and can decrease serum urate levels within 4 hours of administration.

Indications for dialysis include oliguria or anuria, persistent hyperkalemia, hyperphosphatemia-induced symptomatic hypocalcemia, and a calcium phosphate product $\geq$70 mg^2/dL^2 in the setting of AKI. This patient has none of these indications for dialysis.

Urine alkalinization increases the excretion of uric acid by increasing its solubility. However, in the setting of hyperphosphatemia, it can cause precipitation of calcium phosphate crystals in the kidney. Urine alkalinization is not necessary when rasburicase is used, and it role in TLS is controversial.

Allopurinol competitively inhibits xanthine oxidase, blocking the metabolism of hypoxanthine and xanthine to uric acid. Allopurinol effectively decreases the formation of new uric acid and therefore does not affect circulating uric acid. Increasing the dose of allopurinol is therefore not indicated.

KEY POINT

- Patients with tumor lysis syndrome and evidence of uric acid nephropathy require treatment with rasburicase to reduce serum urate levels.

Bibliography
Howard SC, Jones DP, Pui CH. The tumor lysis syndrome. N Engl J Med. 2011 May;364(19):1844-54. [PMID: 21561350]

Item 85   Answer: D
Educational Objective: Manage IgA nephropathy.

Continued observation is the appropriate next step in management in this patient with likely IgA nephropathy (IgAN). IgAN is the most frequent cause of chronic glomerulonephritis, occurs more commonly in men, and most frequently occurs in the second to third decades of life. IgAN involves formation of autoantibodies against structurally abnormal IgA leading to immune complex formation; these immune complexes are deposited in the glomeruli in IgAN or in multiple extrarenal sites in IgA vasculitis (Henoch Schönlein purpura). This young patient has asymptomatic gross hematuria with a nephritic urine sediment without the full nephritic syndrome (hypertension and azotemia are absent). The presence of nephritis with normal or negative serologies (particularly normal complement levels) and improving kidney function and proteinuria suggests IgAN as the most likely diagnosis. IgAN tends to be a chronic condition with a good prognosis in most patients. Factors associated with a worse outcome include hypertension, kidney dysfunction, persistent proteinuria >1000 mg/g, and mesangial and endothelial proliferation with tubulointerstitial damage on kidney biopsy. However, continued observation with serial blood pressure measurements, serum creatinine levels, and urine studies is appropriate in this patient without high-risk features and an improving clinical course.

Treatment with inhibitors of the renin-angiotensin system (such as an ACE inhibitor) slow the rate of progression of most proteinuric chronic kidney diseases and are often used in patients with IgAN with significant proteinuria and high-risk features. However, low-risk patients with minimal proteinuria are usually not actively treated and are followed with continued observation.

Kidney biopsy is usually reserved for patients with high risk for poor outcome. It is not indicated in this patient with no high-risk features of progressive IgAN, such as a urine protein-creatinine ratio >1000 mg/g or a low glomerular filtration rate.

Glucocorticoids are used to treat patients with high-risk disease.

KEY POINT

- Observation with serial blood pressure measurements, urine studies, and serum creatinine levels is appropriate for patients with IgA nephropathy with low-risk features for progression.

Bibliography
Wyatt RJ, Julian BA. IgA nephropathy. N Engl J Med. 2013 Jun 20;368(25):2402-14. [PMID: 23782179]

Item 86   Answer: C

Educational Objective: Manage preeclampsia.

The most appropriate next step in management is delivery of the baby in this woman with preeclampsia without features of severe disease. Preeclampsia is classically defined as new-onset hypertension after 20 weeks of pregnancy with proteinuria (≥300 mg/24 h or a urine protein-creatinine ratio ≥300 mg/g). Delivery of the baby is the definitive treatment for preeclampsia. In patients with preeclampsia and severe disease, generally defined as severe hypertension (systolic blood pressure ≥160 mm Hg or diastolic blood pressure ≥110 mm Hg), thrombocytopenia (platelet count <100,000/μL [100 × 10^9/L]), kidney dysfunction (serum creatinine concentration >1.1 mg/dL [97.2 μmol/L] or doubling of the serum creatinine concentration in the absence of other kidney disease), impaired liver function (elevated blood concentrations of liver aminotransferases to twice the normal concentration), pulmonary edema, or cerebral or visual symptoms, management decisions are usually made based on the balance of fetal and maternal risk with the implications of preterm delivery. In women with preeclampsia without severe features, delivery at 37 weeks has been shown to optimize both maternal and neonatal outcomes (such as

fetal growth restriction, abruption placentae, hemorrhage due to thrombocytopenia, seizures, cerebral hemorrhage, pulmonary edema, and kidney injury) and is the most appropriate next step in managing this patient.

Treatment of mild hypertension in preeclampsia has not been shown to alter the course of disease or improve fetal outcomes. Therefore, antihypertensive treatment is generally reserved for patients with preeclampsia with severe hypertension, which is not present in this patient.

There is evidence that low-dose aspirin therapy may be beneficial in reducing the occurrence of preeclampsia in moderate- to high-risk women. However, it does not have a role in treating preeclampsia or eclampsia.

Glucocorticoids are used to accelerate fetal lung maturation if delivery is contemplated before the 34th week of pregnancy but do not directly affect outcomes in preeclampsia. Therefore, their use is not indicated in this patient.

Because of the benefit of delivery at 37 weeks' gestation in women with preeclampsia, continued monitoring beyond this time is not optimal.

KEY POINT

- Definitive therapy for preeclampsia is delivery of the baby.

Bibliography
Steegers EA, von Dadelszen P, Duvekot JJ, Pijnenborg R. Pre-eclampsia. Lancet. 2010 Aug 21;376(9741):631-44. [PMID: 20598363]

Item 87   Answer: D

Educational Objective: Manage secondary focal segmental glomerulosclerosis.

In addition to starting an ACE inhibitor, weight loss is indicated for this patient with likely secondary focal segmental glomerulosclerosis (FSGS). This patient with obesity, hypertension, and nephrotic-range proteinuria (with normal serum albumin) has FSGS on kidney biopsy. FSGS may be primary (idiopathic) or secondary, and the appropriate therapeutic approach is based on determining the likely cause of the disorder. Primary FSGS involves glomerular injury due to an unclear insult; features suggesting primary FSGS include a low serum albumin level and extensive foot process effacement on kidney biopsy. Patients usually present with hypertension, hypoalbuminemia, and some degree of kidney failure in addition to nephrotic-range proteinuria. Some patients with primary FSGS respond well to immunosuppressive therapy, and this is typically offered to patients with this diagnosis. Secondary FSGS is believed to result from an adaptive response to glomerular hypertrophy or hyperfiltration associated with a number of conditions (including obesity) in which the glomerular filtration rate may be markedly increased; glomeruli on biopsy are often enlarged, reflecting hyperfiltration with only mild foot process effacement. These patients have minimal edema and rarely have the full spectrum of the nephrotic syndrome. In obese patients with likely secondary FSGS, weight loss is sometimes associated with a drop in proteinuria, as is the use of ACE inhibitors or angiotensin receptor blockers, and is the preferred initial therapy.

Immunosuppressive therapy with glucocorticoids or other agents such as the calcineurin inhibitor tacrolimus is not indicated in secondary FSGS.

FSGS is not typically associated with syphilis, and testing for this entity using a rapid plasma reagin test is not indicated.

KEY POINT

- In obese patients with likely secondary focal segmental glomerulosclerosis, weight loss is sometimes associated with a drop in proteinuria, as is the use of ACE inhibitors or angiotensin receptor blockers, and is the preferred initial therapy.

Bibliography

Bose B, Cattran D; Toronto Glomerulonephritis Registry. Glomerular diseases: FSGS. Clin J Am Soc Nephrol. 2014 Mar;9(3):626-32. [PMID: 23990165]

H **Item 88** **Answer:** **B**

Educational Objective: Diagnose atheroembolic kidney disease.

The most likely diagnosis is atheroembolism of cholesterol crystals. Disruption of an atheromatous plaque by instrumentation or anticoagulation during this patient's cardiac catheterization likely caused embolization of cholesterol crystals from the plaque through the arterial circulation distal to the point of disruption. These crystals lodge in capillary beds and cause vascular obstruction but also trigger an inflammatory response. Acute kidney injury (AKI) is a common result of cholesterol embolization, which causes peripheral eosinophilia and hypocomplementemia and shows evidence of inflammation on urinalysis, frequently with eosinophiluria present. Embolization may also lead to digital ischemia or infarction ("blue toe" syndrome) due to digital arterial occlusion or central scotoma due to central retinal artery occlusion. Although not specific for cholesterol atheroembolism, livedo reticularis (areas of lace-like mottled and purplish skin over the legs and thighs) is commonly associated with this disorder. Management is primarily supportive; anti-inflammatory agents (such as glucocorticoids) are not routinely given for treatment of cholesterol atheroembolism.

Acute interstitial nephritis (AIN) should be suspected following the initiation of new medications, although none of the agents this patient is taking has been reported as a cause of AIN. A diffuse rash, but not livedo reticularis, is characteristic of AIN. Eosinophiluria was previously believed to diagnose AIN, but urine eosinophil determination has been shown to be neither sensitive nor specific in the diagnostic evaluation of AIN.

Contrast-induced nephropathy (CIN) is a diagnostic consideration given the dye load associated with cardiac catheterization. However, CIN typically presents as acute tubular necrosis with granular casts, and AKI due to CIN typically peaks at 24 to 72 hours but improves within 5 to 7 days.

Polyarteritis nodosa (PAN) is a necrotizing vasculitis of medium-sized arteries, sometimes associated with hairy cell leukemia or infection with hepatitis B or C. PAN may present with livedo reticularis, as in this patient, but kidney manifestations usually include renal arterial aneurysms with perirenal hematomas and severe hypertension, which findings are missing here. This patient also lacks any of the other neurologic or gastrointestinal manifestations of PAN.

KEY POINT

- Acute kidney injury is a common result of cholesterol embolization, which causes peripheral eosinophilia and hypocomplementemia and shows evidence of inflammation on urinalysis, frequently with eosinophiluria present.

Bibliography

Saric M, Kronzon I. Cholesterol embolization syndrome. Curr Opin Cardiol. 2011 Nov;26(6):472-9. [PMID: 21993354]

Item 89 **Answer:** **C**

Educational Objective: Treat stage 1 hypertension in a black patient.

The thiazide diuretic hydrochlorothiazide is the most appropriate agent for treating hypertension in this 57-year-old patient who is black. He has stage 1 hypertension, defined as a systolic blood pressure of 140-159 mm Hg and/or a diastolic blood pressure of 90-99 mm Hg. Thiazide diuretics (such as hydrochlorothiazide) and calcium channel blockers (such as amlodipine or diltiazem) alone or in combination are effective hypertensive treatment options for black patients and are recommended by the eighth report of the Joint National Committee (JNC 8) as initial therapy in this patient group. However, this patient is already taking a moderate dose of a statin (simvastatin) that undergoes significant metabolism via the cytochrome P450 3A4 (CYP3A4) pathway; lovastatin and, to a lesser extent, amlodipine are also metabolized through this pathway. Several calcium channel blockers inhibit or are metabolized through the CYP3A4 pathway and can increase the risk of statin myopathy in patients taking one of these particular statins. The dihydropyridine agents verapamil and diltiazem and the non-dihydropyridine agent amlodipine have been associated with increased risk with concurrent therapy with these drugs. Thus, hydrochlorothiazide is the most appropriate choice for this patient. The JNC 8 recommends a blood pressure goal of <140/90 mm Hg for black patients (for age ≥60 years, the target is <150/90 mm Hg, regardless of race). Prior recommendations had suggested blood pressure goals of <135/85 mm Hg in black patients given the higher risk of stroke and kidney disease compared with white patients. However, the African American Study of Kidney Disease and Hypertension (AASK) trial (comprised of black patients with hypertension and chronic kidney disease) did not demonstrate any difference in more aggressive (achieved blood pressure of 128/78 mm Hg) or less aggressive (achieved blood pressure of 141/85 mm Hg) blood pressure goals in slowing the rate of glomerular filtration rate decline or other secondary end points. Given his age and race, this patient's blood pressure goal is <140/90 mm Hg, according to JNC 8.

In general, black persons have less blood pressure response to renin-angiotensin system agents than other agents, despite similar plasma renin activity. Therefore, the ACE inhibitor lisinopril is not indicated for this patient.

KEY POINT

- The eighth report of the Joint National Committee recommends a thiazide diuretic or a calcium channel blocker alone or in combination as initial therapy for black patients with hypertension.

Bibliography

Appel LJ, Wright JT Jr, Greene T, et al. AASK Collaborative Research Group. Intensive blood-pressure control in hypertensive chronic kidney disease. N Engl J Med. 2010 Sep 2;363(10):918-29. [PMID: 20818902]

Item 90   Answer: C

Educational Objective: Treat acute ethylene glycol poisoning with intravenous sodium bicarbonate.

The most appropriate additional management intervention in this patient is intravenous sodium bicarbonate therapy. He has findings typical of ethylene glycol intoxication, with evidence of central nervous system depression presumably due to the alcohol, an increased anion gap metabolic acidosis of 28 mEq/L (28 mmol/L), an osmolal gap of 27 mOsm/kg H_2O, and kidney failure likely resulting from deposition of calcium oxalate crystals in the renal tubules. Because the laboratory confirmation of ethylene glycol intoxication may take days, empiric therapy for patients with likely ethylene glycol intoxication is recommended pending confirmation. Treatment usually consists of intravenous hydration, fomepizole (a competitive inhibitor of alcohol dehydrogenase), and hemodialysis to clear both the parent alcohol as well as the toxic metabolites. Intravenous sodium bicarbonate therapy is also recommended in suspected ethylene glycol or methanol ingestion when the blood pH is below 7.30. This is because the toxic metabolites of ethylene glycol (glycolate, glyoxylate, and oxalate) and methanol (formate) penetrate tissues more effectively when in the neutral state, which is increased by an acidic blood pH. Bicarbonate is given to normalize the blood pH and maximize formation of the ionized forms of the associated toxic metabolites.

Both ethylene glycol and methanol are completely absorbed from the gastrointestinal tract, with peak serum levels occurring within 1 to 2 hours of ingestion. Therefore, gastric decontamination, such as with activated charcoal, is not usually performed unless the timing of a large ingestion is known and decontamination can be performed within 1 hour.

Intravenous ethanol was traditionally used as a competitive inhibitor of alcohol dehydrogenase; it is effective because this enzyme has greater affinity for ethanol than for ethylene glycol or methanol. However, fomepizole has been found to be a superior therapy to ethanol, is easier to administer, and has fewer side effects. Although ethanol is a reasonable second-line therapy, there is no benefit to coadministration of fomepizole and ethanol.

Given the patient's possible ingestion of ethylene glycol with an associated low blood pH, not providing bicarbonate therapy would be inappropriate.

KEY POINT

- Empiric therapy with sodium bicarbonate, fomepizole, and hemodialysis is indicated for patients with suspected ethylene glycol intoxication.

Bibliography

Kruse JA. Methanol and ethylene glycol intoxication. Crit Care Clin. 2012 Oct;28(4):661-711. [PMID: 22998995]

Item 91   Answer: C

Educational Objective: Treat secondary hyperparathyroidism in a patient with chronic kidney disease.

The most appropriate next step in management is to begin oral calcitriol. This patient has secondary hyperparathyroidism due to severe chronic kidney disease (CKD). The first priority in treating these patients is to attempt to normalize calcium and phosphorus levels and treat vitamin D deficiency, if present. This patient has normal calcium, phosphorus, and 25-hydroxy vitamin D levels. If vitamin D levels are robust and the phosphorus level is normal, but the parathyroid hormone (PTH) level is elevated above target levels, active vitamin D analogues should be initiated. This is because 1-α hydroxylation of 25-hydroxy vitamin D is impaired in most patients with severe CKD, and these patients should begin oral calcitriol (1,25-dihydroxy vitamin D) or a calcitriol analogue (such as paricalcitol or doxercalciferol) to maintain bone health. Calcitriol directly suppresses PTH production by the parathyroid glands, thereby protecting bones from osteitis fibrosa cystica, which can occur as a result of chronic secondary hyperparathyroidism. Vitamin D analogues should be discontinued in the setting of hypercalcemia or hyperphosphatemia.

Bisphosphonates may be used in the treatment of osteoporosis. However, bisphosphonates may actually worsen some types of bone disease observed in the setting of CKD, especially adynamic bone disease.

Current Kidney Disease Improving Global Outcomes (KDIGO) guidelines do not recommend the routine use of dual-energy x-ray absorptiometry (DEXA) scans in patients with CKD because DEXA has poor predictive value for distinguishing histologic subtypes of bone disease in patients with CKD.

This patient does not have primary hyperparathyroidism, which is typically characterized by inappropriately elevated PTH levels in the setting of hypercalcemia. She has secondary hyperparathyroidism, which is driven by multiple factors, including reduced renal production of calcitriol and factors that are often present in patients with CKD such as hyperphosphatemia and hypocalcemia. Parathyroidectomy is reserved for patients with secondary hyperparathyroidism that is refractory to medical therapy (often referred to as tertiary hyperparathyroidism).

KEY POINT

- Patients with chronic kidney disease and normal calcium and phosphorus levels should be treated with active vitamin D analogues to reduce elevated parathyroid hormone levels and prevent renal osteodystrophy.

Bibliography

Kidney Disease: Improving Global Outcomes (KDIGO) CKD-MBD Work Group. KDIGO clinical practice guideline for the diagnosis, evaluation, prevention, and treatment of chronic kidney disease–mineral and bone disorder (CKD–MBD). Kidney Int Suppl. 2009 Aug;(113):S1-130. [PMID: 19644521]

Item 92   Answer: B

Educational Objective: Diagnose pseudohyponatremia.

The most likely diagnosis is pseudohyponatremia. Plasma osmolality can be measured using the following equation:

$$\text{Plasma Osmolality (mOsm/kg H}_2\text{O}) = 2 \times \text{Serum Sodium (mEq/L)} + \text{Plasma Glucose (mg/dL)}/18 + \text{Blood Urea Nitrogen (mg/dL)}/2.8$$

Using this formula, this patient's calculated plasma osmolality is approximately 266 mOsm/kg H_2O. However, his measured plasma osmolality is in the normal range. In the absence of ingested osmoles such as methanol or ethylene glycol, a normal plasma osmolality in a patient with a low serum sodium level strongly suggests pseudohyponatremia, caused by a laboratory error in the measurement of serum sodium. In normal persons, 93% of plasma is water. Laboratory analysis of serum sodium measures the amount of sodium (and thus the concentration of sodium) dissolved in the plasma water. If a substance is present that decreases the proportion of plasma that is water, such as in laboratories using ion-selective electrodes and indirect potentiometry, the measured serum sodium concentration will be falsely low, resulting in pseudohyponatremia. There are two usual causes of pseudohyponatremia: elevated serum lipid levels or the presence in the serum of abnormal paraproteins such as myeloma proteins. This patient has a medical history, symptoms, and signs suggestive of acute pancreatitis, which can be caused by significant hypertriglyceridemia and may result in pseudohyponatremia.

Patients with adrenal insufficiency may also have hyponatremia, caused by increased antidiuretic hormone (ADH) secretion in response to hypovolemia from urine salt wasting. However, these patients demonstrate a decrease in plasma osmolality rather than a normal plasma osmolality as seen in this patient.

Psychogenic polydipsia, in which patients ingest massive amounts of water, is characterized by hyponatremia with decreased plasma osmolality and decreased urine osmolality to less than the plasma osmolality, indicating maximum suppression of ADH with maximal urine dilution. These findings are not present in this patient.

Patients with the syndrome of inappropriate antidiuretic hormone secretion have hyponatremia with decreased plasma osmolality, which is not seen in this patient.

KEY POINT

- Pseudohyponatremia is caused by a laboratory error in the measurement of serum sodium due to the presence in the serum of elevated serum lipid levels or abnormal paraproteins such as myeloma proteins.

Bibliography

Liamis G, Liberopoulos E, Barkas F, Elisaf M. Spurious electrolyte disorders: a diagnostic challenge for clinicians. Am J Nephrol. 2013;38(1):50-7. [PMID: 23817179]

Item 93   Answer: C

Educational Objective: Treat minimal change glomerulopathy with glucocorticoids.

Glucocorticoids are indicated for this patient who most likely has minimal change glomerulopathy (MCG). MCG is the most common cause of idiopathic nephrotic syndrome in children and accounts for approximately 10% of cases in adults. Although the mechanism of MCG is not well understood, it results in fusion and dysfunction of the epithelial foot processes of the glomerulus, causing significant loss of protein and other macromolecules into the urine. Patients with MCG typically present with acute onset of edema and weight gain due to fluid retention. Urine protein levels tend to be significantly elevated (urine protein-creatinine ratio typically 5000-10,000 mg/g). The abrupt onset of the full nephrotic syndrome, a history of kidney disease in childhood that remitted, negative serologic tests, and a kidney biopsy showing normal light microscopic findings and negative immunofluorescence are diagnostic of MCG. Electron microscopy is confirmatory and usually demonstrates the extensive effacement of the podocyte foot processes. Most patients with MCG are symptomatic, and the disease does not remit spontaneously in the weeks or months after presentation. Treatment with immunosuppressive medications is recommended to prevent complications of severe nephrotic syndrome, including severe symptomatic edema, thromboembolic events, and infections. Glucocorticoids such as prednisone are recommended

CONT.

as first-line therapy unless there are contraindications. More than 80% of patients respond within 16 weeks of treatment. Alternative first-line therapy for patients with contraindications to glucocorticoids (for example, obesity, impaired glucose tolerance or diabetes mellitus, or psychiatric conditions) includes calcineurin inhibitors such as cyclosporine.

Alkylating agents such as cyclophosphamide are reserved for frequently relapsing or glucocorticoid-dependent patients with MCG.

ACE inhibitors such as lisinopril or angiotensin receptor blockers (typically used to inhibit the progression of chronic kidney disease) are typically not indicated to treat MCG because the duration of disease is short with glucocorticoid therapy, and patients are not hypertensive.

Although MCG is not a common cause of end-stage kidney disease in adults, and untreated patients may slowly improve, the nephrotic-range proteinuria of MCG is associated with a significantly increased risk for thromboembolism and infection. Therefore, because most patients treated with glucocorticoid therapy recover with a favorable prognosis, not providing treatment is inappropriate.

KEY POINT

- Glucocorticoids are recommended as first-line therapy in the treatment of minimal change glomerulopathy unless there are contraindications.

Bibliography

Hogan J, Radhakrishnan J. The treatment of minimal change disease in adults. J Am Soc Nephrol. 2013 Apr;24(5):702-11. [PMID: 23431071]

Item 94   Answer: B
Educational Objective: Diagnose thyrotoxic periodic paralysis.

This patient has features of acquired hypokalemic periodic paralysis occurring in association with hyperthyroidism (thyrotoxic periodic paralysis). Hypokalemic periodic paralysis is a rare familial or acquired disorder characterized by generalized flaccid muscle weakness from a sudden intracellular potassium shift precipitated by strenuous exercise or a high carbohydrate meal. Attacks may also occur spontaneously. The acquired form occurs with thyrotoxicosis and is found in men of Asian or Mexican descent. This patient's hyperthyroidism is suggested by the presence of hypertension, tachycardia, palpitations, tremor, heat intolerance, and weight loss. Hypokalemic periodic paralysis resolves with treatment of hyperthyroidism.

Bartter syndrome represents a group of autosomal recessive renal tubular disorders characterized by metabolic alkalosis, hypokalemia, and normal to low blood pressure with mild volume depletion. It is not associated with high blood pressure as seen in this patient.

Primary hyperaldosteronism is associated with hypertension and hypokalemia and is not associated with attacks of sudden weakness or paralysis.

Hypokalemia from Sjögren syndrome occurs in the setting of renal tubular acidosis; in this setting, a hyperchloremic metabolic acidosis with hypokalemia would occur, which is not present in this patient.

KEY POINT

- Hypokalemic periodic paralysis secondary to thyrotoxicosis is characterized by generalized flaccid muscle weakness from a sudden intracellular potassium shift precipitated by strenuous exercise or a high carbohydrate meal.

Bibliography

Falhammar H, Thorén M, Calissendorff J. Thyrotoxic periodic paralysis: clinical and molecular aspects. Endocrine. 2013 Apr;43(2):274-84. [PMID: 22918841]

Item 95   Answer: C
Educational Objective: Manage hypertension during pregnancy.

The most appropriate next step in management is to stop the angiotensin receptor blocker (ARB) losartan and monitor the blood pressure in this patient with hypertension who is attempting to conceive. ARBs, ACE inhibitors, and direct renin inhibitors are all associated with adverse fetal and neonatal outcomes; these agents are absolutely contraindicated during pregnancy and should be stopped prior to conception. Physiologic changes associated with pregnancy cause the systemic blood pressure to fall during most of gestation, and there is evidence that neither the patient nor the fetus appears to be at risk from mildly elevated blood pressure during pregnancy. The 2013 American College of Obstetricians and Gynecologists (ACOG) guidelines recommend treating persistent blood pressure elevations of >160/105 mm Hg in pregnant women with chronic hypertension, with a goal blood pressure with medical therapy in these patients being 120-160/80-105 mm Hg. Because this patient's current blood pressure is well below the recommended goal of therapy and her blood pressure would be expected to decline once she conceives, monitoring her blood pressure once the losartan is stopped is a reasonable approach. If her blood pressure rises into the recommended treatment range, reinstitution of treatment with a medication likely to be safe in pregnancy may be warranted.

Labetalol, a β-blocker with some α-blocking effect, may help preserve placental blood flow and is considered to be relatively safe during pregnancy. However, all antihypertensive medications cross the placenta, and it would be preferable to avoid treatment with any medication during early pregnancy. Because this patient might be able to be managed without medication should she become pregnant, switching to another agent from her ARB is not preferable. However, if further medical therapy is required, labetalol would be an appropriate option.

> **KEY POINT**
> - ACE inhibitors, angiotensin receptor blockers, and direct renin inhibitors are associated with adverse fetal and neonatal outcomes; these medications are absolutely contraindicated during pregnancy and should be stopped prior to conception.

Bibliography

Bullo M, Tschumi S, Bucher BS, Bianchetti MG, Simonetti GD. Pregnancy outcome following exposure to angiotensin-converting enzyme inhibitors or angiotensin receptor antagonists: a systematic review. Hypertension. 2012 Aug;60(2):444-50. [PMID: 22753220]

Item 96   Answer: D

Educational Objective: Diagnose lithium-induced nephrogenic diabetes insipidus using a water restriction test.

The most appropriate diagnostic test to perform next is a water restriction test to evaluate for diabetes insipidus (DI). DI is caused by either an absence of antidiuretic hormone (ADH) secretion (central DI) or renal resistance to ADH (nephrogenic DI), which results in an inability to appropriately concentrate the urine in response to an increase in plasma osmolality. This patient's symptoms of polyuria and polydipsia, in association with long-standing lithium therapy, are suggestive of nephrogenic DI. Lithium is one of the most common causes of nephrogenic DI in adults. On laboratory testing, serum sodium and plasma osmolality are usually high normal or slightly elevated, whereas urine osmolality is lower than plasma osmolality. Like the patient described, most patients with DI do not usually have frank hypernatremia because increased thirst stimulates oral consumption of fluids, which maintains the serum sodium near the upper normal range as long as access to fluids is not impaired. In a water restriction (or deprivation) test, urine volume, urine osmolality, and plasma sodium concentration are measured hourly after complete water restriction. A normal urine osmolality response (usually defined as an increase in urine osmolality above 600 mOsm/kg H_2O) indicates that ADH release and corresponding renal response to ADH are intact. A failure of the urine osmolality to rise despite rising plasma osmolality suggests either central or nephrogenic DI. Desmopressin is then administered. Patients with central DI will respond with increased urine osmolality, whereas in patients with nephrogenic DI (as is likely in this patient), desmopressin will not result in increased urine osmolality after water restriction, confirming the diagnosis.

The cosyntropin stimulation test is used to diagnose adrenal insufficiency, which is manifested by hyponatremia, decreased plasma osmolality, and increased urine osmolality, none of which is seen in this patient.

Hypothyroidism, which is diagnosed by the finding of a high thyroid-stimulating hormone level, can be associated with hyponatremia. In contrast to this patient with DI, patients with hyponatremia secondary to hypothyroidism present with hyponatremia, decreased plasma osmolality, and increased urine osmolality.

A urine sodium measurement is useful in the evaluation of patients with suspected urinary salt wasting, such as those with adrenal insufficiency. Patients with DI have a deficit of free water rather than urinary salt wasting, and as such, urine sodium measurement is not useful in diagnosing DI.

> **KEY POINT**
> - An inadequate response to water restriction (urine osmolality does not rise despite rising plasma osmolality) suggests either central or nephrogenic diabetes insipidus.

Bibliography

Devuyst O. Physiopathology and diagnosis of nephrogenic diabetes insipidus. Ann Endocrinol (Paris). 2012 Apr;73:128-9. [PMID: 22503803]

Item 97   Answer: A

Educational Objective: Treat hyperkalemia using intravenous glucose and insulin to rapidly shift potassium intracellularly.

The most appropriate treatment for lowering this patient's serum potassium level most quickly is intravenous glucose and insulin. He has end-stage kidney disease (ESKD) and presents with hyperkalemia and peaked T waves on electrocardiogram. Hyperkalemia is defined as a serum potassium level >5.0 mEq/L (5.0 mmol/L). Any level >6.0 mEq/L (6.0 mmol/L) can be life-threatening. Signs and symptoms are related to adverse effects of serum potassium on skeletal and cardiac muscle cell membranes, including muscle weakness and cardiac conduction and rhythm abnormalities. Intravenous calcium gluconate stabilizes the myocardium by lowering the threshold potential and is usually administered acutely to decrease the risk of arrhythmias; however, calcium does not have any effect on serum potassium levels. Major underlying causes of persistent hyperkalemia are disorders in which urine potassium excretion is impaired. The most common cause is chronic kidney disease with a glomerular filtration rate <20 mL/min/1.73 m^2 or acute kidney injury. The appropriate treatment for reducing serum potassium quickly in this patient with ESKD and hyperkalemia is both insulin and glucose given intravenously to rapidly shift potassium intracellularly. Insulin effectively drives potassium into cells by increasing activity of the Na-K-ATPase pump in skeletal muscle. Glucose is given to counteract potential hypoglycemia associated with insulin therapy.

High-dose loop and thiazide diuretics increase kidney potassium loss, particularly when combined with saline hydration, in patients with normal kidney function or mild to moderate kidney failure. However, this effect is not immediate, and bumetanide would be ineffective in this patient with ESKD.

Intravenous sodium bicarbonate raises the serum pH and leads to a shift of potassium into cells as part of the buffering process. However, it has not been shown to be an

CONT.

effective or predictable method for producing a hypokalemic response, especially in patients with ESKD.

Oral sodium polystyrene sulfonate in sorbitol binds potassium in the colon in exchange for sodium. It is not useful for acute control of hyperkalemia because its effect on potassium is delayed for at least 2 hours and peaks at 4 to 6 hours. In addition, its effect on hyperkalemia is modest.

KEY POINT

- To quickly lower serum potassium levels related to hyperkalemia, initial treatment involves intravenous glucose (to counteract hypoglycemia) and insulin to rapidly shift potassium intracellularly.

Bibliography

PaPutcha N, Allon M. Management of hyperkalemia in dialysis patients. Semin Dial. 2007 Sep-Oct;20(5):431-9. [PMID: 17897250]

Item 98   Answer: A

Educational Objective: Manage stage 1 hypertension in an older patient.

Addition of the ACE inhibitor lisinopril is appropriate. This 60-year-old patient has stage 1 hypertension. The eighth report of the Joint National Committee (JNC 8) recommends a treatment goal of <150/90 mm Hg for patients with hypertension who are ≥60 years. Given her age and no evidence of cardiovascular or kidney disease and lack of frailty, this patient's treatment goal according to JNC 8 is <150/90 mm Hg. In her circumstance, given a longer expected lifetime than the general population for this age, cautious stepped care for lower blood pressure goals is reasonable. Increasing the dose of one agent is less effective in reducing blood pressure than the addition of a second agent at low dose, which also avoids the risk of side effects more commonly seen at higher doses. In this case, the minor pedal edema may be exacerbated by increasing the amlodipine.

In the absence of any indications for β-blocker therapy (tachycardia, history of angina, or a recent myocardial infarction), metoprolol is not indicated for the initial therapy of hypertension. It can be considered as add-on therapy typically in the setting of vasodilator-induced tachycardia, but given the low resting pulse rate in this patient, an alternative agent should be considered. The Avoiding Cardiovascular Events in Combination Therapy in Patients Living with Systolic Hypertension (ACCOMPLISH) trial demonstrated the benefit of combination therapy with a calcium channel blocker and an ACE inhibitor in reducing cardiovascular events compared with combination therapy using a thiazide diuretic and an ACE inhibitor.

KEY POINT

- The eighth report of the Joint National Committee recommends a blood pressure goal of <150/90 mm Hg for patients with hypertension who are ≥60 years.

Bibliography

James PA, Oparil S, Carter BL, et al. 2014 evidence-based guideline for the management of high blood pressure in adults: report from the panel members appointed to the Eighth Joint National Committee (JNC 8). Erratum in: JAMA. 2014 May 7;311(17):1809. JAMA. 2014 Feb 5;311(5):507-20. [PMID: 24352797]

Item 99   Answer: A

Educational Objective: Diagnose masked hypertension using ambulatory blood pressure monitoring.

Ambulatory blood pressure monitoring (ABPM) is appropriate for this patient who likely has masked hypertension. He has evidence of end-organ manifestations (left ventricular hypertrophy) that is potentially related to hypertension, yet has not presented with blood pressure measurements consistent with hypertension (≥140/90 mm Hg). This raises the possibility of masked hypertension, which is defined as normal office blood pressure measurements but elevated blood pressure (>135/85 mm Hg) in the ambulatory setting. Prior to initiating medical therapy, a more detailed assessment of this patient's blood pressure should be pursued, with ABPM as an appropriate next step. Although ABPM does not carry a formal indication for the diagnosis of masked hypertension, it may be useful in establishing this blood pressure pattern. ABPM-ascertained hypertension is associated with a higher risk of cardiovascular death compared with office or home blood pressure–determined hypertension.

The left ventricular hypertrophy identified by electrocardiogram in this case may be secondary to hypertension but also may be due to other (such as genetic) causes and requires formal echocardiography to further evaluate and guide therapy. Initiating a blood pressure–lowering agent is not appropriate until both blood pressure and the electrocardiogram findings are clarified further with ABPM and echocardiography.

A plasma renin-plasma aldosterone ratio is used to evaluate for hyperaldosteronism as a secondary cause of hypertension and is typically indicated in patients with difficult-to-treat blood pressure elevations and hypokalemia. This patient has not been diagnosed with hypertension and has no electrolyte abnormalities.

Because this patient has evidence of end-organ damage possibly due to hypertension, follow-up assessment of his blood pressures in 6 months might further delay diagnosis and is not appropriate.

KEY POINT

- Ambulatory blood pressure monitoring may be helpful in diagnosing masked hypertension in patients with end-organ manifestations but normal office blood pressure measurements.

Bibliography

Pierdomenico SD, Cuccurullo F. Prognostic value of white-coat and masked hypertension diagnosed by ambulatory monitoring in initially untreated subjects: an updated meta analysis. Am J Hypertens. 2011 Jan;24(1):52-8. [PMID: 20847724]

Answers and Critiques

Item 100 Answer: C

Educational Objective: Diagnose respiratory alkalosis.

The most likely acid-base disorder in this patient is respiratory alkalosis with acute metabolic compensation. This patient has primary acute respiratory alkalosis, likely resulting from a panic attack associated with her anxiety disorder. Acute respiratory alkalosis is evidenced by a low P_{CO_2} and an appropriately reduced serum bicarbonate occurring in response to the lowered P_{CO_2}. For each 10 mm Hg (1.3 kPa) decrease in P_{CO_2}, serum bicarbonate falls acutely by 2.0 mEq/L (2.0 mmol/L) due to intracellular-to-extracellular shift of hydrogen ions as an immediate buffering mechanism. If the respiratory alkalosis is persistent, renal compensation will eventually occur, leading to reduced proximal tubule reabsorption of bicarbonate, and, after 24 to 48 hours, a further decrease in serum bicarbonate totaling 3.0 to 4.0 mEq/L (3.0-4.0 mmol/L) for every 10 mm Hg (1.3 kPa) decrease of P_{CO_2}. The reduction in bicarbonate of 4.0 mEq/L (4.0 mmol/L) for the decrease in P_{CO_2} of 18 mm Hg (2.4 kPa) indicates that renal compensation has not yet occurred. The laboratory studies are not consistent with a primary metabolic alkalosis because the bicarbonate is not elevated.

KEY POINT

- Primary acute respiratory alkalosis is characterized by a low P_{CO_2} and an appropriately reduced serum bicarbonate.

Bibliography
Palmer BF. Evaluation and treatment of respiratory alkalosis. Am J Kidney Dis. 2012 Nov;60(5):834-8. [PMID: 22871240].

Item 101 Answer: C

Educational Objective: Treat metabolic acidosis with alkali therapy to slow progression of chronic kidney disease.

Treatment with oral sodium bicarbonate, 0.5 mEq/kg/d, is appropriate. This patient with chronic kidney disease (CKD) has a normal anion gap metabolic acidosis. Normal anion gap metabolic acidosis may be due to failure of the kidneys to excrete the daily fixed acid load, gastrointestinal loss of bicarbonate, diversion of urine through a gastrointestinal conduit, or retention of hydrogen ions derived from organic anions that are excreted in the urine as sodium salts. The cause is often apparent from the history. This patient's history of analgesic nephropathy, normal anion gap metabolic acidosis, and hyperkalemia suggests the presence of distal (type 4) renal tubular acidosis. Studies have demonstrated that administration of oral alkali to maintain serum bicarbonate levels between 23 and 29 mEq/L (23-29 mmol/L) reduces the risk of progression of CKD. Typical starting doses of alkali for metabolic acidosis due to CKD are 0.5 to 1.0 mEq/kg/d.

The patient has a relatively mild and asymptomatic decrease in serum bicarbonate, and there is no indication for acute administration of intravenous sodium bicarbonate.

Although citrate becomes metabolized to bicarbonate and is therefore considered to be a "bicarbonate equivalent," this patient has hyperkalemia, which is likely due to the decreased ability of the kidneys to excrete potassium in the setting of CKD. Potassium citrate could therefore exacerbate the existing hyperkalemia and should be avoided. Bicarbonate treatment will help correct this patient's hyperkalemia.

Current guidelines suggest treatment with alkali to keep serum bicarbonate levels between 23 and 29 mEq/L (23-29 mmol/L). Therefore, providing no alkali therapy to this patient with a serum bicarbonate level of 18 mEq/L (18 mmol/L) would be inappropriate.

KEY POINT

- Oral alkali therapy to maintain serum bicarbonate levels between 23 and 29 mEq/L (23-29 mmol/L) reduces the risk of progression of chronic kidney disease.

Bibliography
Dobre M, Rahman M, Hostetter TH. Current status of bicarbonate in CKD. J Am Soc Nephrol. 2015 Mar;26(3):515-23. [PMID: 25150154]

Item 102 Answer: A

Educational Objective: Diagnose interstitial nephritis caused by mesalamine therapy.

The most likely diagnosis is interstitial nephritis caused by mesalamine therapy. Interstitial nephritis is characterized by an inflammatory infiltrate into the kidney interstitium that can lead to tubular dysfunction and kidney failure. Interstitial nephritis may be associated with autoimmune diseases and infections but is most commonly caused by drugs. Mesalamine-induced interstitial nephritis is a well-described complication that can be either acute or chronic and may occur months to years after exposure, even in patients who have safely tolerated the medication in the past. Sterile pyuria and leukocyte casts are hallmarks of interstitial nephritis, which can present acutely or may progress indolently and present as chronic kidney disease of unclear duration. Mild subnephrotic proteinuria also can be seen with interstitial nephritis.

Kidney disease in systemic lupus erythematosus is relatively common and may have a variable presentation, often with significant hematuria, proteinuria, and cellular casts. However, lupus nephritis is unlikely in this patient because of the absence of extrarenal lupus manifestations, his male gender, and lack of significant proteinuria or hematuria.

Membranous glomerulopathy primarily affects the glomerulus and is therefore associated with heavy proteinuria and the nephrotic syndrome, making this an unlikely diagnosis for this patient.

Rapidly progressive glomerulonephritis is associated with hematuria and erythrocyte casts and variable proteinuria, usually with other clinical manifestations such as hypertension. In some cases, other systemic symptoms or clinical findings associated with an underlying etiology may be present, such as pulmonary hemorrhage or upper and lower respiratory tract involvement. None of these findings is present in this patient, making this diagnosis unlikely.

KEY POINT

- In patients with interstitial nephritis, the hallmark findings on urinalysis are sterile pyuria and leukocyte casts.

Bibliography

Oikonomou KA, Kapsoritakis AN, Stefanidis I, Potamianos SP. Drug-induced nephrotoxicity in inflammatory bowel disease. Nephron Clin Pract. 2011;119(2):c89-94; discussion c96. [PMID: 21677443]

Item 103   Answer: D

Educational Objective: Diagnose preeclampsia.

The most likely diagnosis is preeclampsia, which is classically defined as new-onset hypertension after 20 weeks of pregnancy with proteinuria ($\geq$300 mg/24 h or a urine protein-creatinine ratio $\geq$300 mg/g). According to new guidelines, preeclampsia can also be diagnosed in patients without proteinuria if the hypertension is accompanied by one of the following conditions: thrombocytopenia (platelet count <100,000/μL [100 × 10^9/L]), kidney dysfunction (serum creatinine concentration >1.1 mg/dL [97.2 μmol/L] or a doubling of the serum creatinine concentration in the absence of other kidney disease), impaired liver function (elevated blood concentrations of liver aminotransferases to twice the normal concentration), pulmonary edema, or cerebral or visual symptoms. Because this patient meets the criteria for blood pressure elevation and also has thrombocytopenia and possibly mild pulmonary edema, the diagnosis of preeclampsia may be made without the presence of proteinuria. She has several risk factors for preeclampsia, including advanced maternal age and first pregnancy. Other risk factors for preeclampsia include family history, diabetes mellitus, obesity, chronic kidney disease, and twin gestation.

Chronic hypertension is defined as systolic pressure $\geq$140 mm Hg and/or diastolic pressure $\geq$90 mm Hg that existed before pregnancy, is present before the 20th week of gestation, or persists longer than 12 weeks postpartum. This patient had normal blood pressures prior to her most recent visit, making chronic hypertension unlikely.

The diagnosis of HELLP (hemolysis, elevated liver enzymes, and low platelets) syndrome requires evidence of hemolysis and abnormal liver chemistry tests in addition to thrombocytopenia.

Normal hemodynamic changes occurring during pregnancy include an increase in cardiac output and reduction in both systemic vascular resistance and systemic blood pressure. Therefore, the significant blood pressure elevation seen in this patient who was previously normotensive is not considered to be a normal change associated with

pregnancy. Crackles, an S$_3$ gallop, and an elevated central venous pressure would not be expected findings during a normal pregnancy and reinforce the diagnosis of preeclampsia.

KEY POINT

- Preeclampsia is classically defined as new-onset hypertension after 20 weeks of pregnancy with proteinuria but can also be diagnosed in patients without proteinuria if the hypertension is accompanied by other end-organ damage.

Bibliography

American College of Obstetricians and Gynecologists; Task Force on Hypertension in Pregnancy. Hypertension in pregnancy. Report of the American College of Obstetricians and Gynecologists' Task Force on Hypertension in Pregnancy. Obstet Gynecol. 2013 Nov;122(5):1122-31. [PMID: 24150027]

Item 104   Answer: D

Educational Objective: Treat hyperphosphatemia in a patient with chronic kidney disease.

In addition to dietary counseling regarding a low phosphate diet, this patient with stage G4/A1 chronic kidney disease (CKD) who now has hyperphosphatemia should begin taking a phosphate binder such as sevelamer. Elevated serum phosphorus levels, particularly exceeding 6.5 mg/dL (2.09 mmol/L), are closely associated with increased mortality. Most patients with severe CKD require oral phosphate binders to be administered with meals. This patient also has known cardiovascular disease and vascular calcification. The Kidney Disease Improving Global Outcomes (KDIGO) guidelines suggest avoiding the use of calcium-containing phosphate binders in patients with known vascular calcification due to the potential for an increase in calcium absorption and worsening calcification of vessel walls. Therefore, a non-calcium–containing phosphate binder such as sevelamer or lanthanum is the preferred agent for this patient. Ferric citrate, another non-calcium–containing phosphorus binder, was recently approved for use in patients receiving dialysis but is not yet approved for patients with non-dialysis CKD.

Although this patient has secondary hyperparathyroidism, administration of calcitriol will increase intestinal absorption of calcium and phosphorus, which will exacerbate the hyperphosphatemia and potentially worsen vascular calcification.

Although administration of oral calcium carbonate will lead to increased absorption of calcium that may treat this patient's mild hypocalcemia and reduce her parathyroid hormone (PTH) levels, it may exacerbate vascular calcium in the setting of severe hyperphosphatemia.

Administration of the calcimimetic cinacalcet will likely decrease this patient's PTH level toward the normal range; however, it will worsen her hypocalcemia and is not an effective treatment for the hyperphosphatemia.

- Patients with chronic kidney disease and hyperphosphatemia should be counseled regarding a low phosphate diet, and most patients require phosphate binders.

Bibliography

Palmer SC, Hayen A, Macaskill P, et al. Serum levels of phosphorus, parathyroid hormone, and calcium and risks of death and cardiovascular disease in individuals with chronic kidney disease: a systematic review and meta-analysis. JAMA. 2011 Mar 16;305(11):1119-27. [PMID: 21406649]

Item 105   Answer: A

Educational Objective: Treat chronic kidney disease-related iron deficiency anemia with intravenous iron.

The most appropriate management of this patient with chronic kidney disease–related iron deficiency anemia is to administer intravenous iron. Iron deficiency is the most common cause of hyporesponsiveness to erythropoietin. It is therefore important to optimize iron stores to maximize the response to erythropoietin. Many patients who receive hemodialysis are unable to maintain adequate iron stores by oral supplementation. The Kidney Disease Improving Global Outcomes (KDIGO) recommendations suggest maintaining transferrin saturation levels of >30% and serum ferritin levels of >500 ng/mL (500 µg/L). In hemodialysis patients, parenteral iron therapy is preferred to oral iron therapy because it is more effective in increasing hemoglobin concentrations and iron stores. Patients treated with intravenous iron are more likely to reduce the dose of erythropoiesis-stimulating agents (ESAs) compared with those taking oral iron. KDIGO guidelines recommend intravenous rather than oral iron replacement among hemodialysis patients who require iron.

As the estimated glomerular filtration rate declines below 30 mL/min/1.73 m^2 (stages G4-G5), anemia can become symptomatic. ESAs are highly effective in raising hemoglobin concentrations and alleviating symptoms, although these medications are associated with risks and are expensive. Once iron stores are replaced, KDIGO guidelines suggest avoiding dosing erythropoietin to achieve a hemoglobin level >11.5 g/dL (115 g/L) unless there are compelling reasons to do so to improve quality of life and the patient agrees to the risks.

There is no role for the routine measurement of erythropoietin levels in the setting of chronic kidney disease because this expensive test does not aid in the diagnosis or guide treatment decisions.

- Iron deficiency is the most common cause of hyporesponsiveness to erythropoietin, and guidelines recommend intravenous rather than oral iron replacement among hemodialysis patients who require iron.

Bibliography

Kidney Disease: Improving Global Outcomes (KDIGO) Anemia Work Group. KDIGO Clinical Practice Guideline for Anemia in Chronic Kidney Disease. Kidney inter Suppl. 2012;2:279-335.

Item 106   Answer: A

Educational Objective: Evaluate a patient for secondary causes of membranous glomerulopathy.

Chest radiography is the most appropriate next diagnostic step. This middle-aged patient presented with the insidious onset of the nephrotic syndrome with membranous glomerulopathy (MG) demonstrated on kidney biopsy. MG may be primary (idiopathic) or secondary to other causes. Primary MG is associated with the antibody to the phospholipase A$_2$ receptor (PLA$_2$R) on the podocyte surface in up to 80% of patients, and the presence of the antibody supports this diagnosis. Testing for anti-PLA$_2$R antibodies may be performed on serum or by staining of kidney biopsy tissue. Secondary causes of MG include malignancies (solid organ cancers, especially lung, colon, and breast), autoimmune diseases (such as lupus or mixed connective tissue disease), infections (hepatitis B and C), and medications (penicillamine, gold, and NSAIDs). Evaluation for potential secondary causes should always be undertaken in patients with MG, especially those who are negative for PLA$_2$R antibodies. Serologic tests for lupus and hepatitis were negative in this patient, and he has not been exposed to potential offending medications. Although MG may be associated with malignancy, an extensive evaluation for cancer is not indicated in patients with a diagnosis of MG beyond age-appropriate cancer screening except for those with symptoms suggestive of a cancer diagnosis (such as weight loss or blood in the stool) or significant risk factors for specific malignancies. Because of this patient's significant smoking history and his associated increased risk for lung cancer, chest radiography should be obtained as part of his evaluation for secondary MG.

Both PET and PET coupled with CT are useful studies in evaluating selected patients with known malignancy, often for staging purposes. However, neither is indicated to initially evaluate for lung cancer. Similarly, whole body CT is of low yield in searching for malignancy.

Although an extensive evaluation for malignancy is usually not indicated in patients with MG beyond age-appropriate cancer screening, this patient's increased risk for lung cancer warrants further evaluation.

- An extensive evaluation for cancer is not indicated in patients with membranous glomerulopathy beyond age-appropriate cancer screening except for those with symptoms suggestive of a cancer diagnosis or significant risk factors for specific malignancies.

Bibliography

Hogan J, Mohan P, Appel GB. Diagnostic tests and treatment options in glomerular disease: 2014 update. Am J Kidney Dis. 2014 Apr;63(4):656-66. [PMID: 24239051]

Item 107 Answer: C

Educational Objective: Protect sites of current or future vascular access in a patient with severe chronic kidney disease.

Placement of a single-lumen catheter in the right internal jugular vein to allow for 6 weeks of intravenous ceftriaxone is appropriate for this patient with severe chronic kidney disease (CKD). This strategy seeks to protect the integrity of peripheral veins. Protecting peripheral veins is an important consideration for all patients with severe CKD or end-stage kidney disease (ESKD) because adequate veins are a prerequisite for the creation of arteriovenous fistulas, which are associated with lower mortality than other forms of vascular access for hemodialysis. Because most patients will require multiple vascular accesses during the course of ESKD therapy, it is critical to protect peripheral veins even if patients already have a functional dialysis access. Small-bore single-lumen catheters placed into the internal jugular vein are less likely to impair venous drainage from the arm than subclavian catheters.

Peripherally inserted central catheter (PICC) lines have a high risk of causing permanent thrombosis or sclerosis to peripheral veins that might otherwise be useful for the creation of vascular access for hemodialysis. PICC lines should be avoided in patients with severe CKD or ESKD who are expected to require future hemodialysis.

Subclavian catheters have a high risk of causing stenosis of the subclavian veins, which can impede return of blood from the arm with arteriovenous dialysis access due to high blood flows. High venous pressure due to subclavian stenosis can lead to arm edema and failure of the arteriovenous access.

The patient's arteriovenous fistula should not be used to administer daily intravenous antibiotics. Inserting needles into a recently created fistula can damage it because the walls of the vein will not have had adequate time to "arterialize," which usually requires at least 2 to 3 months. Dialysis vascular access sites should only be accessed by trained dialysis personnel due to the need to protect against injury and/or infection to the access site. It is also important to avoid inflating blood pressure cuffs on the arm with vascular access to avoid injury or thrombosis.

KEY POINT

- Protection of the peripheral veins for future vascular access is essential in patients with chronic kidney disease.

Bibliography
El Ters M, Schears GJ, Taler SJ, et al. Association between prior peripherally inserted central catheters and lack of functioning arteriovenous fistulas: a case-control study in hemodialysis patients. Am J Kidney Dis. 2012 Oct; 60(4):601-8. [PMID: 22704142]

Item 108 Answer: B

Educational Objective: Identify normal physiologic changes of pregnancy as the cause of decreased serum sodium levels in a pregnant patient.

Normal physiologic changes of pregnancy are the most likely cause of this pregnant patient's decrease in her serum sodium level. While the plasma volume increases during pregnancy, water retention exceeds the concomitant sodium retention, resulting in mild hypo-osmolality and hyponatremia. The plasma osmolality typically decreases by 8 to 10 mOsm/kg H_2O, and the serum sodium decreases by 4.0 mEq/L (4.0 mmol/L). These hormonally mediated changes in plasma osmolality and serum sodium do not require therapy and resolve following delivery.

Cerebral salt wasting can be mistaken for the syndrome of inappropriate antidiuretic hormone secretion (SIADH) and can occur in response to central nervous system disease (particularly subarachnoid hemorrhage) and closed head injury. It is associated with an increased loss of sodium by the kidney, resulting in hyponatremia. However, these changes occur over a longer timeframe than seen in this patient with recent head trauma.

Pituitary apoplexy is acute hemorrhage into the pituitary gland and would be a consideration in this patient. If severe, it may cause headache, vision changes due to ocular nerve compression, and hypopituitarism. All pituitary hormonal deficiencies can occur, including adrenocorticotropic hormone (ACTH) deficiency, which may lead to cortisol deficiency and hypotension if it occurs rapidly. Although the resulting cortisol deficiency may result in mild hyponatremia, this would not occur immediately after injury. Additionally, this patient has a normal blood pressure for pregnancy and no other symptoms or clinical findings suggesting this diagnosis.

Neurologic conditions such as a closed head injury from a motor vehicle accident can cause the SIADH, but hyponatremia would not develop acutely upon initial presentation as in this patient.

KEY POINT

- While the plasma volume increases during pregnancy, water retention exceeds the concomitant sodium retention, resulting in mild hypo-osmolality and hyponatremia; these hormonally mediated changes do not need direct therapy and resolve following delivery.

Bibliography
Cheung KL, Lafayette RA. Renal physiology of pregnancy. Adv Chronic Kidney Dis. 2013 May;20(3):209-14. [PMID: 23928384]

Index

A

NAME AND ADDRESS (Please complete.)

_____
Last Name   First Name   Middle Initial

_____
Address

_____
Address cont.

_____
City   State   ZIP Code

_____
Country

_____
Email address

ACP®
American College of Physicians
Leading Internal Medicine, Improving Lives

Medical Knowledge Self-Assessment Program® 17

TO EARN *AMA PRA CATEGORY 1 CREDITS*™ YOU MUST:

1. Answer all questions.
2. Score a minimum of 50% correct.

==

TO EARN *FREE* INSTANTANEOUS *AMA PRA CATEGORY 1 CREDITS*™ ONLINE:

1. Answer all of your questions.
2. Go to **mksap.acponline.org** and enter your ACP Online username and password to access an online answer sheet.
3. Enter your answers.
4. You can also enter your answers directly at **mksap.acponline.org** without first using this answer sheet.

To Submit Your Answer Sheet by Mail or FAX for a $15 Administrative Fee per Answer Sheet:

1. Answer all of your questions and calculate your score.
2. Complete boxes A–F.
3. Complete payment information.
4. Send the answer sheet and payment information to ACP, using the FAX number/address listed below.

B

Order Number

(Use the Order Number on your MKSAP materials packing slip.)

C

ACP ID Number

(Refer to packing slip in your MKSAP materials for your ACP ID Number.)

COMPLETE FORM BELOW ONLY IF YOU SUBMIT BY MAIL OR FAX

Last Name   First Name   MI

Payment Information. Must remit in US funds, drawn on a US bank.

The processing fee for each paper answer sheet is $15.

☐ Check, made payable to ACP, enclosed

Charge to ☐ **VISA**   ☐ **MasterCard**   ☐ **AMERICAN EXPRESS**   ☐ **DISCOVER**

Card Number _____

Expiration Date _____ / _____   Security code (3 or 4 digit #s) _____
                  MM   YY

Signature _____

Fax to: 215-351-2799

Mail to:
Member and Customer Service
American College of Physicians
190 N. Independence Mall West
Philadelphia, PA 19106–1572

D TEST TYPE

TEST TYPE	Maximum Number of CME Credits
◯ Cardiovascular Medicine	21
◯ Dermatology	12
◯ Gastroenterology and Hepatology	16
◯ Hematology and Oncology	22
◯ Neurology	16
◯ Rheumatology	16
◯ Endocrinology and Metabolism	14
◯ General Internal Medicine	26
◯ Infectious Disease	19
◯ Nephrology	19
◯ Pulmonary and Critical Care Medicine	19

E CREDITS CLAIMED ON SECTION
(1 hour = 1 credit)

Enter the number of credits earned on the test to the nearest quarter hour. Physicians should claim only the credit commensurate with the extent of their participation in the activity.

		.		

F Enter your score here.

Instructions for calculating your own score are found in front of the self-assessment test in each book.

You must receive a minimum score of 50% correct.

_____ %

Credit Submission Date: _____

---

1 Ⓐ Ⓑ Ⓒ Ⓓ Ⓔ
2 Ⓐ Ⓑ Ⓒ Ⓓ Ⓔ
3 Ⓐ Ⓑ Ⓒ Ⓓ Ⓔ
4 Ⓐ Ⓑ Ⓒ Ⓓ Ⓔ
5 Ⓐ Ⓑ Ⓒ Ⓓ Ⓔ

6 Ⓐ Ⓑ Ⓒ Ⓓ Ⓔ
7 Ⓐ Ⓑ Ⓒ Ⓓ Ⓔ
8 Ⓐ Ⓑ Ⓒ Ⓓ Ⓔ
9 Ⓐ Ⓑ Ⓒ Ⓓ Ⓔ
10 Ⓐ Ⓑ Ⓒ Ⓓ Ⓔ

11 Ⓐ Ⓑ Ⓒ Ⓓ Ⓔ
12 Ⓐ Ⓑ Ⓒ Ⓓ Ⓔ
13 Ⓐ Ⓑ Ⓒ Ⓓ Ⓔ
14 Ⓐ Ⓑ Ⓒ Ⓓ Ⓔ
15 Ⓐ Ⓑ Ⓒ Ⓓ Ⓔ

16 Ⓐ Ⓑ Ⓒ Ⓓ Ⓔ
17 Ⓐ Ⓑ Ⓒ Ⓓ Ⓔ
18 Ⓐ Ⓑ Ⓒ Ⓓ Ⓔ
19 Ⓐ Ⓑ Ⓒ Ⓓ Ⓔ
20 Ⓐ Ⓑ Ⓒ Ⓓ Ⓔ

21 Ⓐ Ⓑ Ⓒ Ⓓ Ⓔ
22 Ⓐ Ⓑ Ⓒ Ⓓ Ⓔ
23 Ⓐ Ⓑ Ⓒ Ⓓ Ⓔ
24 Ⓐ Ⓑ Ⓒ Ⓓ Ⓔ
25 Ⓐ Ⓑ Ⓒ Ⓓ Ⓔ

26 Ⓐ Ⓑ Ⓒ Ⓓ Ⓔ
27 Ⓐ Ⓑ Ⓒ Ⓓ Ⓔ
28 Ⓐ Ⓑ Ⓒ Ⓓ Ⓔ
29 Ⓐ Ⓑ Ⓒ Ⓓ Ⓔ
30 Ⓐ Ⓑ Ⓒ Ⓓ Ⓔ

31 Ⓐ Ⓑ Ⓒ Ⓓ Ⓔ
32 Ⓐ Ⓑ Ⓒ Ⓓ Ⓔ
33 Ⓐ Ⓑ Ⓒ Ⓓ Ⓔ
34 Ⓐ Ⓑ Ⓒ Ⓓ Ⓔ
35 Ⓐ Ⓑ Ⓒ Ⓓ Ⓔ

36 Ⓐ Ⓑ Ⓒ Ⓓ Ⓔ
37 Ⓐ Ⓑ Ⓒ Ⓓ Ⓔ
38 Ⓐ Ⓑ Ⓒ Ⓓ Ⓔ
39 Ⓐ Ⓑ Ⓒ Ⓓ Ⓔ
40 Ⓐ Ⓑ Ⓒ Ⓓ Ⓔ

41 Ⓐ Ⓑ Ⓒ Ⓓ Ⓔ
42 Ⓐ Ⓑ Ⓒ Ⓓ Ⓔ
43 Ⓐ Ⓑ Ⓒ Ⓓ Ⓔ
44 Ⓐ Ⓑ Ⓒ Ⓓ Ⓔ
45 Ⓐ Ⓑ Ⓒ Ⓓ Ⓔ

46 Ⓐ Ⓑ Ⓒ Ⓓ Ⓔ
47 Ⓐ Ⓑ Ⓒ Ⓓ Ⓔ
48 Ⓐ Ⓑ Ⓒ Ⓓ Ⓔ
49 Ⓐ Ⓑ Ⓒ Ⓓ Ⓔ
50 Ⓐ Ⓑ Ⓒ Ⓓ Ⓔ

51 Ⓐ Ⓑ Ⓒ Ⓓ Ⓔ
52 Ⓐ Ⓑ Ⓒ Ⓓ Ⓔ
53 Ⓐ Ⓑ Ⓒ Ⓓ Ⓔ
54 Ⓐ Ⓑ Ⓒ Ⓓ Ⓔ
55 Ⓐ Ⓑ Ⓒ Ⓓ Ⓔ

56 Ⓐ Ⓑ Ⓒ Ⓓ Ⓔ
57 Ⓐ Ⓑ Ⓒ Ⓓ Ⓔ
58 Ⓐ Ⓑ Ⓒ Ⓓ Ⓔ
59 Ⓐ Ⓑ Ⓒ Ⓓ Ⓔ
60 Ⓐ Ⓑ Ⓒ Ⓓ Ⓔ

61 Ⓐ Ⓑ Ⓒ Ⓓ Ⓔ
62 Ⓐ Ⓑ Ⓒ Ⓓ Ⓔ
63 Ⓐ Ⓑ Ⓒ Ⓓ Ⓔ
64 Ⓐ Ⓑ Ⓒ Ⓓ Ⓔ
65 Ⓐ Ⓑ Ⓒ Ⓓ Ⓔ

66 Ⓐ Ⓑ Ⓒ Ⓓ Ⓔ
67 Ⓐ Ⓑ Ⓒ Ⓓ Ⓔ
68 Ⓐ Ⓑ Ⓒ Ⓓ Ⓔ
69 Ⓐ Ⓑ Ⓒ Ⓓ Ⓔ
70 Ⓐ Ⓑ Ⓒ Ⓓ Ⓔ

71 Ⓐ Ⓑ Ⓒ Ⓓ Ⓔ
72 Ⓐ Ⓑ Ⓒ Ⓓ Ⓔ
73 Ⓐ Ⓑ Ⓒ Ⓓ Ⓔ
74 Ⓐ Ⓑ Ⓒ Ⓓ Ⓔ
75 Ⓐ Ⓑ Ⓒ Ⓓ Ⓔ

76 Ⓐ Ⓑ Ⓒ Ⓓ Ⓔ
77 Ⓐ Ⓑ Ⓒ Ⓓ Ⓔ
78 Ⓐ Ⓑ Ⓒ Ⓓ Ⓔ
79 Ⓐ Ⓑ Ⓒ Ⓓ Ⓔ
80 Ⓐ Ⓑ Ⓒ Ⓓ Ⓔ

81 Ⓐ Ⓑ Ⓒ Ⓓ Ⓔ
82 Ⓐ Ⓑ Ⓒ Ⓓ Ⓔ
83 Ⓐ Ⓑ Ⓒ Ⓓ Ⓔ
84 Ⓐ Ⓑ Ⓒ Ⓓ Ⓔ
85 Ⓐ Ⓑ Ⓒ Ⓓ Ⓔ

86 Ⓐ Ⓑ Ⓒ Ⓓ Ⓔ
87 Ⓐ Ⓑ Ⓒ Ⓓ Ⓔ
88 Ⓐ Ⓑ Ⓒ Ⓓ Ⓔ
89 Ⓐ Ⓑ Ⓒ Ⓓ Ⓔ
90 Ⓐ Ⓑ Ⓒ Ⓓ Ⓔ

91 Ⓐ Ⓑ Ⓒ Ⓓ Ⓔ
92 Ⓐ Ⓑ Ⓒ Ⓓ Ⓔ
93 Ⓐ Ⓑ Ⓒ Ⓓ Ⓔ
94 Ⓐ Ⓑ Ⓒ Ⓓ Ⓔ
95 Ⓐ Ⓑ Ⓒ Ⓓ Ⓔ

96 Ⓐ Ⓑ Ⓒ Ⓓ Ⓔ
97 Ⓐ Ⓑ Ⓒ Ⓓ Ⓔ
98 Ⓐ Ⓑ Ⓒ Ⓓ Ⓔ
99 Ⓐ Ⓑ Ⓒ Ⓓ Ⓔ
100 Ⓐ Ⓑ Ⓒ Ⓓ Ⓔ

101 Ⓐ Ⓑ Ⓒ Ⓓ Ⓔ
102 Ⓐ Ⓑ Ⓒ Ⓓ Ⓔ
103 Ⓐ Ⓑ Ⓒ Ⓓ Ⓔ
104 Ⓐ Ⓑ Ⓒ Ⓓ Ⓔ
105 Ⓐ Ⓑ Ⓒ Ⓓ Ⓔ

106 Ⓐ Ⓑ Ⓒ Ⓓ Ⓔ
107 Ⓐ Ⓑ Ⓒ Ⓓ Ⓔ
108 Ⓐ Ⓑ Ⓒ Ⓓ Ⓔ
109 Ⓐ Ⓑ Ⓒ Ⓓ Ⓔ
110 Ⓐ Ⓑ Ⓒ Ⓓ Ⓔ

111 Ⓐ Ⓑ Ⓒ Ⓓ Ⓔ
112 Ⓐ Ⓑ Ⓒ Ⓓ Ⓔ
113 Ⓐ Ⓑ Ⓒ Ⓓ Ⓔ
114 Ⓐ Ⓑ Ⓒ Ⓓ Ⓔ
115 Ⓐ Ⓑ Ⓒ Ⓓ Ⓔ

116 Ⓐ Ⓑ Ⓒ Ⓓ Ⓔ
117 Ⓐ Ⓑ Ⓒ Ⓓ Ⓔ
118 Ⓐ Ⓑ Ⓒ Ⓓ Ⓔ
119 Ⓐ Ⓑ Ⓒ Ⓓ Ⓔ
120 Ⓐ Ⓑ Ⓒ Ⓓ Ⓔ

121 Ⓐ Ⓑ Ⓒ Ⓓ Ⓔ
122 Ⓐ Ⓑ Ⓒ Ⓓ Ⓔ
123 Ⓐ Ⓑ Ⓒ Ⓓ Ⓔ
124 Ⓐ Ⓑ Ⓒ Ⓓ Ⓔ
125 Ⓐ Ⓑ Ⓒ Ⓓ Ⓔ

126 Ⓐ Ⓑ Ⓒ Ⓓ Ⓔ
127 Ⓐ Ⓑ Ⓒ Ⓓ Ⓔ
128 Ⓐ Ⓑ Ⓒ Ⓓ Ⓔ
129 Ⓐ Ⓑ Ⓒ Ⓓ Ⓔ
130 Ⓐ Ⓑ Ⓒ Ⓓ Ⓔ

131 Ⓐ Ⓑ Ⓒ Ⓓ Ⓔ
132 Ⓐ Ⓑ Ⓒ Ⓓ Ⓔ
133 Ⓐ Ⓑ Ⓒ Ⓓ Ⓔ
134 Ⓐ Ⓑ Ⓒ Ⓓ Ⓔ
135 Ⓐ Ⓑ Ⓒ Ⓓ Ⓔ

136 Ⓐ Ⓑ Ⓒ Ⓓ Ⓔ
137 Ⓐ Ⓑ Ⓒ Ⓓ Ⓔ
138 Ⓐ Ⓑ Ⓒ Ⓓ Ⓔ
139 Ⓐ Ⓑ Ⓒ Ⓓ Ⓔ
140 Ⓐ Ⓑ Ⓒ Ⓓ Ⓔ

141 Ⓐ Ⓑ Ⓒ Ⓓ Ⓔ
142 Ⓐ Ⓑ Ⓒ Ⓓ Ⓔ
143 Ⓐ Ⓑ Ⓒ Ⓓ Ⓔ
144 Ⓐ Ⓑ Ⓒ Ⓓ Ⓔ
145 Ⓐ Ⓑ Ⓒ Ⓓ Ⓔ

146 Ⓐ Ⓑ Ⓒ Ⓓ Ⓔ
147 Ⓐ Ⓑ Ⓒ Ⓓ Ⓔ
148 Ⓐ Ⓑ Ⓒ Ⓓ Ⓔ
149 Ⓐ Ⓑ Ⓒ Ⓓ Ⓔ
150 Ⓐ Ⓑ Ⓒ Ⓓ Ⓔ

151 Ⓐ Ⓑ Ⓒ Ⓓ Ⓔ
152 Ⓐ Ⓑ Ⓒ Ⓓ Ⓔ
153 Ⓐ Ⓑ Ⓒ Ⓓ Ⓔ
154 Ⓐ Ⓑ Ⓒ Ⓓ Ⓔ
155 Ⓐ Ⓑ Ⓒ Ⓓ Ⓔ

156 Ⓐ Ⓑ Ⓒ Ⓓ Ⓔ
157 Ⓐ Ⓑ Ⓒ Ⓓ Ⓔ
158 Ⓐ Ⓑ Ⓒ Ⓓ Ⓔ
159 Ⓐ Ⓑ Ⓒ Ⓓ Ⓔ
160 Ⓐ Ⓑ Ⓒ Ⓓ Ⓔ

161 Ⓐ Ⓑ Ⓒ Ⓓ Ⓔ
162 Ⓐ Ⓑ Ⓒ Ⓓ Ⓔ
163 Ⓐ Ⓑ Ⓒ Ⓓ Ⓔ
164 Ⓐ Ⓑ Ⓒ Ⓓ Ⓔ
165 Ⓐ Ⓑ Ⓒ Ⓓ Ⓔ

166 Ⓐ Ⓑ Ⓒ Ⓓ Ⓔ
167 Ⓐ Ⓑ Ⓒ Ⓓ Ⓔ
168 Ⓐ Ⓑ Ⓒ Ⓓ Ⓔ
169 Ⓐ Ⓑ Ⓒ Ⓓ Ⓔ
170 Ⓐ Ⓑ Ⓒ Ⓓ Ⓔ

171 Ⓐ Ⓑ Ⓒ Ⓓ Ⓔ
172 Ⓐ Ⓑ Ⓒ Ⓓ Ⓔ
173 Ⓐ Ⓑ Ⓒ Ⓓ Ⓔ
174 Ⓐ Ⓑ Ⓒ Ⓓ Ⓔ
175 Ⓐ Ⓑ Ⓒ Ⓓ Ⓔ

176 Ⓐ Ⓑ Ⓒ Ⓓ Ⓔ
177 Ⓐ Ⓑ Ⓒ Ⓓ Ⓔ
178 Ⓐ Ⓑ Ⓒ Ⓓ Ⓔ
179 Ⓐ Ⓑ Ⓒ Ⓓ Ⓔ
180 Ⓐ Ⓑ Ⓒ Ⓓ Ⓔ